Healthcare in Early Medieval Northern Italy

STUDIES IN THE EARLY MIDDLE AGES

Previously published volumes in this series are listed at the back of the book.

VOLUME 26

Healthcare in Early Medieval Northern Italy

More to Life than Leeches?

by

Clare Pilsworth

BREPOLS

British Library Cataloguing in Publication Data

Pilsworth, Clare, author.
Healthcare in early medieval Northern Italy : more to life than leeches.
-- (Studies in the early Middle Ages ; 26)
1. Medical care--Italy, Northern--History--To 1500.
2. Medicine, Medieval--Italy, Northern.
3. Social medicine--Italy, Northern--History--To 1500.
I. Title
II. Series
362.1'09451'09021-dc23

ISBN-13: 9782503528557

D/2014/0095/132
ISBN: 978-2-503-52855-7
Printed in the EU on acid-free paper

In memory of

Great-Auntie Elsie
(Hawkins, née Greenfield)
who loved history and always wanted to be a teacher

and

Grandad (Arthur) Carroll
who liked getting books out from the library on obscure subjects –
hope you would have appreciated this one!

Contents

List of Illustrations

Figures

Maps

Tables

Acknowledgements

This book is based upon the research project 'Between the mountains and the sea: the transmission and use of medical miscellanies in the trans-alpine regions' (no. 070693) and an extension grant for further work on xenodochia, both funded by the Wellcome Trust. I am very grateful for the Trust's continued support and advice.

I wish to thank the staff at Manchester University Library, John Rylands University library, Manchester, Cambridge University Library, the British Library, London, the Archivio Capitolare, Modena, the microfilm department of the Biblioteca Apostolica Vaticana, and the Stiftsbibliothek, St Gallen.

During the course of writing this book I have moved from one 'home', the Centre of the History of Medicine (CHSTM), Manchester University, to another, the Classics and Ancient History department in the same university. At CHSTM I wish in particular to thank Mick Worboys, Gillan Mawson, Neil Pemberton, Aya Homei, and Carsten Timmerman. A constant source of support, advice, and friendship has been Penny Gouk, formerly of CHSTM.

I have been made very welcome in my new department, and would like to thank in particular David Langslow, Paul Fouracre, Kate Cooper, Luca Larpi, Martin Ryan, all members of the Centre of Late Antiquity, and former members of the university Caroline Petit, Sarah Tatum, Alex Ralston, Julia Hillner, Conrad Leyser, and Poul-Martin Pedersen.

As an early medieval history of medicine specialist the advice and support of others scattered across the world has also been vital. Peregrine Horden has become a much valued friend and colleague, and has also lived with this book far too long! I am also grateful to Monica Green, Debby Banham, April Harper, Iona McCleery, Catherine Rider, Rebecca Flemming, Marianne Elsakkers, Sally Crawford, Brigitta Hoffmann, and Eliza Glaze. Over the years I've also benefitted much from the help and advice of Eddie Coleman, Tom Brown, Chris Wickham, Rosamond McKitterick, Ross Balzaretti, Julia Barrow, Felice Lifshitz, Trish Skinner, Marios Costambeys, Nick Everett, Helmut Reimitz, Max Diesenberger, Klaus-Dietrich Fischer, and Thomas Granier, and all those who have commented and responded to my papers of work in progress at Dublin, Edinburgh, Oxford, and the Leeds International Medieval Congress.

I am also grateful for the hard work of Sam Koon, Luca Larpi, Alex Ralston, and above all Frances Parton and Sam Ottewill-Soulsby for library and research assistance. Thank you also to Martin Crampin for drawing the Italy map, and Elizabeth Tyler and Laura Napran for friendly and efficient editing and proof-reading.

It is my family and friends, however, who have lived longest with 'the damn book': thanks to Clara East and family, Helen Evans and Elina Screen for Cambridge friendship and accommodation. My biggest debt, however, is to the amazing 'Team Coulborn/Pilsworth': my mother-in-law Norma Coulborn, husband Neil Coulborn, and above all to my parents Janice and Robert Pilsworth. Without their help, support, and whip-cracking, this book would have taken even longer to finish, if at all. Without our son Christopher and daughter Emma this book would have been finished somewhat more quickly, but who have brought much so joy (and organised chaos) to our lives!

Abbreviations

AASS	*Acta sanctorum* (Brussels, 1643–1940)
ChLA	*Chartae Latinae antiquiores*, ed. by A. Bruckner and R. Marichal (Olten and Lausanne, 1954–)
ChLA	*2nd ser. Chartae Latinae Antiquiores, 2nd series*, ed. by G. Cavallo and G. Nicolaj (Dietikon-Zurich, 1997–)
CLA Codices	*Latini Antiquiores*, ed. by E. A. Lowe (Oxford, 1934–71)
Justinian, *Digest Corpus Iuris Civilis*, I.2	*Digesta*, ed. by T. Mommsen, 9th edn (Berlin, 1902); trans. by A. Watson, *The Digest of Justinian*, 4 vols (Philadelphia, 1985)
Justinian, *Institutes*	Thomas, J. A. C., *The Institutes of Justinian, Text, Translation and Commentary* (Oxford, 1975)
MGH	*Monumenta Germaniae Historia*
AA	*Auctores Antiquissimi* (Berlin, 1887–)
Concilia	*Concilia* (Hannover, 1893–)
Epistolae	*Epistolae* (Berlin, 1891–)
Leges	*Leges* (Hannover, 1835–89)
SRL	*Scriptores rerum langobardicarum et italicarum saec. VI–IX* (Hannover, 1878)
SRM	*Scriptores rerum merovingicarum* (Hannover, 1885–1920)

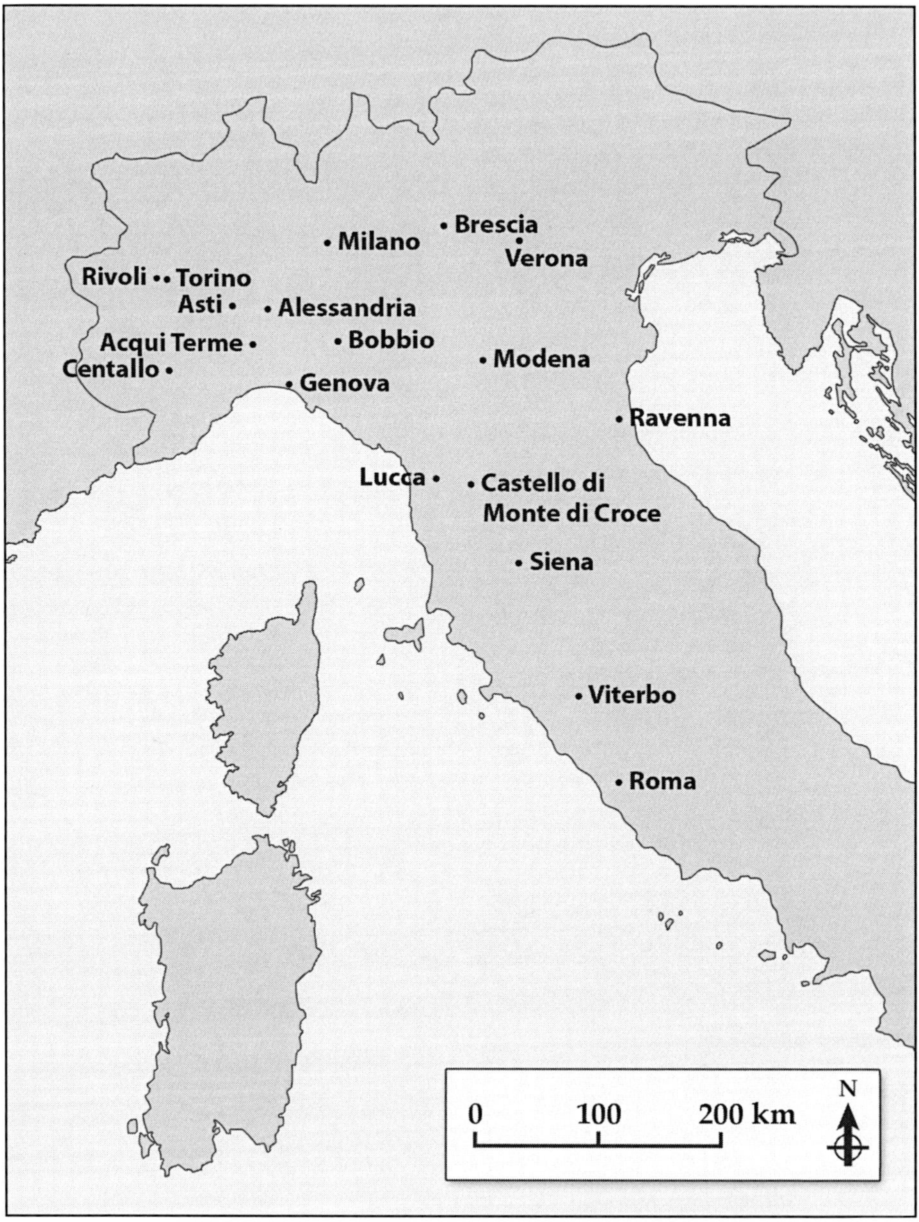

Map 1. Map of Italy.
Drawn and reproduced with kind permission of Martin Crampin.

Preface: More to Life than Leeches? Medicine in Post-Roman Italy

Outside of a small academic circle, most people are still surprised to discover that there was any medicine at all being practiced in Europe between around 500 and 900 AD. If pressed, the most popular images people associate with premodern Western medicine tend to involve unskilled practitioners with poor personal hygiene inflicting copious bloodletting (with or without leeches) on their hapless patients, while muttering dark magical incantations. Medical teaching and textbooks, and a weighty legal framework in which doctors (or 'leeches' in Anglo-Saxon) worked as respected members of the community are conspicuously absent from this enduring view of early medieval European medicine.[1]

Academics (alongside their institutions and funding bodies) must shoulder part of the blame for this state of affairs. Work on early medieval European medicine remains largely patchy and specialized, despite the pioneering efforts of Loren McKinney in the 1930s, followed by substantial contributions from Beccaria, Sigerist, Green, Fischer, and Horden, amongst others in subsequent decades.[2] Even among academics, early medieval medicine remains the undera-

[1] On Anglo-Saxon medicine, see, for example, A. Meaney, 'The Practice of Medicine in England about the Year 1000', *Social History of Medicine*, 13 (2000), 221–37.

[2] L. MacKinney, *Early Medieval Medicine: With Special Reference to France and Chartres* (Baltimore, 1937); A. Beccaria, *I codici di medicina del periodo presalernitano* (Roma, 1956); H. E. Sigerist, *Studien und Texte zur frühmittelalterlichen Rezeptliteratur* (Leipzig, 1923); M. Green, ed., *The Trotula: An English Translation of the Medieval Compendium of Women's Medicine* (Philadelphia, 2002); M. Green, *Making Women's Medicine Masculine: The Rise of*

chieving sibling, with Gerhard Baader declaring early medieval medical knowledge and practice as 'deplorable'.[3]

Perhaps partly in response to these overwhelmingly negative views of early medieval medicine — both popular and academic — research has tended to focus either on high end medical manuscripts and legal frameworks for medicine and medical practice, or unashamedly embrace the magical, social, and religious aspects of illness and health.[4] What is largely missing is an attempt to gain a holistic view of early medicine, one that takes account of both magical and ritualistic practices and learned medical texts.

The body of material for the study of pre-1000 AD medicine in Western Europe certainly does not make this a straightforward task. Given the relative paucity of surviving sources from this period, archaeological evidence, medical and legal texts, scribbled recipes, and saints' lives all have to be pressed into service, notwithstanding their individual difficulties of interpretation. Early medieval medicine itself is complicated, multifaceted, and often contradictory: instructions for medico-magical incantations involving the body parts of vultures jostle for space with bureaucratic documents on liability for work-related injuries.[5]

Nowhere is this more true than for early medieval Italy, but this is precisely what makes the Italian peninsula such a unique, and surprisingly underused resource for capturing the complexity and nuances of medical practice and attitudes to health and illness before 900 AD in Western Europe. If any region of Europe can counter the 'eye of newt' reputation of premodern medicine it is Italy.[6] The Italian peninsula, as one might expect as the former powerhouse of

Male Authority in Pre-Modern Gynaecology (Oxford, 2008); K.-D. Fischer, 'Praenostica — Die Rezeption des Prognostikons im Frühmittelalter', in *La science médicale antique: nouveaux regards*, ed. by V. Boudon-Millot and others (Paris, 1980), pp. 183–220; P. Horden, *Hospitals and Healing from Antiquity to the Later Middle Ages* (Aldershot, 2008).

[3] G. Baader, 'Early Medieval Latin Adaptations of Byzantine Medicine in Western Europe', in *Symposium on Byzantine Medicine*, ed. by J. Scarborough (Washington, DC, 1985), pp. 251–59 (p. 251).

[4] Two examples at either end of the spectrum could be A. Niederhellmann, *Arzt und Heilkunde in den frühmittelalterlichen Leges: Eine wort- und sachekundliche Untersuchung* (Berlin, 1983) and V. Flint, *The Rise of Magic in Early Medieval Europe* (Princeton, 1991).

[5] On vulture medicine and the contradictions of early medieval medicine, see P. Horden, 'What's Wrong with Early Medieval Medicine?', *Social History of Medicine*, 24.1 (2011), 5–25.

[6] For this phrase, see A. Van Arsdall, 'Challenging the "Eye of Newt" Image of Medieval Medicine', in *The Medieval Hospital and Medical Practice*, ed. by B. Bowers (Aldershot, 2007), pp. 195–205.

the Roman Empire, had the strongest Roman traditions in post-Roman Europe. A key part of this Roman legacy was the preservation of literally thousands of original charters and other legal documents from the sixth century onwards, not to mention hundreds of manuscripts, carefully stored largely in churches, cathedrals, and monasteries across the peninsula.

It was also in Italy, in the former Roman capital of Ravenna on the North East coast, where learned medical schools almost certainly continued the longest, and where Greek medical texts continued to be copied and translated long after the formal end of the Roman Empire in the West in 476 AD.[7] Whatever the significance of that precise date, for several centuries thereafter the Italian peninsula was partitioned in a dizzying revolving-door series of combinations between assorted so-called barbarian generals or leaders and Eastern Roman (Byzantine) emperors. Kingdoms which comprised either part or all of Northern and Central Italy include those of Odoacer (476–93), the Ostrogoths (493–552/3), the Lombards (568–774), the Byzantines (554–751 (in the North), and the Franks (Carolingians) from North of the Alps from 773–74 onwards.[8]

[7] On the end of the Roman Empire, see, for example, A. Cameron, *The Mediterranean World in Late Antiquity AD 395–600* (London, 1993), pp. 33–36; C. La Rocca, ed., *Italy in the Early Middle Ages, 476–1000* (Oxford, 2002), pp. 15–17. On Ravenna and the translation of Greek medical texts, see: N. Palmieri, 'Nouvelles remarques sur les commentaires à Galien de l'école médicale de Ravenne', in *Docente Natura: Mélanges de médicine ancienne et médiévale offerts à Guy Sabbah*, ed. by N. Palmieri and A. Debru (Saint-Étienne, 2001), pp. 209–46; I. Mazzini and N. Palmieri, 'L'école médicale de Ravenne: Programmes et méthodes d'enseignement, langue, hommes', in *Les écoles médicales à Rome*, ed. by P. Mudry and H. Pigeaud (Geneva, 1991), pp. 285–310; G. Cavallo, 'Libri e continuità della cultura antica in età barbarica', in *Magistra barbaritas: I barbari in Italia*, ed. by G. P. Carratelli (Milano, 1984), pp. 603–62 (pp. 628 and 633); J. Jouanna, 'Remarques sur la valeur relative des traductions latines pour l'édition des texts hippocratiques', in *Le Latin Médical: la constitution d'un langage scientifique, réalités et langage de la medicine dans le monde romain*, ed. by G. Sabbah (Saint-Étienne, 1991), pp. 11–26; I. Mazzini, 'I caratteri comuni a tutto: Ippocrate latino tardo-antico e conseguenti considerazioni su alcuni emendamenti al texto', in *I Testi di medicina latini antichi: problemi filologici e storici*, ed. by I. Mazzini and F. Fusco (Roma, 1985), pp. 65–74; A. M. Ieraci Bio, 'La cultura medica a Ravenna nel VI secolo', *Atti dell'Accademia Pontaniana*, 43 (1994), 279–308. For a sceptical view, see M. E. Vázquez Buján, 'Problemas generales de las antiuguas traducciones médicas latinas', *Studi Medievali*, 3rd ser., 25 (1984), 641–80.

[8] See N. Christie, *The Lombards: The Ancient Longobards* (Oxford, 1995); T. S. Brown, *Gentlemen and Officers: Imperial Administration and Aristocratic Power in Byzantine Italy AD 554–800* (Roma, 1984); R. McKitterick, *The Frankish Kingdoms under the Carolingians 751–987* (London, 1983); La Rocca, *Italy*, particularly chapter one: W. Pohl, 'Invasions and Ethnic Identity', in *Italy in the Early Middle Ages, 476–1000*, ed. by C. La Rocca (Oxford,

The result of these multiple invasions was a complex social, ethnic, and political patchwork, across which, nevertheless, people, manuscripts, and goods continued to move. Ravenna continued as capital for both the Ostrogothic and subsequently Byzantine regimes in Italy up to 751 AD. This is why the city has been seen as a bridge between both the West and East, and the Roman and medieval worlds.[9] Really, though, the whole of Italy can be characterized as the glue binding — however tenuously and fractiously — East and West, North and South, Roman and 'Barbarian', Christian, Jewish, and Islamic traditions together in early medieval Europe.

Patricia Skinner's 1997 book on health and medicine in early medieval Southern Italy sought to capture the resulting diversity and vitality of medical culture south of Rome, but no comparative study exists for points north.[10] Yet, as any visitor even today in the age of globalization will tell you, Northern Italy remains distinct from the South whether you are talking in terms of affluence, politics, landscape, or even culinary traditions. For the purposes of this book, 'early medieval' will cover the period between *c.* 500 and *c.* 900 AD and 'Northern Italy' will be broadly defined as the lands and kingdoms North of Rome. Unlike Southern Italy, in early medieval Northern Italy Jewish and Muslim influence on cultural and political life is slight, but links with both the East and the North were obviously strong. Frankish and Alammanic immigrants leave their mark in the legal evidence.[11] Cities such as Lucca in present day Tuscany were vital in preserving charters detailing legal transactions, on which I shall draw throughout the book, but particularly in chapter six, as we explore the role and social status of doctors in early medieval Northern Italy.

This book has grown out of my Wellcome Trust funded research project on manuscripts containing medical and non-medical material in what is now Northern Italy and Switzerland in the early Middle Ages. It soon became clear, however, that these manuscripts could not be studied in a vacuum — they needed contextualizing in the light of the rich legal, literary, and archaeological evidence of early medieval Italy. The overall aim of the project, however,

2002), pp. 11–33. See also T. S. Brown, 'Byzantine Italy, *c.* 680–*c.* 876', in *The New Cambridge Medieval History*, 7 vols (Cambridge, 1995–2005), II: *c. 700–c. 900*, ed. by R. McKitterick (1995), pp. 320–48, and P. Delogu, 'Lombard and Carolingian Italy', in *The New Cambridge Medieval History*, II, pp. 290–319.

[9] A. Carile, ed., *Storia di Ravenna*, 3 vols (Ravenna, 1990–92).

[10] P. Skinner, *Health and Medicine in Early Medieval Southern Italy* (Leiden, 1996).

[11] E. Hlawitschka, *Franken, Alemannen, Bayern und Burgunder in Oberitalien, 774–962* (Freiburg im Breisgau, 1960).

remained the same — to move beyond 'high end' manuscripts to every day, 'workhorse' manuscripts, and to demonstrate the diversity of early medieval medicine in Italy North of Rome.[12] The relatively high survival rate of manuscripts and legal documents, not to mention archaeological evidence, means that we can outline concepts of health, illness, and medical thought in early medieval Italy.

I shall begin with the way disease was viewed and treated in Part I, drawing on surviving contemporary manuscripts from the region, before turning to people and places of healing in Part II. Precisely who was performing healing and where was a source of great anxiety for early medieval rulers and ecclesiastical writers. Similarly, certain diseases such as leprosy and rabies seemed to excite and alarm writers and manuscript compilers a good deal more than the more mundane conditions such as arthritis or vitamin deficiencies, even though the last named two were almost certainly much more a feature of the majority of peoples' everyday lives. This obviously also poses considerable challenges for historians attempting to understand health and disease in early medieval Europe, the subject of Part I.

Chapter one explores how illness is portrayed in the legal sources, while in contrast Chapter two explores the other side of the coin, individuals' actual health and life expectancy through the archaeological evidence. Chapter three draws on both legal and medical texts, particularly herbals, to assess how illnesses might have been treated. Interestingly, leeches do not appear to have been one of the options! The opening chapter of Part II focuses on shrines and healing, but questions just how significant a role this played in healthcare in early medieval Northern Italy. Virtually all treatment and healing would actually have taken place in the home, the subject of chapter five, together with an exploration of the role of unsanctioned healers and *xenodochia*, hostels, in

[12] For work on early medieval medical manuscripts, see Baader, 'Early Medieval Latin Adaptations', 251–59; F. E. Glaze, 'The Perforated Wall: The Ownership and Circulation of Medical Books in Medieval Europe, *ca.* 800–1200' (unpublished doctoral thesis, Duke University, 1999); K.-D. Fischer, 'Der Liber medicinalis des Pseudo-Democritus', in *Tradición e innovación de la medicina latina de la antigüedad y de la Alta Edad Media*, ed. by M. E. Vázquez Buján (Santiago de Compostela, 1994), pp. 45–56; K.-D. Fischer, 'Dr Monk's Medical Digest', *The Year 1000: Medical Practice at the End of the First Millennium, Social History of Medicine*, 13.2 (2000), 239–51, and K.-D. Fischer, 'Ad glauconem', in *Galenismo e medicina tardoantica: fonti greche, latine e arabe*, ed. by I. Garofolo and A. Roselli (Napoli, 2003), pp. 283–346; Vázquez Buján, 'Problemas generales', pp. 641–80; F. Wallis, 'The Experience of the Book: Manuscripts, Texts and the Role of Epistemology in Early Medieval Medicine', in *Knowledge and the Scholarly Medical Traditions*, ed. by D. Bates (Cambridge, 1995), pp. 101–26.

healthcare. The final chapter is devoted to the most visible group of healers, doctors. I shall show that the figure of the doctor remained important in legal and popular imagination, and that the local doctor was a respected fixture in many early medieval towns. The aim of this book is therefore simple: to show that there was indeed much more to early medieval medicine than 'leeches' in both senses of the word, as a blood-sucking animal or the stereotype of the avaricious doctor.

Part I

Illness, Disease, and Treatment

Introduction

Blood and Ink: Health, Medicine, and the Body in Early Medieval Northern Italian Books

The art of medicine was invented as a good greater than wealth and a source of benefit to our lives. It professes to effect, preserve, and maintain the health of the body; through this, a wide experience of things beneficial accrues to mankind, the arts endure, and every sort of training and instruction and even, in fact, the workings of the soul itself, are carried out. Perhaps, indeed, if they are to be developed or devised at all, all things require health of the body.[1]

Whether these were the exact words of the lecturer Agnellus in sixth-century Ravenna, delivered to rapt (or gently snoozing) medical students we will never know: this introduction to a commentary on the works of Galen now exists only in a ninth-century manuscript of a supposed contemporary transcription.[2] What is not in doubt, however, is that this is a

[1] 'Bonum aliquid divitiarum et oportunum vite nostre inuenta est ars medicine. Sanitatem enim operari et conseruare promittit et exercere corpori; per quam magna bonorum hominibus additur peritia et artes constant et omnis meditatio et disciplina procedit et ipse animae operationes.' Agnellus of Ravenna, Prologue to commentary on *De Sectis*, in Agnellus of Ravenna, *Lectures on Galen's 'De sectis'*, ed. by L. Westerink and others (Buffalo, 1981), p. 3.

[2] Milano, Biblioteca Ambrosiana, G 108 inf. See Beccaria, *I codici*, pp. 288–91. For a discussion of this manuscript's contents, the Ravennate origin of the texts it contains, and a transcription of the commentary on *Ad glauconem*, see N. Palmieri, 'Un antico commento a Galeno della scuola medica di Ravenna', *Physis*, 23.2 (1981), 196–295. See also Glaze, 'The Perforated Wall', p. 45. The text is edited and translated in Ieraci Bio, 'La cultura medica'. See

sophisticated early medieval Northern Italian reflection on the relationship between good health, good medicine, and 'good' society. Medicine here, however, is much more about prevention of illness and maintenance of health than treatment and cure. This echoes much more ancient ideas about health, illness, and the functioning of the body.

The Rise and Rise of Humoral Theory

Based on the ideas of Hippocrates, a healthy body is essentially one where the four humours — black bile, red/yellow bile, blood, and phlegm — are in balance.[3] The ancient medical sect the Methodists proposed an alternative theory that acknowledged the existence of humours but which focused on blockages of the pores of the body to explain ill health.[4] The fifth-century North African Caelius Aurelianus did include Methodist material in his compilation *Acute and Chronic Illnesses* based on the work of Soranus.[5] However, to what degree this work, if at all, was known in early medieval Italy or Western Europe is a mystery, as the earliest complete manuscript of this work dates only to the sixteenth century.[6] A copy of at least part of the volume on Chronic diseases is recorded in an early medieval library catalogue at the monastery of Lorsch North of the Alps, so it may have been circulating in Italy too, but if so, was likely to have been rare. Only extracts from some of Aurelius's other texts, such as the *Responsiones*, were certainly known in Northern Italy as an early ninth-century

also B. Cavarra, 'La cultura medica a Ravenna fra VI e VII secolo', *Medicina nei secoli*, 5.3 (1993), 345–59.

[3] For a summary of humoral theory see V. Nutton, 'Medicine in the Greek World, 800 BC to 50 BC', in *The Western Medical Tradition 800 BC to AD 1800*, ed. by L. Conrad and others (Cambridge, 1995), pp. 11–38 (pp. 23–25). On Hippocratic definitions of health and disease see J. Jouanna, *Hippocrates*, trans. by M. DeBevoise (Baltimore, 1999), pp. 323–47.

[4] V. Nutton, 'Roman Medicine 250 BC to AD 200', *The Western Medical Tradition 800 BC to AD 1800*, ed. by L. Conrad and others (Cambridge, 1995), pp. 39–70 (p. 41).

[5] Caelius Aurelianus, *Akute Krankheiten: Buch I–III; Chronische Krankheiten: Buch IV–V*, ed. by G. Bendz, trans. by I. Pape, 2 vols (Berlin, 1990). See also M. Frede, 'The Method of the So-Called Methodical School of Medicine', in *Science and Speculation: Studies in Hellenistic Theories and Practice*, ed. by J. Barnes and others (Cambridge, 1982), pp. 1–23. The degree to which the work is a straight translation or adaptation of Soranus is debated — see V. Nutton, 'Medicine in Late Antiquity and the Early Middle Ages', in *The Western Medical Tradition 800 BC to AD 1800*, ed. by L. Conrad and others (Cambridge, 1995), pp. 71–88 (p. 82).

[6] K.-D. Fischer and others, eds, *Bibliographie des textes médicaux latins* (Saint-Étienne, 1983), p. 43.

copy, probably written, according to Bernhard Bischoff, at or near Verona, is now preserved in Karlsruhe, Germany.[7]

It was instead humoral theory that became dominant in early medieval thinking and culture.[8] This in no small part was thanks to the second-century doctor and systematizer of Hippocratic theory, Galen (129–*c.* 210 AD), whose works Agnellus was busy elucidating in late antique Ravenna. Galen's *oeuvre* (and works attributed to him) came to tower over the medical landscape for the next one and half thousand years in Western Europe.[9] In a few works Galen mentions 'seeds' of disease, for example in relation to the plague, but it was only one possible factor, and health still depended largely on the constitution of the individual.[10] He states in his *Ars Medica* that 'a body is healthy in the general sense when it has from birth a good mixture of the simple, primary parts, and good proportion in the organs which are composed of these'. A morbid (unhealthy) body has a 'bad mixture in the homogeneous parts'. This is not a simple binary distinction, however, as according to Galen a third category exists, where a body is neither healthy nor morbid, but shares characteristics of both.[11]

[7] Karlsruhe, Staatsbibliothek, MS Aug. Perg. 120. See B. Bischoff, *Katalog der festländischen Handschriften des neunten Jahrhunderts*, 2 vols (Wiesbaden, 1998–2004), I (1998), 345. See also A. Holder, *Die Reichenauer Handschriften*, 3 vols (Leipzig, 1906–18), I (1906), pp. 304–07; K.-D. Fischer, 'Unberücksichtigte Handscriftenfunde zur Überlieferung der Werke des Caelius Aurelianus', in *Le traité des Maladies aiguës et des Maladies chroniques de Caelius Aurelianus: nouvelles approches*, ed. by P. Mudry (Nantes, 1999), pp. 161–70, and Fischer, 'Dr. Monk's Medical Digest'.

[8] See V. Nutton, *Ancient Medicine* (London, 2004), p. 6. See also I. Müller, *Humoralmedizin: physiologische, pathologische und therapeutische Grundlagen der galenistischen Heilkunst* (Heidelberg, 1993).

[9] See N. Siraisi, *Medieval and Early Renaissance Medicine: An Introduction to Knowledge and Practice* (Chicago, 1990), pp. 4–6; A. Wear, 'Galen in the Renaissance', in *Galen: Problems and Prospects*, ed. by V. Nutton (London, 1981), pp. 229–62.

[10] V. Nutton, 'The Seeds of Disease: An Explanation of Contagion and Infection from the Greeks to the Renaissance', *Medical History*, 27.1 (1983), 1–34 (pp. 1–8).

[11] 'Salubre simpliciter corpus est, quod ab ipso quidem simplicibus ac primis partibus probe temperatum est; in organis vero, quae ex illis componuntur, est commoderatum.' *Claudii Galeni opera omnia*, ed. by K. G. Kühn, 20 vols (Leipzig, 1821–33; repr. Hildesheim, 1964–65), I (1964), ch. 2, p. 309–10; 'quod ab ortu vel similaribus partibus intemperatum', ch. 2, pp. 310; and 'quia utriusque contrariorum ex aequo est particeps', ch. 1, p. 309. Translated in *Galen: Selected Works*, ed. and trans. by P. Singer (Oxford, 1997), pp. 345–48 and pp. 374–76. *Claudii Galeni opera omnia*, Kühn, I, ch. 2, p. 309–10; *Claudii Galeni Pergameni scripta minora*, ed. by G. Helmreich, I. Marquardt, and I. Mueller, 3 vols (Leipzig, 1884–93), III (1893). See also D. Gourevitch, 'The Paths of Knowledge: Medicine in the Roman World', in *Western*

Galen's *Ars medica* was certainly known in early medieval Northern Italy, since it was one of the works commented on by the elite medical teacher Agnellus we encountered earlier, along with Galen's *De sectis*, *De pulsibus*, and *Ad glauconem*. In the final Galenic commentary of the four contained in the ninth-century Milanese medical codex which preserves Agnellus's lectures, the only commentary not containing a subscription ascribing it to Agnellus is on Galen's *Ad glauconem philosophum*. In this work, the idea that health is very individual is clearly outlined.[12] According to Galen, the commentator writes, everyone has their own temperament (combination of humours): 'some are dry, others moist, others hot, others cold.'[13]

The diffusion of the concept of the humours and how it affects health, however, extend well beyond medical texts and/or advice for the wealthy. In a model letter for the appointment of the *comes archiatrorum*, chief doctor and as such, a high ranking official in the Ostrogothic regime in the first half of the sixth century in Northern and Central Italy, its author, the Roman senator Cassiodorus, states that 'the health of men is too obscure, based upon a mixture consisting of opposing humours: when whatsoever of those should have grown, it immediately leads the body to illness'.[14] It might be expected that a powerful, educated man such as Cassiodorus, active in Ravenna in the period when medical texts were being translated from Greek into Latin at Ravenna, and commentaries composed, would have at the very least a basic understanding of the humoral system. Ideas about the humoral system even seep into penitentials, that is, handbooks for priests and bishops when handing out penances for their sinful flock. Preserved in a late ninth-century manuscript copied in Northern

Medical Thought from Antiquity to the Middle Ages, ed. by M. Grmek (Cambridge, MA, 1998), pp. 125–29.

[12] The other two commentaries, apart from those on the *Ars medica* and *Ad glauconem* are on *De sectis ad eos qui introducuntur* (fols 2^r–48^r) and on *De pulsibus ad Tirones* (fols 92^r–114^r). See Palmieri, 'Un antico commento', pp. 204–05. Klaus-Dietrich Fischer has prepared a new edition of *Ad Glauconem*: Galen, *Ad glauconem*, ed. by K.-D. Fischer, in *Galenismo e medicina tardoantica: fonti greche, latine e arabe*, ed. by I. Garofolo and A. Roselli (Napoli, 2003), pp. 283–346.

[13] 'Aliquibus enim sicca est, aliis humida, aliis calida, aliis frigida, hoc est temperantia propriam dixit.' Milano, Biblioteca Ambrosiana, G 108 inf, fol. 114^v, lines 16–18, transcribed in Palmieri, 'Un antico commento', p. 233.

[14] 'obscura nimis est hominum salus, temperies ex contrariis umoribus constans: ubi quicquid horum excreuerit, ad infirmitatem protinus corpus adducit', Cassiodorus, *Variarum Libri XII: De anima*, ed. by A. Fridh (Turnhout, 1973), VI, XIX, p. 249. Thanks to Sam Koon for discussion of this translation: any infelicities remain my own.

Italy, it is stated that a woman who is menstruating should 'not be prevented from entering the church or taking communion, because (periods) result from a superfluity of nature for which she is not responsible'.[15]

Health, Self, and the Environment

In the light of humoral theory in which all patients were unique, treatments to maintain balance to the body therefore had to be tailored to the individual as well. The first-century Roman writer Celsus declares that a variety of activity is essential for the (well-off) healthy individual: he should alternate between town and country, take exercise, but also rest and go to the baths.[16] Celsus's *De medicina* was copied both by the monks of Sant'Ambrogio in Milan and Nonantola in the course of the ninth century.[17] The archetype for both derives, according to Billanovich, from the sixth or seventh centuries.[18]

Texts outlining recommended diet and lifestyle to maintain health (a regimen) were, given the dangers and uncertainty of many treatments, understandably popular. The idea of regimen played a key role in works of the Hippocratic

[15] 'Si mulier menstruo patitur, ab aecclesia et a communione non repellatur, quia superfluitas naturae ei in culpa non reputatur.' Merseburg A Penitential (V23), *Paenitentialia Franciae, Italiae et Hispaniae saeculi VIII–IX*, ed. by R. Kottje, *Paenitentialia minora Franciae et Italiae saeculi VIII–IX* (Turnhout, 1994), lines 1085–92, p. 152. The Italian copy of this text is Città del Vaticano, Biblioteca Apostolica Vaticana, MS Vaticani latini 5751 (V23): see *Paenitentialia minora*, Kottje, p. xxxiii. The penitential retains the link between menstruation and pollution, however, by adding that a woman who refuses communion while menstruating out of veneration for Christ is to be praised: 'et si pro veneratione Christi corporis non communicat, laudanda est.' Merseburg A (V23), lines 1096–1100, p. 152.

[16] On the medicine of Celsus, see, for example, G. Sabbah and P. Mudry, eds, *La Médecine de Celse: aspects historiques, scientifiques et littéraires* (Saint-Étienne, 1994). This particular passage is cited in P. Horden, 'Travel Sickness: Medicine and Mobility in the Mediterranean from Antiquity to the Renaissance', in *Rethinking the Mediterranean*, ed. by W. V. Harris (Oxford, 2005), pp. 179–99 (p. 182), but see also Horden's article on the importance of the 'non-naturals' (sleep, exercise, and diet) for the maintenance of health: P. Horden, 'A Non-Natural Environment: Medicine without Doctors and the Medieval European Hospital', in *The Medieval Hospital and Medical Practice*, ed. by B. Bowers (Aldershot, 2007), pp. 133–45.

[17] G. Billanovich, 'Milano, Nonantola, Brescia', in G. Billanovich and M. Ferrari, 'La trasmissione dei testi nell'Italia nord-occidentale', *La cultura antica nell'occidente latino dal VII all'XI secolo*, Settimane di studio del Centro Italiano di Studi sull'Alto Medioevo, 22 (Spoleto, 1975), pp. 321–52 (pp. 326 and 332). The Nonantola manuscript is now preserved at the Vatican archive: Città del Vaticano, Biblioteca Apostolica Vaticana, MS Vaticani latini 5951.

[18] Billanovich, 'Milano', p. 337.

corpus, as did an acute awareness of the influence of environment on health.[19] The ninth-century Milanese manuscript containing the transcriptions of Agnellus's musings on Galen begins with three Hippocratic texts, including *Airs, Waters, and Places*.[20] This work argues that the environment in which people live affects the type of diseases they suffer from.[21] A manuscript, now preserved in Sweden but copied in ninth-century Northern Italy, also contains a text on the relationship between place, lifestyle, and disease.[22] Another ninth-century manuscript, copied in Nonantola, contains the first-century writer Cornelius Celsus's *De medicina*, in which he warns his readers, concerning pestilence, that: 'Such then are the things to be done in pestilence of all sorts, and particularly in one brought by south winds. And the same precautions are needed by those who travel, when they have left home during an unhealthy season, or when entering an unhealthy district.'[23]

The environment, however, can also be part of the solution. In Aurelius's writings on stomach ailments he advises patients to swim in the sea and other water-based cures.[24] Food was also seen as crucial in maintaining health. In Agnellus of Ravenna's lectures on Galen's *De Sectis*, he emphasizes the importance of 'fine and digestible' (*subtiles et digestibiles*) food for the young and convalescents.[25] Even here, though, environment plays a role since the traveller is advised to eat cold and moist foods when travelling to hot and dry countries.[26] 'Diet' also does not simply signify food, but a regimen for the sick: Agnellus

[19] Nutton, 'Medicine in the Greek World', p. 26.

[20] The three texts are: *Prognosticon* (1^r–3^v, 15–19^v); *De septimanis* (4^r–15^r, 3^v); *De aere, aquis, locis* (19bis^r–21^v). See Beccaria, *I codici*, pp. 288–91.

[21] Nutton, *Ancient Medicine*, p. 75.

[22] Uppsala, K Universitetsbiblioteket, C. 664 (med. 6), 10. (p. 25) *De situs locorum, ubi infirmus iacere debeat*. See Beccaria, *I codici*, p. 346.

[23] 'Cum vero haec in omni pestilentia facienda sint, tum in ea maxime, quam austri excitarint. Atque etiam peregrinantibus eadem necessaria sunt, ubi gravi tempore anni discesserunt ex suis sedibus, vel ubi in graves regiones venerunt.' Celsus, *De medicina = On Medicine*, trans. by W. G. Spencer, 3 vols (Cambridge, MA, 1935–38), I (1935), ch. 10, pp. 79–81.

[24] 'Tunc aegrotantes maritima natatione exercendi atque cataclysmo curandi, hoc est aquarum illisione, suppositis partibus patientibus. animo praeterea securo atque facili esse convenit curandos et aquarum naturalium usum adhibere, ut sunt in Italia, quae Cotiliae sunt appellatae et Nepesinae.' Caelius Aurelianus, *Tardae Passiones*, II section II, ch. 45, p. 704.

[25] *Agnellus of Ravenna*, Westerink, pp. 28–29.

[26] *Agnellus of Ravenna*, Westerink, pp. 28–29.

states that 'whatever can be done for a sick patient is diet, whereas nourishment is either food or drink'.[27]

Categorizing Disease

Despite the emphasis on the individual and avoiding imbalance and hence illness, Classical writers and their early medieval readers maintained also a strong sense of the identity of specific named diseases and conditions. Ancient and early medieval medical writers did distinguish between acute and chronic conditions: Caelius Aurelianus, following Hippocrates' distinction between sudden and short illnesses and more intractable ailments, divided his massive fifth-century medical compendium into books on acute (*celeres*) and chronic (*tardae*) illnesses, although as discussed above this particular work was probably very rare.[28] Many of the problems he describes, such as lung and breathing problems (asthma, for example), diabetes, epilepsy, or liver disease, are still considered long-term, chronic conditions today. However, in ancient and medieval medicine, this division does not always necessarily equate with modern medical definitions of 'acute' and 'chronic' conditions or stages of an illness. Four centuries before Aurelianus, Cornelius Celsus, whose work definitely was circulating in early medieval Northern Italy, dismissed a simple binary distinction between acute and chronic diseases:[29]

> Having dealt with all that pertains to whole classes of diseases taken together, I come to the treatment of diseases one by one. Now the Greeks divided these into two species, terming some acute, others chronic. But because maladies did not always respond in the same way to treatment, some of the Greek writers have placed among the acute what others have placed among the chronic; from this it is clear that there are more than two classes. For some diseases are certainly of short duration, which carry off the patient quickly, or themselves come quickly to an end; some are chronic, in which neither recovery is near at hand nor death; and there is a third class, at one time acute, at another time chronic, and that occurs not only in fevers, where it is most frequent, but in other affections also. And besides the above

[27] 'Quicquid potest fieri circa egrotum dieta dicitur, adescatio vero cibus aut potus.' *Agnellus of Ravenna*, Westerink, pp. 42–44.

[28] *Caelius Aurelianus*, Bendz and Pape.

[29] Firenze, Biblioteca Medicea Laurenziana, Plutei LXXIII codex 1, Beccaria, *I codici*, no. 88, p. 278; Città del Vaticano, Biblioteca Apostolica Vaticana, MS Vaticani latini 5951, Beccaria, *I codici*, no. 102, p. 312.

> there is a fourth class which cannot be said to be acute, because it is not fatal, nor really chronic, because if treated it is readily cured.[30]

Unlike humoral theory this debate appears to have had virtually no impact whatsoever outside of medical 'textbooks'. One criticism of early medieval medicine is that the theoretical aspects of Classical medical thought have been gutted, leaving only the meagre fillet of practice behind. This survey of surviving medical manuscripts copied in early medieval Northern Italy shows that not to be entirely true, although obvious gaps — such as significant works on surgery — are apparent. To what extent do most patients, however, then or now, care how an illness is categorized or described? One of the reasons that the idea of the four humours was so enduring in Western medical thought and popular imagination is that it simultaneously provides both an explanation for illness and its solution — by restoring balance. Anything else is literally academic.

It is also a case of 'mind the gap' when comparing the illnesses and diseases described and discussed by medical writers and lawmakers, and those experienced by their readers and subjects. Is this simply a result of looking at two very different types of evidence, textual and archaeological, or does this have something to tell us about the way health and illness were viewed and managed in early medieval Northern Italy? Chapter one on legal codes and disease, and the following chapter on health, disease, and life expectancy will explore these issues. Chapter three outlines the principal treatments available to the inhabitants of the Italian peninsula between 500 and 900 AD.

[30] 'Hos autem in duas species Graeci diviserunt, aliosque ex his acutos, alios longos esse dixerunt. Idemque quoniam non semper eodem modo respondebant, eosdem alii inter acutos, alii inter longos rettulerunt; ex quo plura eorum genera esse manifestum est. 2 Quidam enim breves utique sunt, qui cito vel tollunt hominem, vel ipsi cito finiuntur; quidam longi, sub quibus neque sanitas in propinquo neque exitium est; tertiumque genus eorum est, qui modo acuti, modo longi sunt, idque non in febribus tantummodo, in quibus frequentissimum est, sed in aliis quoque fit. 3 Atque etiam praeter hos quartum est, quod neque acutum dici potest, quia non peremit, neque utique longum, quia, si occurritur, facile sanatur.' Celsus, *De Medicina*, Spencer, Book III, ch. 1, p. 219.

Chapter 1

Disease, Medicine, and the Law

> If the *schultheis* [Lombard legal official] before whom the case is brought is ill or is known to be in another district on his own business, he shall be awaited until he returns or until he convalesces from his illness. And when he has returned or recovered from his illness, if he delays to do justice within the established four days, the schultheis himself, as has just been said, shall pay six solidi as composition to him who brought the case and a like six solidi to his judge.[1]

So decreed the eighth-century Lombard king Liutprand. As today, there were many reasons as to why someone may not be able to participate in normal social activities due to physical or mental impairment or illness. Firstly, there were congenital conditions which a person would have coped with all their lives. Secondly, a disability could result from an accident or the after-effects of a disease. Finally, a person could become temporarily unwell due to a specific ailment, and be expected either to die or make a full recovery. Early medieval writers, particularly the compilers of legal codes, recognized all of these different categories, which is why law codes are such an important source

[1] 'Et si forsitan ille, super quem reclamavit, infirmus est, aut pro utilitatem sum in alia civitatem esse nuscitur, expectit eum dum revertitur, aut de infirmitate sua convaliscit. Et dum regressus fuerit aut de infirmitate convaluerit, si intra statutus quattuor dies menime eum ad iustitiam faciendum distrinxerit, conponat ipse sculdahis, sicut iam dictum est, cuius causa est, solidos numero sex et iudici suo similiter solidos sex.' *Leges Liutprandi regis*, in MGH Leges, 4, ed. by F. Bluhme (Hannover, 1868; repr. 1984), 25, VII, p. 119; *The Lombard Laws*, trans. by K. Fischer Drew (Philadelphia, 1973), pp. 155–56.

for the social history of medicine in early medieval Northern Italy, and warrant an entire chapter devoted to them.

As well as understanding different types and categories of illness and disability, lawmakers also recognized, as Liutprand's edict hints, the difficulty of determining if someone is genuinely ill or simply seeking to either avoid their responsibilities and/or take advantage of someone else's illness. I shall argue that lawmakers sought to 'normalize' most illnesses and, where possible, to protect and integrate the genuinely sick into society rather than excluding them or placing them on the edge of social interaction.[2] The principal legal traditions of early medieval Northern Italy — both Lombard and Roman — should be seen as a two way mirror, both shaping and reflecting attitudes towards illness, injury, and disability.

In discussing disease lawmakers also had to grapple with the issue of how to name and describe certain conditions. For us, as Jon Arrizabalaga has pointed out in his analysis of the historiography of disease, a 'double translation' is involved: we are studying premodern diseases described by writers before the advent of germ theory.[3] As discussed in the introduction to Part I, humoral theory also emphasizes the individual character of any ailment, dependent on age, gender, disposition, and location. Nevertheless, neither were ancient and medieval writers early social deconstructionists: they described pandemics in which individuals shared common symptoms, and they confidently label specific ailments.[4] I have therefore followed, wherever possible, contemporary nomenclature, without making a definitive judgement as to whether, in biomedical terms, it equates to a specific named modern disease or not.

Whether termed as a generic 'illness' or 'infirmity', a named disease or an impairment, a loss of health (even when temporary) then, as now, has an impact far beyond the physical. It has economic, theological, social, and moral impli-

[2] R. Van Dam, *Leadership and Community in Late Antique Gaul* (London, 1985), p. 1.

[3] J. Arrizabalaga, 'Problematizing Retrospective Diagnosis in the History of Disease', *Asclepio*, 54.1 (2002), 51–70 (p. 67).

[4] D. Harley, 'Rhetoric and the Social Construction of Sickness and Healing', *Social History of Medicine*, 12.3 (1999), 407–35. See also J. Lachmund and G. Stollberg, eds, *The Social Construction of Illness: Illness and Medical Knowledge in Past and Present* (Stuttgart, 1992) and the debate in the journal, *Sociology of Health and Illness*, between Nicolson, McLaughlin and Bury: M. Bury, 'Social Constructionism and the Development of Medical Sociology', *Sociology of Health and Illness*, 8 (1986), 137–69; N. Nicolson and C. McLaughlin, 'Social Constructionism and Medical Sociology: A Reply to M. R. Bury', *Sociology of Health and Illness*, 9 (1987), 107–26; M. Bury, 'Social Constructionism and Medical Sociology: A Rejoinder to Nicolson and McLaughlin', *Sociology of Health and Illness*, 9 (1987), 439–41.

cations. It is these connections I wish to explore in this chapter, beginning with an outline of the confusing forest of legal codes, and responses to illness and impairment within them. This will be followed by an analysis of those conditions — such as leprosy, rabies, or the plague, which did provoke fear and exclusion. Despite the ostensibly very different preoccupations of the various lawcodes in force in early medieval Northern Italy, I shall demonstrate that they shared key concerns surrounding the issues of illness, injury, rights, and responsibilities.

Lawcodes in Early Medieval Italy

Early medieval legal codes have been described as a 'temptingly systematised source [...] in the face of irregular and unevenly distributed charter evidence'.[5] This is particularly true for mid-seventh-century Lombard Italy, for example, in the absence of surviving charter material.[6] For a start, however, in early medieval Italy, from the second half of the sixth century onwards, which legal code you were subject to at least partly depended on whether you identified yourself (or were identified) as Roman, Lombard, Alamannic, or Frankish.[7] Before that date — even under the Ostrogoth Theodoric — Roman law was in force.[8] Theodoric was careful to issue only edicts rather than laws.[9] These various Roman and 'barbarian' codes continued to be revised by subsequent rulers, and were supplemented, after the Carolingian invasion of Northern/Central Italy in 773–74, by Frankish capitularies (in theory at least applicable to all living in Carolingian controlled areas).[10] Even after the Frankish invasion, though, Lombard law largely remained until the eleventh century.[11]

[5] P. Skinner, *Women in Medieval Italian Society, 500–1200* (Harlow, 2001), p. 35.

[6] Skinner, *Women*, p. 35.

[7] La Rocca, *Italy*, p. 28; Skinner, *Women*, pp. 10–11. See also Drew, *Lombard Laws*, pp. 12–13, and B. Pohl-Resl, 'Legal Practice and Ethnic Identity in Lombard Italy', in *Strategies of Distinction: The Construction of Ethnic Communities, 300–800*, ed. by W. Pohl and H. Reimitz (Leiden, 1998), pp. 205–19.

[8] On descriptions of Theoderic as a 'romanus princeps', see J. Moorhead, *Theoderic in Italy* (Oxford, 1992), pp. 44–51. On Alemannic law, see C. Schott, *Lex Alamannorum: Das Gesetz der Alemannen*, 2 vols (Augsburg, 1993) and Hlawitschka, *Franken*.

[9] Moorhead, *Theoderic*, p. 48 and pp. 75–77. For the edicts, see *Edictum Theoderici regis*, ed. by F. Bluhme, in MGH Leges, 5 (Hannover, 1889; repr. 1987), pp. 145–79.

[10] Skinner, *Women*, p. 11.

[11] Drew, *Lombard Laws*, pp. 21–22.

It has been argued that legal codes reflect the aspirations and ideals of rulers as much as the actual practice of law, and we often have no way of knowing which laws were still in force (and enforced) and which just quietly lapsed without ever being removed from the legal codes.[12] This is particularly true for the vast body of Roman law, which, in theory at least, applied to all those identifying themselves as Roman throughout the Italian peninsula. The *Theodosian Code* was originally issued in 438, but there was also the legal compendia of the Emperor Justinian, who conquered parts of North East and Southern Italy in the sixth century to form the kingdom of Byzantine Italy. These, issued between 529 and 534 included the *Codex Justinianus*, the *Digest* or *Pandects* — a compilation of judgements and law from Roman authors — and the *Institutes* (largely drawn from the Roman *Institutionem* of Gaius).

Although the extracts comprising the *Digest* were presumably chosen for their continuing possible relevance in at least some parts of sixth-century Italy, this cannot be assumed, and it was compiled primarily for teaching purposes.[13] It does mean, however, that those administering the law were at least familiar with these concepts, no matter to what degree they actually applied to or were used for their particular city or region. Further, there is a tantalizing fragment of manuscript evidence to support the *Digest*'s inclusion in this study as legally relevant: Halberstadt, Bibliothek des Domgymnasiums (not numbered) contains a fragment of the *Codex Theodosianus*, together with sixth-century cursive paragraphs of the Justinian code, originally copied in the second half of the fifth century in Northern Italy and then reused for another text at the turn of the eighth century.[14] This palimpsest therefore demonstrates that the Justinian code was circulating — and being cross-referenced with earlier Roman law — in sixth-century Italy at least, in however a limited way.

In this respect, the Lombard law codes are far more specific both in terms of the geographical area and individuals which they are intended to cover, and when they are issued: subsequent Lombard kings supplement and alter

[12] Skinner, *Women*, p. 35. For general studies on early medieval law, see K. F. Drew, *Law and Society in Early Medieval Europe* (London, 1988); A. Arjava, *Women and Law in Late Antiquity* (Oxford, 1996); and J. Brundage, *Medieval Canon Law* (London, 1995). On early medieval Byzantine law, see *The Digest of Justinian*, trans. by A. Watson, 4 vols (Philadelphia, 1985), and Brown, *Gentlemen*.

[13] See above, n. 12.

[14] See *Codices latini antiquiores: A Palaeographical Guide to Latin Manuscripts Prior to the Ninth Century*, ed. by E. A. Lowe (Oxford, 1959), VIII, no. 1212, p. 53.

the original code.[15] The manuscript tradition for Lombard law is also richer: Rothari's seventh-century Lombard law code for example, is fairly contemporary, and an insight into what rulers felt they should be legislating about or what they believed their subjects were concerned about, whether or not it was ever enforced, is still valuable.[16] Further, lawcodes arguably still trace the basic contours and features of early medieval society: for example, secular doctors, *medici*, feature more heavily in Mediterranean 'barbarian' law codes than in their more Northerly counterparts, a distinction that is supported by the contemporary charter evidence discussed in chapter six.[17] The Alamannian code is also relevant since individuals identifying themselves as Alamans (settled in much of what is now Switzerland) appear in early medieval Italian charters.[18] The earliest version of this code, the *Pactus Alamannorum* dates to the first half of the seventh century, and therefore is probably slightly more ancient than Rothari's edict.[19]

All these codes, however, as we shall see, have their own particular preoccupations when it comes to legislation concerning illness and ill-health. This is what makes their comparison so telling: they are all concerned with the same geographical space, the Italian peninsula, but legislate on often quite different aspects of illness and injury. This can be viewed both ways: as proof that legal codes operate in a bubble detached from the early medieval inhabitants' concerns, or that the codes were tailored to reflect and address the particular culture and anxieties of each ethnic group. Or, perhaps it is only when we view all the codes alongside each other that we begin to get a more rounded picture of the relationship between health, disease, and legislation on the Italian peninsula. After all, both the lawcodes and the populations of the various Italian kingdoms had to operate alongside each other, in varying degrees of (dis)harmony.

[15] Drew, *Law and Society*, and Drew, *Lombard Laws*.

[16] La Rocca, *Italy*, p. 193 and see also G. Russo, 'Leggi longobarde nel codice O.I.2 della Biblioteca Capitolare di Modena', in *Longobardi e Lombardia: Aspetti di civilità Longobarda, Atti del 6 congresso internazionale di studi sull'alto medioevo* (Spoleto, 1980), pp. 607–21.

[17] A. Niederhellmann, *Arzt*, p. 86.

[18] See Hlawitschka, *Franken*.

[19] Niederhellmann, *Arzt*, p. 12.

Business as Usual? Illness, Impairment, and the Law

Sensory and Mental Impairment in Roman Law

In Justinian's lawcode a key theme is the rights and responsibilities of the deaf, dumb, and blind. 'A dumb man cannot be appointed as a tutor, since he cannot give authorization. 3. Most authorities [...] are of the opinion that a deaf man cannot be appointed as a tutor, since a tutor's duty is not only to speak, but also to listen.'[20] It is interesting here that the compilers acknowledge that there is legal disagreement concerning whether a deaf man can be a guardian (tutor) or not. The emphasis is on the oral, but obviously if both parties were literate communication could still take place, which is perhaps why the legal judgements were not unanimous on this point. One way round the problem of speaking or listening is for a relative to stand in for you. Book Forty, concerning the freeing of slaves, states that 'the son of a deaf or dumb father can manumit by his command, but the son of a lunatic cannot manumit'. The implication here surely is that the deaf or dumb are assumed to be of sound mind and capable of making important decisions, while the insane are not.[21] It is not specified, in the case of a deaf or dumb father and his son, how exactly they are envisaged as communicating. It is assumed, legally speaking, however, that the son can accurately represent the father's wishes. In any case the deaf or dumb man is represented as taking part, albeit through an intermediary, in normal social transactions from marriage to manumitting slaves. This clause also assumes that the person concerned is a property owner who has slaves on his estate.

In Justinian's codes, however, the central concerns arguably are the legal rights and responsibilities of an individual, and their ability to participate in normal social, legal, and financial transactions. In this context, therefore, soundness of mind and the possession of all faculties become much more significant than communicable diseases. In the *Digest*, for example, one clause discusses what should happen if a concubine who is a freedwoman becomes 'insane' — 'furere coeperit'.[22] It is stated in this case that the man involved

[20] 'Mutus tutor dari non potest, quoniam auctoritatem praebere non potest. Surdum non posse dari tutorem plerique et Pomponius libro sexagesimo nono ad edictum probant, quia non tantum loqui, sed et audire tutor debet.' Justinian, *Digest*, Book 26, 1, 1.2–3.

[21] 'Surdi uel multi patris filius iussu eius manumittere potest: furiosi uero filius non potest manumittere.' Justinian, *Digest*, Book 40, 2, 10.

[22] 'Si patronus libertam concubinam habens furere coeperit [...].' Justinian, *Digest*, Book 25, 7, 2.

effectively has a duty of care, as 'it is more humane to say that she is still his concubine'.[23] The central concern of Justinian law in regard to mental health is the implications for the management of someone's financial affairs while they are unwell. A guardian (curator) is to be appointed. Interestingly though, the remit of a curator is envisaged to be broader than just financial oversight: 'the curator's concern and care should extend over the health and well-being of the lunatic as well as the property.'[24] Unfortunately no mention is made of what exactly the legal compilers thought care for the 'health and well-being' of the person concerned should ideally involve (or how such a provision could ever be enforced). Legally speaking, financial extravangance is depicted as analogous to insanity:

> Today, however, praetors and governors, if they encounter persons who have set neither time limits nor boundary to their expenditure, but squandered their substance by extravagance or dissipation are accustomed to appoint a curator for them on the analogy of a lunatic. They remain in care, the lunatic until he regains his health of mind, the other until he comes to his senses; when this happens, they automatically cease to be in their curator's power.[25]

In other words, to be in good mental health, according to the *Digest*, is to be in control, of one's finances as much as one's emotions. Control is an issue that also resonates in contemporary medical commentaries: in Agnellus of Ravenna's sixth-century commentary on Galen's *De sectis*, he comments that: '[When] rational understanding dominates the organism, then our bodies are well governed; when violent passions prevail, then our bodies are governed wrongly, as they are overcome by passions.'[26] There is also an intriguing literary parallel in Byzantine Rome where, as in Roman law, it is the disruption of order and control which is the central concern. In an episode related by Gregory the Great a

[23] 'Si patronus libertam concubinam habens furere coeperit, in concubinatu eam esse humanius dicitur.' Justinian, *Digest*, Book 25, 7, 2.

[24] 'Consilio et opera curatoris tueri debet non solum patrimonium, sed et corpus ac salus furiosi.' Justinian, *Digest*, Book 27, 10, 7.

[25] 'Sed solent hodie praetores uel praesides, si talem hominem inuenerint, qui neque tempus neque finem expensarum habet, sed bona sua dilacerando et dissipando profudit, curatorem ei dare exemplo furiosi: et tamdiu erunt ambo in curatione, quamdiu uel furiosus sanitatem uel ille sanos mores receperit: quod si euenerit, ipso iure desinunt esse in potestate curatorum.' Justinian, *Digest*, Book 27, 10, 1.

[26] '<Quando> rationabilis sensus obtinet animal, tunc bene gubernantur corpora nostra; quando furia nos obtinet, tunc male gubernantur.' *Agnellus of Ravenna*, Westerink, pp. 54–55.

priest called Amantius is said by the Bishop Floridus to have healed an insane man in a 'domus infirmorum' in an unidentified location in Rome:

> I had him brought to me to stay for a few days in the house of the sick [*in infirmorum domo*], where, if he had a gift [*gratia*] for healing, it could quickly be verified. For among the other sick people there lay a madman (*mente captus*), the sort whom medicine calls by the Greek word *freneticus*. One night the insane man (*insanus*) let out great cries and disturbed the other patients with his immense clamour, so that none could get any sleep there. What a wretched business; because one person was very ill everyone grew worse.[27]

Amantius prayed over him and the man recovered, no longer disturbing the others. As Peregrine Horden has rightly highlighted, this passage raises all sorts of pertinent questions about the origins of the care of the sick in general, and the mentally ill in particular, in early medieval Western Europe.[28] However, it also demonstrates that the Justinian *Digest* was in step with both Classical medical thought and contemporary views on mental illness rather than simply an irrelevant teaching tool.

The Lombard law codes, in contrast, tend to group mental health problems together with diseases such as leprosy, and pay little attention to visual or auditory impairment other than where it occurs as a result of an assault and restitution needs to be paid to the victim. They are, however, together with the Ostrogothic and Carolingian edicts and decrees which preceded and succeeded the Lombard regime respectively, still concerned with the fundamental issues of order and individual rights and responsibilities.

[27] Cited in P. Horden, 'The Late Antique Origins of the Lunatic Asylum?', in *Transformations of Late Antiquity: Essays for Peter Brown*, ed. by P. Rousseau (Aldershot, 2009), pp. 259–78 (p. 261). 'Quem tantae uirtutis uirum ipse etiam uidere curaui, eumque ad me deductum in infirmorum domo paucis diebus manere uolui, ubi, si qua adesset curationis gratia, citius probari potuisset. Ibi autem quidam inter aegros alios mente captus iacebat, quem medicina graeco uocabulo freneticum appellat. Qui nocte quadam cum magnas uoces scilicet insanus ederet, cunctosque aegros inmensis clamoribus perturbaret, ita ut nulli illic capere somnum liceret, fiebat res ualde miserabilis, quia unde unus male, inde omnes deterius habebant.' Gregory the Great, *Dialogues*, ed. by A. de Vogüé, 3 vols (Paris, 1978–80), II (1979), Book 3, Chapter 35.3, pp. 404, 406.

[28] Horden, 'The Late Antique Origins', p. 262.

Courts, Inheritance, and Illness in 'Barbarian' Law

In non-Roman, 'Barbarian', law, it was the rights of the sick and dying rather than deaf, dumb, or blind which took precedence. It is also telling that in the eyes of the lawmakers patients were more often than not in need of protection above all from their own families. An edict of the Ostrogothic king Theodoric in the early sixth century outlines what should happen if someone is unable to sign their own will because they are either 'ignorant of letters' (illiterate) or 'close to death'.[29] In these cases eight witnesses are required, whose faith cannot be doubted.[30] Two centuries later the Lombard kings Liutprand and Aistulf, are similarly concerned that the wishes of ill or dying individuals should be both expressed and then fully carried out after their death. In the first year of Liutprand's reign (713) he states that:

> If a Lombard, suffering from human infirmity, is ill, even though he is confined to his bed he has the right, while he lives and is able to speak rationally, to make decisions on behalf of his soul or to dispose of his property in whatever manner and to whatever extent is pleasing to him. And that which he decides shall remain firmly in effect.[31]

Making sure legal provisions made before death would 'stick' was obviously an ongoing problem, since in 755 Aistulf states that:

> We know that many unscrupulous men have acted contrary to the wishes of their dead relatives who, for the well-being of their souls, distributed their property to sacred places and gave outright liberty together with some property to their dependents. Acting with cleverness, the heirs remove [the freed slaves] from their huts and replace them in servitude, so that they lose their liberty as well as their property. Therefore we decree, in order to correct this evil practice, that the desire and command of the dead be carried out: if any Lombard, whether in sickness or in health, arranged by charter that holy places shall have his property and that the household servants by whom that property is served are to be free in order that

[29] 'Quod si testator aut litteras ignorando aut per necessitatem vicinae mortis propriam subscriptionem non potuerit commodare.' *Edictum Theoderici regis*, Bluhme, 29, p. 155.

[30] 'Tunc octavus testis pro testatore adhibeatur huiusmodi, de cuius fide dubitari omnino non possit.' *Edictum Theoderici regis*, Bluhme, 29, p. 155.

[31] 'Si quis Langobardus, ut habens casus humanae fragilitatis egrotaverit, quamquam in lectolo reiaceat, potestatem habeat, dum vivit et recte loqui potest, pro anima sua iudicandi vel dispensandi de rebus suis, quid aut qualiter cui voluerit; et quod iudicaverit stabilem debeat permanere.' *Leges Liutprandi regis*, Bluhme, VI, p. 109; Drew, *Lombard Laws*, p. 146.

> they may make a return [i.e. pay rent] to those holy places, these things shall be observed to all time by a man's heirs as was established.[32]

Aistulf adds that when a man dies suddenly, if his wishes were for a slave to be freed upon his death, this should be carried out, even if the formal procedure for the granting of freedom had not been done before his or her master's death.[33] Whether or not this was a frequent problem is not clear: Aistulf certainly uses this opportunity to present himself as a pious and merciful ruler: 'Because of our compassion [...] it seems to us to be a good thing that slaves be given their freedom from servitude since our Redeemer himself deigned to become a slave in order that He might make us free.'[34]

Another problem that legislators considered was what should happen when someone, 'either because of age or other infirmity, despairs of ever having children and therefore transfers his property to someone else', but who then goes on

[32] 'Cognovimus multotiens perfidos homines contra voluntatem defunctorum suorum parentum agere, dum ipsi pro animabus suis per loca venerabilia res suas distribuebant, et pertinentibus suis simplicem libertatem cum rebus quibuslibet donabant, et cum ipsis hominibus per astutia agebant, et eos ad suis cespitibus removentis in suum servitium replicabant, postmodum libertatem simul et res amittebant. Ideo previdimus, hanc resecare malitiam, ut voluntas et ordinatio inpleatur defuncti. Et ita sancimus, ut si quis Langobardus per cartola, in sanitatem aut egritudinem suam, res suas ordinaverit, et dixerit, eas habere loca venerabilia, et familias, per que res ipsas excoluntur, liberas esse dixerit, ut in ipsis religiosis locis redditum faciant: secundum ipsius statute reddant omni in tempore iuxta domini sui preceptionem ipsi et filii filiorum illorum.' *Leges Ahistulfi regis*, in MGH Leges, 4, ed. by F. Bluhme (Hannover, 1868; repr. 1984), 12, III, pp. 199–200; Drew, *Lombard Laws*, p. 233.

[33] 'Nam si ad finis mortis properaverit, ita ut nec thingare hominem suum possent, neque in manu sacerdotis traderint circa altario liberum dimittendum, propter subitanea morte, et instituerit, ut post eius obitum per manum sacerdotes, qualem designaverit, circa sacro altario deduci debeatur: causa miserationis decrevimus, ut sicut dominus eorum preceperit, ita inpleatur, et sacerdotes, quem designaverit, eum absque cuiuscumque contradictionem absolvat, et liber permaneat.' *Leges Ahistulfi regis*, Bluhme, 12, III, p. 200; If a man has hastened to his end so that he, on account of his sudden death, was not able to free one of his men by the formal procedure (*gairethinx*) and could not hand him over to a priest to set him free before an altar, but he did order that after his death the slave whom he designated should be led around the sacred altar by the hand of the priest: because of our compassion we decree that it shall be done as the slave's lord ordered and the priest shall free that man whom his lord designated without any contradiction, and this man shall then remain free, Drew, *Lombard Laws*, p. 233.

[34] 'Quia maxima merces nobis esse videtur, ut de servitio servi ad libertatem ducantur, eo quod redemptor noster servus fieri dignatus est, ut nos libertatem donarit.' *Leges Ahistulfi regis*, Bluhme, 12, III, p. 200; Drew, *Lombard Laws*, p. 233.

to make a miraculous recovery (or acquire a young wife) and beget an heir.[35] In these cases, the Lombard king Rothari decrees, 'the gift which was made before the children were born is broken and the one or more legitimate sons who were born afterwards shall be the heirs of the father in all things'.[36] According to this edict, daughters and illegitimate children are also entitled to their share.[37]

Despite such complications, wills would appear to have continued to be seen as a 'good thing' by all of Northern Italy's many rulers between the sixth and tenth centuries and beyond. This was almost certainly because of their potential to simplify disputes about inheritance, and the conquerors of much of Italy in 773–74, the Carolingians, were keen that as many people as possible, whether poor and/or ill, should have access to will making. Lothar, a grandson of Charlemagne's, and co-emperor with his father Louis the Pious from 815, legislates for orphans and the poor who cannot afford scribe's fees for the drawing up of documents.[38] He states that the scribes must do it free of charge. In cases where someone is 'required to make a journey or has a grave infirmity' he refers them to a statute of his father's, Louis the Pious, which deals with the making of wills in various circumstances.[39]

Another capitulary, again issued by Lothar for Italy in 822–23, states that scribes/clerks (*cancellarii*) should:

[35] 'Si quis se disperaverit aut propter senectutem aut propter aliquam infirmitatem corporis, filius non possit habere, et res suas alii thingaverit posteaque eum contegerit, filius legitimus procreare.' *Edictus Rothari*, ed. by F. Bluhme, in MGH Leges, 4, ed. by F. Bluhme and A. Boretius (Hannover, 1868; repr. 1984), 4, ch. 171, p. 39, Drew, *Lombard Laws*, p. 82.

[36] 'Omne thinx quod est donatio, quod prius fecerat, rumpatur, et filii legitimi unus aut plures, qui postea nati fuerint, heredes in omnibus patri succedant.' *Edictus Rothari*, Bluhme and Boretius, ch. 171, pp. 39–40; Drew, *Lombard Laws*, ch. 171, p. 82.

[37] 'Si autem filias legitimas una aut plures, seu filios naturales unum aut plures post thinx factum habuerit, habeant et ipsi legem suam, sicut supra constitutem est, tamquam si nihil alii thingatum fuisset.' *Edictus Rothari*, Bluhme and Boretius, ch. 171, p. 40; Drew, *Lombard Laws*, p. 82.

[38] 'De orfanis autem vel ceteris pauperibus, qui exsolvere hoc non possunt, in providentia comitis sit, ut nequaquam inde aliquid accipiat.' Hlotharii capitulare papiense Feb 832, in *MGH: Capitularia regum Francorum*, ed. by A. Boretius and V. Krause, 2 vols (Hannover, 1883), II, no. 201, ch. 13, p. 62.

[39] 'Si vero necessitas itineris aliquem compulerit aut infirmitas gravis, secundum capitulare genitoris nostri faciat.' *MGH: Capitularia regum Francorum*, Boretius and Krause, II, ch. 13, p. 62. On the reference to Louis's capitulary, see Azarra and Moro, *I capitolari*, n. 46, p. 161, and Capitula legibus Addenda, 818–19, in *MGH: Capitularia regum Francorum*, Boretius and Krause, I, no. 136, ch. 6, p. 282.

> come to sick men and according to the law draft a will, to be strengthened by witnesses. It should immediately be written up in a charter and shown to the bishop, counts, judges and other citizens [...] in order to be truly recognised (as legitimate).[40]

This provision could be dismissed as simply a pious hope rather than a reflection of contemporary, effective, legislation. However, some eighty years later a certain Petrus, 'called Spoletino', a *sculdassius* (legal official) in the Carolingian administration, is doing something very similar to that envisaged by Lothar, in order that his last testament would be carried out according to his wishes.[41] Extremely unusually, the charter, dated 898, explicitly states that Petrus had the document drawn up while he was 'lying in bed, ill' ('in egritudine lectulo iacente'), and that he had already made a will previously.[42] Further, rather than use the 'usual suspects', his preferred local/family witnesses as in his previous legal transactions, he makes sure he has the most high powered witnesses he can muster, including a judge, to help ensure that his wishes are carried out to the letter after his death.[43]

Petrus had obviously enjoyed a relatively long life, and there is no indication that his illness was in any way connected with his official legal role in the

[40] 'De cancellariis qui veraces electi sunt: ad homines infirmos veniant et secundum legem instrumenta conscribant, et a testibus roborentur; et statim cum scripta fuerit cartula, ostendant eam episcopo, comiti, iudices vel civariis aut in plebe, ut vera agnoscatur esse.' 158. Hlotharii capitularia italica, Memoria Olannae comitibus data. 822–23, in *MGH: Capitularia regum Francorum*, Boretius and Krause, I, no. 15, p. 319. An Italian translation with facing Latin is given in *I capitolari italici: storia e diritto della dominazione carolingia in Italia*, ed. and trans. by C. Azzara and P. Moro (Roma, 1998), p. 117.

[41] On Petrus and his career see F. Bougard, 'Pierre de Niviano, dit le Spolétin, sculdassius, et le gouvernement du comté de Plaisance à l'époque carolingienne', *Journal des savants* (1996), 291–337. This article is also available as a free download on the *Reti Medievali* website <http://centri.univr.it/RM/>: click on Biblioteca and then under Scaffale on B for the downloadable articles of F. Bougard, accessed 14 April 2014. On Carolingian administration in Italy in general see F. Bougard, *La justice dans le royaume d'italie: de la fin du* VIIIe *siècle au début du* XIe *siècle* (Roma, 1995). See also P. Bonacini, 'Giurisdizione pubblica ed amministrazione della giustizia nel territorio piacentino altomedievale', *Civiltà padana: Archeologia e storia del territorio*, 5 (1994), 43–98.

[42] 'in egritudine lectulo iacente', *Chartae Latinae Antiquiores, 2*nd *series,* ed. by G. Cavallo and G. Nicolaj (Dietikon-Zurich, 1997–), Part 67, Italy 39, Piacenza 4, ed. by G. Cavallo and G. Nicolaj (Zürich, 2005), no. 15, Piacenza, Archivio capitolare di S. Antonino, Diplomatico, Atti private, busta 3, n. 370 (formerly C/52), 30 April 898 at Niviano, new cursive, p. 55, line 2.

[43] I discuss this case at more length in C. Pilsworth, 'Beyond the Medical Text: Health and Illness in Early Medieval Italian Sources', *Social History of Medicine*, 24.1 (2011), 26–40 (pp. 33–35).

Carolingian administration of Italy. A common concern for both Lombard and Roman legislators, however, was what we might term today occupational injuries, an area little explored in previous studies of law or medicine in early medieval Italy.

Accidents Will Happen: Occupational Hazards

Accidents at work, even in modern Western societies, with the weight of modern health and safety legislation and litigation, remain a feature of everyday life. It is certainly a topic that recurs throughout the various lawcodes in force in early medieval Northern Italy. Justinian's *Digest*, for example, includes a very modern sounding discussion of liability for accidents at work (all that is missing are personal injury lawyers):

> Nanusa says if I lend you a slave to plaster a wall, and he falls down from a scaffold, the risk is mine. I think, however, that this is true only where I lent him to you for the purpose of working on a scaffold; but if he should do his work on the ground, and you caused him to get up on a scaffold; or if, through some defect in the latter which was not built properly, even though not fastened by the party in question, or it happened through the age of the ropes or poles; I say that the party himself who requested the loan, must be responsible for the accident which occurred through his negligence. Mela stated that if a slave was lent to a stone-cutter and was killed by the fall of a scaffold, the artisan is liable to an action on loan, because he built the scaffold in a careless manner.[44]

The focus here is effectively on the damage or loss of property (the slave), and no mention is made of compensation to the slave's family, or what happens if the slave survives but is unable to work anymore.

Similarly, when pruning trees, certain steps need to be taken (health and safety measures in modern terms!) to avoid liability: if near a public way, a verbal warning needs to be given:

> If again, anyone, in pruning a tree, by letting a bough fall, kills your slave who is passing, and this takes places near a public way, or a way belonging to a neighbour,

[44] 'Nam et si seruum tibi tectorem commadauero et de machina ceciderit, periculum meum esse Namusa ait: sed ego ita hoc uerum puto, si tibi commodaui, ut et in machina operaretur; ceterum si ut de plano opus faceret, tu eum inposuisti in machine, aut si machinae culpa factum minus diligenter non ab ipso ligatae uel funium perticarumque uetsutate, dico periculum, quod culpa contigit rogantis commodatum, ipsum praestare debere: nam et Mela scripsit, si seruus lapidario commodatus sum machina perierit, teneri fabrum commodati, qui neglegentius machinam colligauit.' Justinian, *Digest*, Book 13, 6, 5.7.

> and he has not cried out to make persons take care, he is in fault; but if he has called out, and the passer-by would not take care, he is not to blame. He is also equally free from blame if he was cutting far from any public way, or in the middle of a field, even though he has not called out, for by such a place no stranger has a right to pass.[45]

Again, the legislator seems to have death rather than injury in mind, and there is no discussion of what should occur if a free man is killed, although the implication is that the liability would still be with the tree-cutter if adequate warning had not been given. This statute also assumes, however, that a witness could state whether a warning had been given or not.

The Lombard laws, in contrast, nearly a century later than the sixth-century Justinian legal compendia (but partly based on older Lombard customs and Roman law) focus much more on non-fatal injuries to freemen caused deliberately rather than accidentally to slaves in the course of their work. Further, the Lombard edicts start with the assumption that it is obvious who is responsible or liable for the injury. In other words, there is less concern for the causes or circumstances of an accident or injury, and more emphasis on the effects of an incident, both for the individual and the community. Indeed, an abiding concern of Lombard law codes is to limit or avoid blood feuds between families as a result of injury or death to another, whether accidental or deliberate. Rothari's *Edict* therefore states that:

> If anyone breaks a freeman's arm above the elbow, which bone is the *murioth*, he shall pay twenty solidi as composition. If moreover, the break is below the elbow, which bone is *trene*, he shall pay sixteen solidi as composition. If he breaks the leg above the knee, which bone is *lagi*, he shall pay twenty solidi as composition. If below the knee, which is the tibia, he shall pay sixteen solidi as composition. If indeed the limb was mutilated or crippled, he shall pay a fourth part of the *wergild*, as is read in this edict, as composition.[46]

[45] 'Item si putator ex arbore deiecto ramo servum tuum transeumtem occiderit, si prope viam publicam aut vicinalem id factum est neque praeclamavit, ut casus evitari possit, culpae reus est: si praeclamavit neque ille curavit cavere, extra culpam est putator. Aeque extra culpam esse intellegitur, si seorsum a via forte vel in medio fundo caedebat, licet non praeclamavit, quia eo loco nulli extraneo ius fuerat versandi.' *The Institutes of Justinian: Text, Translation and Commentary*, ed. and trans. by J. A. C. Thomas (Oxford, 1975), Book IV, III, *The Lex Aquilia*, 5, p. 270.

[46] 'De brachio, coxa seu tibia rupta. Si quis homini libero brachium super gubitum, hoc est murioth, ruperit, conponat solidos vigenti; si autem subtus gubitum, quod est treno, conponat solidos sedecim; si coxa ruperit super genuculum, quod est lagi, conponat solidos sedecim. Si

What is significant about this edict is its precision in naming each individual bone, and giving the Lombard vernacular name as well as the Latin. The sliding scale of payments appears to be based on the size of the bone broken but this system perhaps also reflects the time it takes for bones of different sizes to heal or for at least some level of function to return.[47] Unlike the Justinian statutes discussed above, the possibility of long term disability is considered: implicitly in this edict a simple break is expected to heal (although no explicit mention of a bonesetter is made) but for a 'mutilated or crippled' limb a quarter of the victim's *wergild* is to be given. This is presumably due to the assumption by the compilers of this edict that this disability would at least potentially limit the type of work an individual could do, depending on the limb damaged and original occupation. The careful labelling of individual bones also presumes some basic anatomical knowledge, at least on the part of those expected to read and administer this edict. The level of detail suggests that the edict was designed to avoid conflict or confusion about the correct amount of compensation to be paid to the victim.

The emphasis in the legal codes on accidental and occupational injuries does not accord the same attention by medical writers, but many herbal recipes, discussed in chapter three on medical recipes, seek to aid wounds and breaks. Further, the surviving archaeological evidence supports the prevalence of accidents and injuries in early medieval Northern Italian communities. In the Piedmontese cemeteries of Centallo, Rivoli, and Acqui, in the far Northwest of Italy at the foot of the Alps, fractures of the ulna (forearm) are fairly common. At Centallo, all three cases are male, but at Acqui one is female, and another female at Acqui had a broken femur (thigh bone).[48] Fractures of the tibia (shinbone) can also be found at all three sites. All these injuries could be acquired from falls, work-related accidents, or fights.

One injury probably caused deliberately in the course of a fight or dispute is a severely damaged skull belonging to a male buried at Rivoli. As the excavators note, there is no evidence of cranial regrowth, so the unlucky man died imme-

vero semus aut clodus fuerit, conponat sicut in hoc edictum legitur, quartam partem pretii.' *Edictus Rothari*, Bluhme and Boretius, ch. 384, p. 89. Drew, *Lombard Laws*, p. 128.

[47] Niederhellmann, *Arzt*, p. 9.

[48] F. Mallegni and others, 'Su alcuni gruppi umani del territorio piemontese dal IV al XVIII secolo: aspetti di paleobiologia', in *Archeologia in Piemonte*, ed. by M. V. Gambari, L. Mercando, and E. Micheletto (Torino, 1998), III: *Medioevo*, ed. by L. Mercando and E. Micheletto, pp. 233–61 (p. 252).

diately or soon after the attack.[49] In the eleventh-century cemetery at Monte di Croce, an adult male was buried who had suffered a cut which had penetrated through to the hip bone.[50] He survived, however, for several weeks, which points to some form of care, however basic or inept.[51] Whether this man sustained his injury in the course of a battle, a brawl, or an occupational accident, must remain a moot point. Once more then, legal provisions are responding to causes of ill-health and death in early medieval Italian society.

Moral Contagion and Disease

It is much less certain, however, if the majority of the population experienced rabies, 'lepra', or even pestilence outside of specific epidemics more than any other illness or condition. It could be argued, however, that legislators were meeting a psychological and emotional rather than practical need in focusing on the most feared diseases. While 'lepra' and rabies feature above all in Lombard legislation, however, the disease arguably causing the greatest loss of life during an outbreak was pestilence. Yet pestilence appears to have been much more a concern for medical writers and chroniclers and modern historians than for early medieval lawmakers. I outline responses to all three of these most feared diseases to attempt to explain this contradiction.

Lepra

It has been suggested that leprosy, for example, is prominent in the written sources due to a combination of the ubiquity of skin conditions and the horror with which it was viewed.[52] Modern leprosy is caused by the mycobacterium leprae, but 'biblical' leprosy is apparently not analogous, since the term is applied to inanimate objects as well as humans.[53] 'Lepra' appears in the

[49] Mallegni, 'Su alcuni gruppi', p. 252.

[50] G. Fornaciari, S. Giusiani and A. Vitiello, 'Paleopatologia del cimitero signorile del castello di monte di croce (1st fase, XI secolo)', *Atti del III Congresso Nazionale di Archeologia Medievale, Salerno* (Salerno, 2003), pp. 716–19 (p. 719).

[51] Fornaciari, 'Paleopatologia', p. 719.

[52] Skinner, *Health and Medicine*, pp. 59–61. See also Niederhellmann, *Arzt*, p. 56 and Siraisi, *Medieval and Early Renaissance Medicine*, p. 130.

[53] Nutton, *Ancient Medicine*, p. 29. E. Leiber, 'Old Testament "Leprosy", Contagion and Sin', in *Contagion: Perspectives from Pre-Modern Soceties*, ed. by L. Conrad and D. Wujastyk

Hippocratic corpus (literally 'scaly disease') and is discussed in some detail by the Roman author Caelius Aurelianus.[54] It was also linked with sexual misconduct and sin.[55] It receives most attention in the Lombard law code of Rothari, from 643:

> If anyone is afflicted with leprosy and the truth of the matter is recognized by the judge or by the people and the leper is expelled from the district (*civitas*) or from his house so that he lives alone, he shall not have the right to alienate his property or give it to anyone. Because on the day that he is expelled from his home, it is as if he had died. Nevertheless, while he lives he should be nourished on the income from that which remains.[56]

This clause is obviously concerned with separating the leper, physically and legally, from the rest of the community. It is significant that although in Lombard law a *medicus* is called to treat certain injuries, there is no mention of a medical examination here. Instead, it is a *iudex* or 'the people' who decide whether someone should be expelled or not from the village or town. It would appear from this that Rothari envisages a situation where popular pressure due to fear of contagion or extreme physical deformity could force an individual to leave. However, it also makes provision to support the sufferer in what was obviously recognized as, potentially at least, a long term condition. This clause also does not explicitly equate leprosy with sinfulness.[57]

(Aldershot, 2000), pp. 99–136, especially at pp. 99–100. See also M. D. Grmek, *Diseases in the Ancient Greek World* (Baltimore, 1989), pp. 152–76. In contrast, on the origins of leprosy from a bio-medical viewpoint see M. Monot and others, 'On the Origin of Leprosy', *Science*, 308.5724 (2005), 1040–42. On the medieval period and beyond see L. Demaitre, *Leprosy in Pre-modern Medicine: A Malady of the Whole Body* (Baltimore, 2007) and C. Rawcliffe, *Leprosy in Medieval England* (Woodbridge, 2006).

[54] Cited in Nutton, *Ancient Medicine*, p. 30.

[55] For example, elephantiasis. See Niederhellmann, *Arzt*, p. 56. On sin and leprosy see P. Skinner, 'A Cure for a Sinner: Sickness and Healthcare in Medieval Southern Italy', in *The Community, the Family, and the Saint: Patterns of Power in Early Medieval Europe*, ed. by J. Hill and M. Swan (Turnhout, 1998), pp. 297–307. On the debate concerning the links between sin and disease in general see J. Kroll and B. Bachrach, 'Sin and the Etiology of Disease in Pre-Crusade Europe', *Journal of the History of Medicine and Allied Sciences*, 41.4 (1986), 395–414.

[56] 'De lebroso. Si quis leprosus effectus fuerit, et cognitum fuerit iudici vel populo certa rei veritas, et expulsus foris a civitatis aut casum suam, ita ut solus inhabitet, non sit si licentia res suas alienare aut thingare cuilibet personae. Quia in eadem diae, quando a domo expulsus est, tamquam mortuus habetur. Tamen dum advixerit. De rebus quas reliquerit, pro mercedis intuitu nutriatur.' *Edictus Rothari*, Bluhme and Boretius, ch. 176, p. 41; Drew, *Lombard Laws*, p. 83.

[57] Patricia Skinner views this clause as blaming the sufferer for their condition, but I see it

A later clause in Rothari's edict, however, does specifically link sin and leprosy:

> If it happens that after a girl or woman has been betrothed she becomes leprous or mad or blind in both eyes, then her husband shall receive back his property and he shall not be required to take her to wife against his will. And he shall not be guilty in this event because it did not occur on account of his neglect but on account of her weighty sins and resulting illness.[58]

Sin, in this context, however, is not simply associated with particular illnesses or conditions, but is strongly gendered, applying only to the woman who becomes unwell. As Patricia Skinner has argued, the issue here is sexual purity before marriage, which was only considered necessary for the woman.[59] However, the issue at stake is also — from the point of view of the betrothed woman as a commodity — one of 'defective goods'.

This concept is even more clearly expressed in Rothari's edict in the section concerning bondsmen who are identified as having leprosy after they are sold:

> If anyone buys a bondsman and afterwards he turns out to be a leper or mad, then the seller, if he is accused, shall offer oath alone that he did not know of this infirmity when he sold the bondsman. [And if he can so swear], he shall not be further liable.[60]

For both the betrothed woman and the bondsman no treatment or financial support is mentioned. Therefore status played a role in how a sufferer was treated as well as gender or the type of disease. There are scattered references in the early medieval period in Europe to hostels (*xenodochia*) specifically for those suffering from leprosy. Gregory of Tours claims that Bishop Agricola of Châlon (535–80) founded a 'exsinodochium (*sic*) leprosum' and in the ninth cen-

much more as what might be termed a 'community protection' issue. See Skinner, *Health and Medicine*, p. 60.

[58] 'Si puella sponsata lebrosa apparuerit. Si contigerit, postquam puella aut mulier sponsata fuerit, lebrosa aut demoniaca aut de ambos oculos excecata apparuerit, tunc sponsus recepiat res suas, et non conpellatur ipsam invitus tollere ad uxorem, nec pro hac causa culomnietur; quia non neclicto dimisit, sed peccatum eminente et egritudine superveniente.' *Edictus Rothari*, Bluhme and Boretius, ch. 180, p. 42; Drew, *Lombard Laws*, pp. 84–85. See also Niederhellmann, *Arzt*, p. 53.

[59] Skinner, *Health and Medicine*, p. 60.

[60] 'De mancipis lebroso. Si quis conparaverit mancipium, et postea lebrosus aut demoniosus apparuerit, tunc vinditor si pulsatus fuerit, preveat sacramentum singulus, quod in conscientia ipsius de ipsa infirmitate non fuissit, quando eum vindedit, et amplius non calomnietur.' *Edictus Rothari*, Bluhme and Boretius, ch. 230, p. 57.

tury just across the Alps from Northern Italy Bishop Otmar was said to have founded an institution to care for leprosy patients.[61] As I discuss in chapter five, *xenodochia* in general were designed to care for travellers and the poor, so it is probable that these leprosy *xenodochia* were used predominantly by those who did not have sufficient means to support themselves without working. It is therefore possible that similar institutions existed in early medieval Northern Italy, but, to date, I have not found any reference to *xenodochia* specifically for leprosy sufferers in the surviving documents.

Further, leprosy is not mentioned in either Ostrogrothic edicts or later Lombard legislation. It is also not prominent in Justinianic (Roman) legal codes and is mentioned only briefly in the Carolingian capitularies. In a general edict of Charlemagne's from 789 it is simply stated that those with leprosy should not mix with the rest of the population. No mention is made of sin: on the surface the issue would appear to be one of contagion and the public health implications. However, the capitulary is so laconic we cannot be sure: equally it could be argued that it is moral contagion Charlemagne is concerned about.[62]

The relative lack of attention to the spectrum of diseases labelled 'leprosy' in the majority of lawcodes in force in early medieval Northern Italy obviously does not mean that leprosy and other skin conditions were not a problem, and archeological evidence supports the presence of actual leprosy in early medieval populations.[63] It does, though, suggest that the evidence from Rothari's edict should not be overstated. Indeed, in the majority of clauses discussed above leprosy is grouped with madness or blindness. This suggests that leprosy is functioning in Rothari's edict, rhetorically speaking, both as a 'serious disfiguring illness' from which one is not expected to recover, but also possibly as a warning to his people to avoid sin.

[61] Gregory of Tours, *Liber in gloria confessorum*, in MGH SRM, 1, 2 vols (Hannover, 1885–1951; repr. 1969–92), II, ed. by B. Krusch (1885; repr. 1969, 1988), pp. 294–370, translated as Gregory of Tours, *Glory of the Confessors*, trans. by R. Van Dam (Liverpool, 1988), ch. 85; J. Duft, *Sankt Otmar: die Quellen zu seinem Leben, lateinisch und deutsch* (Zürich, 1959), p. 26, both cited in Niederhellmann, *Arzt*, p. 56. In Byzantium the saint Zoticos is said to have cared for those with leprosy — see H.-J. Stiker, *A History of Disability* (Ann Arbor, 2000), p. 73. I am grateful to Peregrine Horden for pointing out the parallel with Zoticos.

[62] Duplex legationis edictum, 23 March 789, 36. De leprosis: ut se non intermisceant alio populo, *Capitularia regum Francorum*, I, no. 20, p. 69.

[63] Siraisi, *Medieval and Early Renaissance Medicine*, p. 130. See also Niederhellmann, *Arzt*, pp. 52–54, and the recent article by J. L. Boldsen, 'Leprosy in the Early Medieval Lauchheim Community', *American Journal of Physical Anthropology*, 135.3 (2008), 301–10.

In an intriguing footnote, over a century after Rothari issued his *Edict*, Pope Stephen III, in 770–71, opposed the Frank Charlemagne's proposed marriage to a daughter of the Lombard king Desiderius on the basis that the Lombards are related to lepers.[64] This is obviously, as Cristina La Rocca has argued, a term of abuse, and the Pope is vitriolic on the whole subject, but it is not clear why this particular word was used. Is it simply a term of abuse implying sexual impurity or were the Lombards and leprosy generally closely associated with each other by contemporaries, however erroneously or maliciously? Could this explain why Lombard rulers, above all others in the Italian peninsula, were concerned to legislate on this subject? An alternative explanation is perhaps that visual purity was perhaps particularly prized, or even that personal hygiene was particularly low, leading to a myriad of skin complaints.

The Fear of Water: Rabid Dogs and Men

Another iconic — and much feared — condition in the early medieval sources was when a person became 'rabiosa'.[65] This was an illness that was apparently known in the ancient world as it was discussed in both the Hippocratic corpus and Aristotle's book on animals.[66] However, as with leprosy, the terms used by contemporary writers potentially cover more than one disease, as they often focus on one particular symptom, fear of water. This symptom is not unique to people who were 'rabiosa'.

In Isidore's *Etymologies* — a popular text in early medieval Northern Italy — the definition is as follows:[67]

[64] *Codex Carolinus*, in MGH Epistolae, 3, ed. by W. Grundlach (Berlin, 1892; repr. 1994), ep. no. 45, p. 561, cited in La Rocca, *Italy*, p. 29.

[65] C. Lewis and C. Short, eds, *A Latin Dictionary* (Oxford, 1969) defines the adjective 'rabiosus' as raving, fierce, mad, or rabid, p. 1520.

[66] Aristotle (fourth century BC), *History of Animals*, Book 8, ch. 22 discusses rabies that causes dogs to go mad, but he states it is not fatal in humans. In the first-century AD apocryphal letter of Hippocrates to Democritus, however, it is described as affecting humans too. Cited in J. Théodoridès, *Histoire de la rage: cave canem* (Paris, 1986), p. 26 and p. 28 respectively.

[67] Karlsruhe, Staatsbibliothek, Aug. Perg. 229, ninth century, Chieti area; Città del Vaticano, Biblioteca Apostolica Vaticana, MS Vaticani latini 5763, eighth century, Northern Italy; Modena, Archivio Capitolare, O.I.17, second half eighth century, Northern Italy; Cesena, Biblioteca Comunale Malatestiana, Codex Sinistro XXI, ninth century, with tenth century Italian additions. See M. Ferrari, 'La biblioteca del monastero di S. Ambrogio: episodi per una storia', in *Il Monastero di S. Ambrogio nel Medieovo: convegno di studi nel XII centenario*

> Hydrophobia is fear of water, for the Greeks call water ὕδωρ and fear φοβος; hence Latin speakers also call this lymphaticus from fear of water. It is caused either by the bite of the rabid dog or from its froth cast upon the ground. If a human or beast should touch this foam he is either filled with madness or becomes rabid.[68]

Illness resulting from the bite of a dog is also discussed in several Classical and late antique medical works copied in Northern Italy before the tenth century. Soranus of Ephesus (first–second century AD) mentions it, while the first-century writer Celsus states that the bite of a dog can infect an individual with venom, which, untreated, will kill the victim.[69] Celsus's *De medicina*, as mentioned in the introduction to Part I, was copied in the first half of the ninth century at the monastery of Nonantola in Northern Italy, in a manuscript now preserved at the Vatican library, Città del Vaticano, MS Vaticani Latini 5951.[70] Another ninth-century manuscript, of uncertain origin, was annotated in the tenth century — alongside Isidore's *Etymologies* — by Rather of Verona with a fragment of Quintus Serenus's poem, *Liber medicinalis*.[71] In this poem a dog bite results in the body being poisoned.[72] He recommends the herbal remedy of

784–1984 (Milano, 1988), pp. 82–104; B. Bischoff, 'Verbreitung der Werke Isidors von Sevilla', in his *Mittelalterliche Studien: Ausgewählte Aufsätze zur Schriftkunde und Literaturgeschichte*, 3 vols (Stuttgart, 1966–81), I (1966), 171–94; C. Codoñer Merino, 'La medicina en algunos manuscritos de Isidoro de Sevilla', in *Isidorus medicus: Isidoro de Sevilla y los textos de medicina*, ed. by A. Ferraces Rodriguez (Coruña, 2005), pp. 65–84.

68 'Id esta aquae metus. Graeci enim ὕδωρ aquam, φοβον timorem dicunt, unde et latini hunc morbu ab aquae metu lymphaticum vocunt. Fit autem (aut) ex canis rabidi moreu, aut ex aeris spuma in terra proiecta, quam si homo vel bestia tetigerit. Aut dementia repletur aut in rabiem vertitur.' Isidore of Seville, *Etymologiae*, ed. by W. M. Lindsay (Oxford, 1985), IV, 6, 15. *The Etymologies of Isidore of Seville*, trans. by S. Barney and others (Cambridge, 2006), p. 110. On Isidore and medical sources see Ferraces Rodriguez, *Isidorus medicus*.

69 Celsus, *De medicina*, Book V, paragraph 27, cited in Théodoridès, *Histoire*, p. 35. For an edition and translation of the text see Spencer, *Celsus*.

70 See Beccaria, *I codici*, no. 102, pp. 312–13.

71 Cesena, Biblioteca Comunale Malatestiana, Codex Sinistro XXI.5, fols 52ʳ–53ᵛ. See Beccaria, *I codici*, no. 87, pp. 276–77. The transcribed section of Serenus's poem in this manuscript comprises the Preface and chapters I–VIII. Since Serenus's work is arranged traditionally, from head to foot, these chapters are concerned only with problems relating to the head, hair and skin rather than bites which are dealt with much later in the work. However, this transcription demonstrates that Serenus's poem was circulating in Northern Italy before 1000 AD.

72 'XLIV Hominis vel simiae morsu. Siue homo seu similis turpissima bestia nobis Vulnera dente dedit, virus simul intulit atrum.' Quintus Serenus, *Liber medicinalis*, ed. and trans. by R. Pépin (Paris, 1950), ch. XLIV, p. 43. See also Théodoridès, *Histoire*, p. 37.

betony in wine to treat it, or the application of boiled horseradish (raphanus) on the wound.[73]

In Agnellus's commentary on Galen's *De Sectis*, students are even taught to recognize a rabid dog:

> How can we know if the dog which bit was rabid? We reply that we must know if it was done during the dog-days, which derive their name from that star, that is, the Dog Star. If the dog which bit had reddened eyes, that is bloodshot, and its tongue was hanging from its jaws, its tail curled away from the neck, if exceedingly shaggy, foaming about the mouth, threatening other dogs around it, we say that the dog is clearly rabid.[74]

A question that is little considered by historians, however, is to what extent are the Classical medical definitions of 'rabies', its causes and treatments, reflected in contemporary non-medical sources? Section 323 of Rothari's edict is entitled 'In homine rabioso', which Kathleen Fischer-Drew translates as 'on madmen'.[75] The edict goes on to say that 'if a man, because of his weighty sins, becomes *rabiosus* or possessed and does damage to man or beast, nothing shall be required from heirs'.[76] On the face of it there is nothing in the edict itself to explicitly state that this 'madness' is connected with the bite of a dog. No distinction appears to be made between madness caused by demons or by other means. Indeed, the illness is attributed to the sins of the victim. However, the immediate context of the edict *does* strongly suggest a link with rabid dogs: edict 323 is just one among a whole raft of measures concerning dogs, all listed

[73] 'Vettonicam ex duro prodest absumere Baccho, Nec non et cortex raphani decocta medetur, Si trita abmorsis fuerit circumlita membris.' Quintus Serenus, *Liber medicinalis*, Pépin, XLIV, p. 43. See also Théodoridès, *Histoire*, p. 37.

[74] 'Unde possumus scire si canis rabidus fuit ille qui morsit? Et dicimus quia debemus scire si in quinocaumate factum est; quinocaumata dicitur propter illum astrum, id est stella Canis; et ipse canis qui morsit si habuerit oculus rubeus, id est sanguineus, et linguam foris pendentem et caudam a ceruicem replectam et pilos ericiosos et circa labia spumam habentem et alios canes circa se minantes, dicimus, Manifeste canis rabidus est.' *Agnellus of Ravenna*, Westerink, pp. 76–77.

[75] Drew, *Lombard Laws*, p. 115.

[76] My translation, lightly adapted from Drew, *Lombard Laws*. Drew's translation actually reads: 'If a man, because of his weighty sins, goes mad or becomes possessed and does damage to man or beast, nothing shall be required from heirs.' The original Latin reads: 'Si peccatis eminentibus homo rabiosus aut demoniacus factus fuerit, et damnum fecerit in hominem aut in peculium, non requiratur ab heredibus; et ei ipse occisus fuerit, simili modo non requiratur.' *Edictus Rothari*, Bluhme and Boretius, ch. 323, p. 74.

consecutively.[77] For example, the edict that immediately follows the one on 'rabiosus' individuals states that: If a dog or horse or any other animal goes mad and does damage to man or beast, nothing shall be required from its owner. And from him who kills such an animal, likewise nothing shall be required, as above.[78]

Edict 326 is even more explicit:

> If a horse injures a man with its hoof, or an ox injures a man with its horn, or a pig injures a man with its tusks, or if a dog bites a man — except in the case where the animal is mad (*rabiosus*) as above — he whose animal it is shall pay the composition (*wergild*) for the killing or damage [...].[79]

There is therefore a clear understanding of the link between the bite of rabid dog and a human becoming 'rabiosus' themselves. What is missing is any discussion on hydrophobia or treatments, but this would have been irrelevant in this context, since the object of these laws is to outline the boundaries of legal and criminal responsibility for acts carried out by rabid humans and dogs alike.

Pestilence

In early medieval sources pestilence (plague), like leprosy and insanity, is a visible, feared illness with rich biblical overtones.[80] Much discussion has centred on precisely what the plague or pestilence — as described by many early medieval writers — was. In the first century AD Cornelius Celsus gives advice on how to act during an episode of 'pestilence':

[77] See *Edictus Rothari*, Bluhme and Boretius, chs 322–29, pp. 74–75; Drew, *Lombard Laws*, pp. 115–16.

[78] 'Si canis aut caballus aut quislibet peculius rabiosus factus fuerit, et damnum fecerit in hominem aut in peculium, non requiratur a domino, et qui ipsum occiderit, simili modo non requiratur, ut supra.' *Edictus Rothari*, Bluhme and Boretius, ch 324, p. 74; Drew, *Lombard Laws*, p. 115.

[79] 'Si caballus cum pede, si boues cum corno, si porcus cum dentem hominem intrigauerit, aut si canis morderit, excepto ut supra si rabiosus fuerit, ipse conponat homicidium aut damnum, cuius animals fuerit.' *Edictus Rothari*, Bluhme and Boretius, ch. 326, p. 75; Drew, *Lombard Laws*, p. 117.

[80] For an overview on plague, see the collected essays in L. Little, ed., *Plague and the End of Antiquity: The Pandemic of 541–750* (Cambridge, 2007). On pestilence in general see D. Stathakopoulos, *Famine and Pestilence in the Late Roman and Early Byzantine Empire* (Aldershot, 2002).

> There are also observances necessary for a healthy man to employ during a pestilence, although in spite of them he cannot be secure. At such a time, then, he will do well to go abroad, take a voyage; when this cannot be, to be carried in a litter, walk in the open before the heat of the day, gently, and to be anointed in like manner; further as stated above he should avoid fatigue, indigestion, cold, heat, venery, and keep all the more to rule, should he feel any bodily oppression. At such a time he should not get up early in the morning nor walk about barefoot, and least so after a meal or bath. Neither on an empty stomach nor after a meal should he provoke a vomit, or set up a motion; indeed if the bowels tend to be loose, they are to be restrained.[81]

It is perhaps significant that Celsus focuses entirely on prevention rather than suggesting that any cure could be efficacious. 'Pestilence' is of course a very general term that could cover many different infectious diseases: smallpox, typhus, and measles are other possible candidates for ancient episodes of 'plague' or 'pestilence'.[82] That having been said, certainly some sort of pandemic hit Italy (along with many other parts of Western Europe) in the 540s. As I shall discuss below, the analysis of the surviving strains of the bacterium *Yersinia Pestis* and related types of bacteria leads Robert Sallares to conclude that the Justinianic plague of the 540s onwards was the first episode of bubonic plague, as it not a particularly ancient pathogen.[83] It is certainly true that bubonic plague is extremely distinctive due to the buboes (swellings) in the groin, armpits, or neck.[84] Isidore of Seville's description of the 'pestilence' is that it spreads

[81] 'Est etiam observatio necessaria, qua quis in pestilentia utatur adhuc integer, cum tamen securus esse non possit. Tum igitur oportet peregrinari, navigare, ubi id non licet, gestari, ambulare sub diu ante aestum leniter eodemque modo ungui; et, ut supra (ch. 9, 1–3, 6) comprensum est, vitare fatigationem, cruditatem, frigus, calorem, libidinem, multoque magis se continere, si qua gravitas in corpore est. Tum neque mane surgendum neque pedibus nudis ambulandum est, minime post cibum aut balineum; neque ieiuno neque cenato vomendum est, neque movenda alvus; atque etiam, si per se mota est, conprimenda est.' Celsus, *De medicina*, Spencer, Book I, ch. 10, pp. 78–79.

[82] See L. Little, 'Life and Afterlife of the First Plague Pandemic', in *Plague and the End of Antiquity: The Pandemic of 541–750*, ed. by L. Little (Cambridge, 2007), pp. 3–32 (p. 4); R. Sallares, 'Ecology, Evolution and Epidemiology of Plague', in *Plague and the End of Antiquity: The Pandemic of 541–750*, ed. by L. Little (Cambridge, 2007), pp. 231–89 (pp. 245–46) and P. Horden, 'Mediterranean Plague in the Age of Justinian', in *The Cambridge Companion to the Age of Justinian*, ed. by M. Maas (Cambridge, 2005), pp. 134–60.

[83] Sallares, 'Ecology', pp. 246–48. Sylvatic plague in rodents, however, he concludes, may be more ancient — see Sallares, 'Ecology', pp. 285–86.

[84] Little, 'Life and Afterlife', pp. 3–4. Other forms of plague, pneumonic and septicemic,

quickly, is caused by corrupt air, and its principal symptom is swellings (*inguen*) in the groin area.[85] Procopius's *History* includes a description of a disease with black pustules which could become enlarged.[86] Paul the Deacon, writing at the end of the eighth century about events in Italy in the mid-sixth century states that 'there appear in the groins of men [...] a swelling of the glands, after the manner of a nut or date, presently followed by an unbearable fever'.[87] The late sixth-century Greek writer Evagrius from Antioch, however, may be writing about possibly two diseases, as one has swellings and fever similar to that described by Paul and Procopius, but he also includes diarrhoea and bloody eyes as symptoms, and sees it not as a disease from a particular year but ongoing for several decades.[88] However, he may be writing about two forms of the plague: modern clinical descriptions distinguish between bubonic plague — the principal symptoms of which are a high fever, buboes, muscle pain, head aches, and even seizures — and septicaemic plague, which is characterized by abdominal pain, diarrhoea, vomiting, and organ failure.[89] We should also not assume that symptoms are necessarily identical between all patients, let alone between time periods.

There are also obvious difficulties in the interpretation of all these sources — Paul the Deacon is writing centuries after the events he describes, and for all

are less distinctive, particularly in the early stages of the disease. See Sallares, 'Ecology', p. 235.

[85] 'Pestilentia est contagium, quod dum unum adprehenderit, celeriter ad plures transit. Gignitur enim ex corrupto aere, et in visceribus penetrando innititur. Hoc etsi plerumque per aerias potestates fiat, tamen sine arbitrio omnipotentis Dei omnino non fit. Dicta autem pestilentia, quasi pastulentia, quod veluti incendium depascat, ut (Virgil, *Aeneid*, 5, 683): Toto descendit corpore pestis. Idem et contagium a contingendo, quia quemquem tetigerit, polluit. Ipsa et inguina ab inguinum percussione.' *Etymologiae*, 4.6.17–18; Barney, *Etymologies*, p. 110.

[86] Procopius VI xx, 21, cited in Christie, *From Constantine*, p. 458. Robert Sallares sees this as Septicemic plague — see Sallares, 'Ecology', p. 235.

[87] Paul the Deacon, *Historia Langobardorum*, in MGH SRL, ed. by L. Bethmann and G. Waitz (Hannover, 1878), Book II, ch. 4, p. 74; translated as, *History of the Langobards*, trans. by W. Fouke (Philadelphia, 1907); cited in P. Horden, 'Mediterranean Plague', pp. 134–60 (p. 146).

[88] Cited in Horden, 'Mediterranean Plague', p. 142. On Frankish sources and their discussion of the plague, see A. Stoclet, 'Consilia humana, ops divina, superstitio: Seeking Succor and Solace in Times of Plague, with Particular Reference to Gaul in the Early Middle Ages', in *Plague and the End of Antiquity: The Pandemic of 541–750*, ed. by L. Little (Cambridge, 2007), pp. 135–49.

[89] The third form is pneumonic plague, with a severe cough, bloody sputum, and breathing difficulties. See <http://www.emro.who.int/health-topics/plague > accessed 25 January 2013.

the authors their statements need to be viewed in the context of the intended aims and audience for their works. For example, for Paul, as for many writers — taking their cue from the Old Testament — plague could be seen as a punishment, and its disappearance a sign of forgiveness and repentance: in Rome Paul describes how the pandemic ended once an altar to St Sebastian was created in the church of St Pietro in Vincolo.[90] In the absence of any compelling archaeological evidence, however, such as mass grave pits securely attributed to an epidemic, it is on such accounts that historians have based their debate as to the nature of this early medieval 'plague'.[91] Further, unlike in early modern Europe a thousand years later, there does not appear to have been a flowering of anti-plague literature, or if there was, it did not survive.[92] Obviously vast social differences — not least literacy levels and the invention of the printing press — separate the two periods, but for sustained pandemics one might have expected some sort of response in herbal recipe collections at least. That having been said, the first-century writer Cornelius Celsus, whose work circulated in early medieval Northern Italy, does discuss the difficulty of treating 'pestilence':

> Among fevers the case of pestilence demands special consideration. In this it is practically useless to prescribe fasting or medicine or clysters. If strength permits of it, blood-letting is best, and especially if there is fever with pain: but if that is hardly safe, after the fever has either declined or remitted, the chest is cleared by an emetic. But in such cases the patient requires to be taken to the bath earlier than in other affections, to be given hot and undiluted wine, and all food glutinous, including that sort of meat.[93]

[90] Paul the Deacon, *Historia Langobardorum*, VI, ch. 5, cited in Skinner, 'A Cure', p. 298.

[91] Christie, *From Constantine*, p. 501. Michael McCormick is currently undertaking a study of possible mass plague burials: see M. McCormick, 'Towards a Molecular History of the Justinianic Pandemic', in *Plague and the End of Antiquity: The Pandemic of 541–750*, ed. by L. Little (Cambridge, 2007), pp. 290–312 (p. 298) and M. McCormick, *Origins of the European Economy: Communications and Commerce AD 300–900* (Cambridge, 2002), especially at p. 39 and p. 169.

[92] On the plague and plague treatises in early modern England, for example, see P. Slack, *The Impact of Plague in Tudor and Stuart England* (London, 1985); R. Keiser, 'Two Medieval Plague Treatises and their Afterlife in Early Modern England', *Journal of the History of Medicine and Allied Sciences*, 58.3 (2003), 292–324. See also J. Arrizabalaga, 'Facing the Black Death: Perception and Reactions of University Medical Practitioners', in *Practical Medicine from Salerno to the Black Death*, ed. by L. García-Ballester and others (Cambridge, 1994), pp. 237–88 and V. Nutton, ed., *Pestilential Complexities: Understanding Medieval Plague, Medical History*, Supplement, 27 (London, 2008), pp. 1–16.

[93] 'Desiderat quoque propriam animadversionem in febribus pestilentiae casus. In hac utile

This may not be bubonic plague, however (although pneumonic is a possibility), as the treatment of buboes is not mentioned. Partly because of the difficulties of interpreting ancient and early medieval sources through the prism of modern clinical definitions of the various forms of plague, historians and archaeologists have increasingly turned their attention towards the possibilities offered by the ever more sophisticated analysis of DNA from ancient and medieval cemeteries.

Both Robert Sallares and Michael McCormick, in a recent collection of articles edited by Lester Little on the plague pandemic 540–750 AD, discuss the disease from a bio-medical approach. *Yersinia pestis* has been found in some skeletons, but the results are currently contradictory: the degradation of DNA over time and the risk of contamination from modern DNA are all difficulties which molecular biologists have to grapple with.[94] The authors of a 2005 investigation into the DNA of two sixth-century female skeletons found in what is now Upper Bavaria were confident, however, that the *Yersinia pestis* DNA they recovered had not occurred as a result of contamination.[95] As far as the host of the vector of the plague — rats — are concerned Sallares, *contra* Horden, has found scattered references to the deaths of rats during the Justinianic plague.[96] Of course, since a link was not made at that time it may not have been thought significant or relevant.[97] It is therefore not possible to say definitively whether it is precisely the same disease as that of the Black Death in the High Middle Ages, plague in early modern Europe, or nineteenth-century pandemics in China.[98]

minime est aut fame aut medicamentis uti, aut ducere alvum. Si vires sinunt, sanguinem mittere optimum est, praecipueque si cum dolore febris est: si id parum tutum est, ubi febris aut tenuata est aut levata est, vomitu pectus purgare. Sed in hoc maturius quam in aliis morbis ducere in balineum opus est, vinum calidum et meracius dare, et omnia glutinosa; inter quae carnem quoque generis eiusdem.' Celsus, *De medicina*, Spencer, I, Book III, ch.7, pp. 262–63.

[94] McCormick, 'Towards a Molecular History', pp. 293–96.

[95] I. Wiechmann, and G. Grupe, 'Detection of Yersinia pestis DNA in Two Early Medieval Skeletal Finds From Aschheim (Upper Bavaria, 6th Century AD)', *American Journal of Physical Anthropology*, 126 (2005), 48–55 (p. 52).

[96] Nicephorus Gregoras, *Historiae Byzantinae*, 16.1, in *Patrologiae cursus completus: series graeca*, ed. by Jacques-Paul Migne, LXXIV, cols 517–18, and John of Ephesus in Pseudo Dionysios of Tel-Mahre, *Chronicle*, p. 87, cited in Sallares, 'Ecology', p. 269. For a more sceptical view, see Horden, 'Mediterranean Plague', p. 151. On rat populations and the plague, see M. McCormick, 'Rats, Communications, and Plague: Toward an Ecological History', *Journal of Interdisciplinary History*, 34.1 (2003), 1–25.

[97] Sallares, 'Ecology', p. 270.

[98] See J. Shrewsbury, *A History of Bubonic Plague in the British Isles* (Cambridge, 1971);

Even if we assume that it is, as the bulk of the evidence currently appears to suggest, different strains could have varying degrees of virulence, making connections all the more difficult.[99]

As Peregrine Horden has argued, however, the exact origin and nature of the mid-sixth-century pandemic is not necessarily important from a historical point of view: it is more a question of its perception and impact on social and economic life.[100] Jo Hays, however, argues that while diseases are 'socially constructed' in many ways they also are a 'pathological reality' and that modern clinical definitions can help historians understand the spread, decline or disappearance of a particular disease.[101] Given the scanty data available on this pandemic, however, it is not surprising that there is equal disagreement as to the 'plague's' impact on sixth-century Italy. Rouche, Liebeschutz, Brown, and Sallares have all emphasized the devastating consequences of plague, but Wickham, Harris, and Durliat have argued for a more limited effect.[102] Horden and Christie do not discount a significant impact, but point to the problems involved in drawing conclusions from insufficient or indirect evidence.[103] Both Sallares and McCormick suggest that acquired immunity in rats may explain the plague's abeyance in the mid-eighth century in Europe.[104]

G. Twigg, *The Black Death: A Biological Reappraisal* (London, 1984); and S. Cohn, *The Black Death Transformed: Disease and Culture in Early Renaissance Europe* (London, 2003), and rebuttal by Sallares, 'Ecology'.

[99] Cf. McCormick, 'Towards a Molecular History', p. 305.

[100] Horden, 'Mediterranean Plague', p. 151.

[101] J. Hays, 'Historians and Epidemics: Simple Questions, Complex Answers', in *Plague and the End of Antiquity: The Pandemic of 541–750*, ed. by L. Little (Cambridge, 2007), pp. 33–58 (p. 45).

[102] M. Rouche, 'Europe Accumulates its First Gains: Sixth to Ninth Centuries', in *The Cambridge Illustrated History of the Middle Ages*, 3 vols (Cambridge, 1986–97), I: *350–950*, ed. by R. Fossier, trans. by J. Sondheimer (Cambridge, 1989), pp. 474–529; J. Liebeschuetz, *The Decline and Fall of the Roman City* (Oxford, 2001); T. S. Brown, 'The Transformation of the Mediterranean 400–900', in *The Oxford Illustrated History of Medieval Europe*, ed. by G. Holmes (Oxford, 1988), pp. 1–62; C. Wickham, *Land and Power: Studies in Italian and European Social History 400–1200* (London, 1994); W. V. Harris, ed., *The Transformations of Urbs Roma in Late Antiquity*, Journal of Roman Archaeology Supplementary Series, 33 (1999); J. Durliat, 'La peste de 6e siècle', in *Hommes et richesses dans l'empire Byzantin*, ed. by C. Abadie-Reynal and others, 2 vols (Paris, 1989–1991), I: *IVe–VIIe siècles* (1989), pp. 107–25. Cited in Christie, *From Constantine*, pp. 501–04. See also Sallares, 'Ecology', especially at p. 273.

[103] See Horden, 'Mediterrean Plague', pp. 154–56 and Christie, *From Constantine*.

[104] Sallares, 'Ecology', p. 289 and McCormick, 'Towards a Molecular History', p. 310.

Certainly a lack of a response in the legal codes of the Italian peninsula might suggest a lesser impact in the early medieval Italian kingdoms than was previously thought. After all, just a few centuries later it was Italy which was to be in the vanguard of the development of public health measures to attempt to restrict the spread of the plague throughout early modern Europe.[105] Alternatively, perhaps lawmakers, whether Roman, Lombard, or Frank, focused on those illnesses or conditions about which 'something could be done', or be predicted. This may explain lawmakers' silence on fevers/malaria for example, despite the fact that malaria was almost certainly prevalent in a number of regions in early medieval Italy.[106]

Conclusion

Then, as now, illness, injury, and impairment was a fact of life, and the responses to it complex. Depending on the law to which you were subject and the injury or condition, you or your family could either be compensated, or, at the other end of the spectrum, be ostracized if your illness was identified as 'lepra'. Legal allowances in all law codes had to be made to accommodate the sick and impaired and to attempt, however ineffectually, to carry out their wishes after death. Certain diseases, such as 'lepra', the pestilence, and becoming 'rabiosa' have received a disproportionate amount of attention in both the legal and literary sources (not to mention in modern historiography). This was due to a combination of the fear in which they were held, and the broad range of conditions which they could in actuality cover.

The lack of attention to plague and epidemic diseases in general in the legislation indicates that, unlike Italy in later centuries, legislators did not see a major role for themselves in managing or responding to such disasters. It may also show that great epidemics were actually few and far between, and therefore, unlike the plethora of skin complaints likely to be deemed 'lepra', had little impact on either the lawmakers or their subjects.

Although the Roman and Lombard law codes, Ostrogothic edicts, and Carolingian capitularies all differed in terms of the diseases, conditions, or injuries they discussed most, not to mention their responses to them, all shared

105 On the plague in early modern Europe see Cohn, *The Black Death*.

106 The word malaria (from the Italian *mal aere*, bad air) is only attested from the fifteenth century, but different types of fever, treated as individual illnesses, were well known to ancient and medieval authors. See R. Sallares, *Malaria and Rome: A History of Malaria in Ancient Italy* (Oxford, 2002), pp. 7, 14 and 18.

core concerns. These were, perhaps unsurprisingly for rulers, a desire to see swift, uncomplicated resolutions to disputes, but also to enable as many people as possible, whether the 'deserving' sick, poor or minors, to participate and benefit from, the legal process.

The fact remains, however, that unless you were unfortunate enough to have a work-related, accident, a skin complaint, or disease identified as leprosy or rabies, or were savvy enough to make a will or charter, the average early medieval inhabitant would have had little contact with the legal process in relation to health. They were much more likely, however, to have suffered from vitamin deficiencies, joint problems, headaches, and upset tummies, none of which feature in any of the law codes. For these, we need to look beyond the legal and literary evidence, to herbal recipes, and archaeological evidence, as discussed in chapters two and three.

Chapter 2

LIVE, EAT, DIE: HEALTH, DIET, AND LIFE EXPECTANCY

> Italy is a land of ailments and produces unwholesome foods; wherefore you must watch with the most careful consideration as to what, when, in what manner, and with whom you eat; and especially to avoid drunkenness for it is from the heat of wine that ardent fevers are accustomed to attack those who are not cautious.[1]

So writes the Anglo-Saxon Alcuin, who despite forging his career over the Channel in Francia obviously considered the Italian climate and diet in comparison to be 'foreign', exotic, and potentially dangerous. This sentiment is also found, however, in the late antique commentary of the elite medical teacher Agnellus on Galen's *De sectis*. He states that 'men, through eating too many different kinds of food, contract various illnesses'.[2] Citing Hippocrates, he also makes the age old point that one man's meat can, literally, be another man's poison: 'there are some natures which digest barley-gruel and [do not digest meat], while others may digest meat but not gruel.'[3] Even at a macro-level, just

[1] 'Italia infirma est patria, et escas generat noxias; idcirco cautissima consideratione videas, quid, quando, vel qualiter, vel quibus utaris cibis, et maxime ebrietatis assiduitatem devita, quia ex vini calore febrium ardor ingruere solet super incautos.' Alcuin, Ep. 281, ed. by E. Dümmler, MGH Epistolae, 4, Karolini Aevi II (Berlin, 1895), p. 439. Cited in MacKinney, *Early Medieval Medicine*, p. 86 and p. 183 n. 157.

[2] 'Homines plures cibos utendo varias egritudines incurrunt.' *Agnellus of Ravenna*, Westerink, pp. 8–9.

[3] 'Sunt nature hominum que sucus ptysane digerent et carnes que <***> contra carnes digerent et sucus non digerent.' *Agnellus of Ravenna*, Westerink, pp. 62–63.

as there was no political unity on the Italian peninsula in the Middle Ages, so too no single early medieval 'Italian diet' can be outlined, even within regions. Substantial differences in diet — and health — also existed between different cultural and climatic zones on the peninsula, not to mention differences engendered by social status and age.[4]

At least, however, we are no longer completely reliant on written sources like Alcuin's warning on the dangers of the Italian *dolce vita*, when attempting to piece together the population's health, diet, and life expectancy. In recent decades technological developments in scientific analysis have meant that more and more attention has been paid to archaeological evidence for information about health, disease, and diet.[5] This evidence is of two main types: either it is osteo-archaeological, that is derived from the analysis of teeth and bones from contemporary cemeteries, or it is archeo-botanical, based on samples taken from early medieval settlements. For both types, however, the data can be interpreted often in many different ways. For example, as far as disease is concerned, evidence of mass burials at a cemetery may point to a rapid epidemic but also to a massacre.[6] Equally, though, several burials in an identical stratum may also indicate an infectious disease progressively ravaging a population.[7]

Further, the sites from which the data is drawn are not evenly distributed geographically, and tend to favour higher status burials. The data is also weighted according to the type of cemeteries and sites excavated by archaeologists: Christie points out that there is proportionately more information on Lombard cemeteries than native Roman sites — the latter tend to be uncovered in the course of 'rescue' archaeology during modern construction work.[8] Further,

[4] One recent study of the impact of age and sex on diet on those buried at the Roman necropolis at Portae Romae, on the coast south of Rome, is T. Prowse and others, 'Isotopic Evidence for Age Related Variation in Diet from Isola Sacra, Italy', *American Journal of Physical Anthropology*, 128 (2005), 2–13. I am grateful to Brigitta Hoffmann for the reference and a copy of this article.

[5] A great introduction to the possibilities of osteo-archaeological analysis is R. Fleming, 'Bones for Historians: Putting the Body Back into Biography', in *Writing Medieval Biography: Essays in Honour of Frank Barlow*, ed. by D. Bates, J. Crick, and S. Hamilton (Woodbridge, 2006), pp. 29–48. I am grateful to Peregrine Horden for introducing me to this article. See also C. Roberts and M. Cox, *Health and Disease in Britain* (Stroud, 2003), especially pp. 165–89.

[6] See, for example, D. Soren and N. Soren, *A Roman Villa and a Late Roman Infant Cemetery: Excavation at Poggio Gramignano, Lugnano in Teverina* (Roma, 1999), p. 463.

[7] Soren and Soren, *A Roman Villa*, p. 463.

[8] N. Christie, *From Constantine to Charlemagne: An Archaeology of Italy* AD *300–800* (Aldershot, 2006), p. 153.

more bone analysis has been done on rural rather than urban populations in early medieval Italy.[9] Chronologically, less burial sites from the eighth and ninth centuries in Italy have been excavated in comparison with the preceding centuries.[10]

All sites also need to be viewed in the context of how we view disease and disability. Irina Metzler has argued, for the high Middle Ages, that a distinction needs to be made between physical impairment and a socially disabling condition.[11] One does not always follow the other, and Sally Crawford has shown in the Anglo-Saxon burial evidence that physical impairment can be associated with wealth as well as with relative poverty.[12] Conversely, archaeological evidence for the survival of those with serious physical impairment which would have required care by others does not necessarily equate with the impaired individual being cared *about* or being a valued member of the community. The degree to which an individual could play a social and economic role in their communities also depends on the precise nature of the impairment together with their social status. For example, in a family where every member had to undertake physical labour to feed and cloth themselves, the loss of the use of one or more limbs could be devastating. In a wealthy family, however, a child with limited mobility might be sent to a monastery where they could undertake vital roles as a scribe, a teacher to oblates, and/or to pray for the souls of the family. Further, osteological evidence of a vitamin deficiency may not have been severe enough to affect someone's everyday life. These sorts of questions therefore stretch the limits of the archaeological evidence. Archaeological and epigraphical evidence (from gravestones and inscriptions) can, however, tell us more about how long someone lived. I therefore begin with the 'baseline' of life

[9] Christie, *From Constantine*, p. 250.

[10] Christie, *From Constantine*, p. 153.

[11] I. Metzler, *Disability in Medieval Europe: Thinking about Physical Impairment during the High Middle Ages, c. 1100–1400* (London, 2006), p. 9.

[12] In H. Härke, '"Warrior Graves?" The Background of the Anglo-Saxon Weapon Burial Rite', *Past and Present*, 126.1 (1990), 22–43 (p. 36), Härke argues that weapons are included in grave goods even when they would not have been used by an individual due to physical impairment. He gives as an example a skeleton from Berinsfield, Oxfordshire, who had spina bifida but who nevertheless was buried with a shield and spear. However, in the subsequent publication of the Berinsfield cemetery, A. Boyle and others, eds, *Two Oxfordshire Anglo-Saxon Cemeteries: Berinsfield and Didcot* (Oxford, 1995), p. 55, it is made clear that this is a case of spina bifida occulta, which in most cases does not cause any physical symptoms. I am grateful to Sally Crawford for the references, and for alerting me to this point. On spina bifida occulta see <http://www.nhs.uk/conditions/spina-bifida/Pages/Introduction.aspx>, accessed 18 January 2013.

expectancy, before looking in more detail at diet in the literary and archaeological sources. I shall argue that type of settlement, in particular whether a community is secular or monastic, was less important in determining diet than the economic status of its inhabitants.

Demography and Life Expectancy

Even attempting a ballpark figure for life expectancy in early medieval Northern Italy is tricky, given the difficulties outlined above of uneven excavation data from mainly elite cemeteries.[13] Some cemeteries would have served particular sections of society, such as soldiers or a farming settlement.[14] Further, the bones of children and women are smaller, more fragile, and, particularly in the case of neo-nates and babies, buried separately, not necessarily even in a formal cemetery.[15] Ginatempo argues that we are a long way from being able to talk about socio-economic demography in the Middle Ages. However, Giovannini does analyse available archaeological evidence from Italy between the sixth and eleventh centuries, and argues that the traditional picture of famine, hardship, and early death needs to be revised.[16] He argues that infant mortality probably did not exceed 30% — although this needs to be considered in the light of separate burial areas for young children as mentioned above — and that at least 15–20% of the population is likely to have survived beyond the age of 50.[17] This arguably might be expected, though, if the data is mainly taken from elite cemeteries. Interestingly, in the light of my discussion in the previous chapter on pestilence, Giovannini does not see evidence for famine or epidemics being common in early medieval Italy.[18] In contrast, Del Panta and others, in their study of the Italian population from the Middle Ages to the twentieth century, see both contagious diseases and a precarious diet as factors in high infant mortality, ranging between fifteen and fifty per cent in the first year of life.[19]

[13] M. Ginatempo, 'Corpi e uomini tra scienza e storia: studi di osteo-archeologia umana per l'italia medievale', *Archeologia Medievale*, 15 (1988), 7–64 (p. 8).

[14] Ginatempo, 'Corpi e uomini', p. 8.

[15] Ginatempo, 'Corpi e uomini', p. 10. On one cemetery dedicated to infants, see Soren and Soren, *A Roman Villa*.

[16] F. Giovannini, *Natalità, Mortalità e Demografia dell'Italia Medievale sulla Base dei Dati Archeologici* (Oxford, 2001), p. 112.

[17] Giovannini, *Natalità*, p. 112.

[18] Giovannini, *Natalità*, p. 112.

[19] L. Del Panta, ed., *La Popolazione Italiana dal medioevo a oggi* (Roma, 1996), p. 25.

The broad spectrum of mortality, however, reveals how varied the data which we do have can be, and the impossibility of coming up with a single figure. It is therefore perhaps more productive to look at mortality rates on a cemetery by cemetery basis: even though they are not necessarily a representative sample of all strata of society, they do at least relate to a limited geographical area.

Right at the end of the early medieval period, in present-day Northern Tuscany, evidence from the child-dominated cemetery of Castello di Monte di Croce shows that the majority of adults here died between the ages of forty and fifty-nine years old.[20] Since the cemetery mainly consists of child burials, however, it could be that the aged were grouped with children but younger men and women were buried elsewhere. Still, it demonstrates that a minority, at the very least, if not of low status, could hope to reach forty or even fifty years of age. At birth, however, your life expectancy could be considerably shorter, since, of the children buried here, over 80% died before their fifth birthday.[21]

The other evidence for life expectancy is epigraphic. A sixth-century Dacian Imperial bodyguard called Martinianus was buried at St Vittore al corpo in Milan, and his inscription stated that he had served as a protector for forty five years, which would make him at least in his late fifties or early sixties when he died.[22] It could be argued that this was recorded in the now lost inscription precisely because it was so unusual. Was it unusual because of the soldier's age, though, or rather was it the long service which was more exceptional? The same site, however, was also the original home for the fourth-century inscription of a certain Probus, who served for twenty five years as a member of the clergy, and was meant to have died at eighty.[23] It is of course possible that this figure has been rounded up, and simply denotes someone who was considered extremely old.

[20] Fifty-five skeletons were sufficiently well conserved to determine approximate age of death, of which fifteen were adult — see G. Fornaciari, S. Giusiani, and A. Vitiello, 'Paleopatologia del cimitero signorile del castello di monte di croce (1st fase, XI secolo)', *Atti del III Congresso Nazionale di Archeologia Medievale, Salerno* (2003), pp. 716–19 (p. 717).

[21] 82.5% of the forty children's skeletons analysed for age range at death. Fornaciari, 'Paleopatologia', p. 717.

[22] M. Sannazaro, 'Attestazioni di militari e militaria a milano', in *Miles Romanus: dal Po al Danubio nel tardoantico: atti del convegno internazionale, Pordenone-Concordia Sagittaria*, ed. by M. Buora (Pordenone, 2002), pp. 65–80 (p. 70).

[23] Milan, Museo della Scienza e della Tecnica, 368 AD:

B(onae) Probus m(emoriae)
praesb(yter) qui an(nos) (viginti quinque) in clerio labora
vit vix(it) an(nos) (octoginta) et cum virginia sua fecit
an(nos) (triginta) depos(itus) (tertia die) non(as)

Another epitaph, though, this time from the rural hinterland of Milan, suggests that living into your eighties if you were a healthy male was certainly possible. One Adeodatus, a priest, died in 525 AD at the ripe old age of eighty-five. He was certainly exceptional, but Sannazaro has found that five out of thirty fourth- and fifth-century epitaphs from Northern Italy of clergy and their families record individuals in their sixties.[24] Again, lower status individuals do not warrant epitaphs, so like much of the cemetery evidence it privileges those of higher status.

Nevertheless, rural clergy are by no means the aristocracy, and although they would have done less manual work than the average early medieval Italian inhabitant, they are still likely to have had to be physically active, as their families would have been, in their everyday lives. Six further fourth- and fifth-century individuals in the same region — described on their epitaphs by the Roman honorifics 'spectabiles' or 'inlustres' — also lived into their fifties or sixties.[25] This having been said, however, in all groups Sannazaro analysed, the majority were younger than forty: among clergy and their families, six out of thirty died in their twenties, and four were younger than twenty.[26]

Both the epigraphic and archaeological evidence therefore suggest that if you were male, survived childhood, and were of middling or high status you could, with luck, expect to reach forty years old or more. We should certainly not overplay a contrast between the Roman and early medieval period, as Scheidel's study of disease and death in Rome in antiquity shows.[27] For the majority however, in either ancient Rome or early medieval Italy, life expectancy would appear to be considerably less than forty plus, particularly taking into account the high mortality levels of children under five. Status, diet, and occupation obviously also could play an important role in longevity, and it is these factors on which I now focus.

Martias Valentini
ano iterum et Valente
cons(ulibus).

Milano capitale dell'impero romano 286–402 D.C. (Milano, 1990), p. 113.

[24] M. Sannazaro, 'Chiese e comunita cristiane rurali nelle fonti epigrafiche dell'italia settentrionale', in *Chiese e insediamenti nelle campagne tra V e VI secolo*, ed. by G.P. Brogiolo (Mantova, 2003), pp. 39–55 (p. 49).

[25] Sannazaro, 'Chiese e comunita', p. 49.

[26] Sannazaro, 'Chiese e comunita', p. 49.

[27] W. Scheidel, 'Germs for Rome', in *Rome the Cosmopolis*, ed. by C. Edwards and G. Woolf (Cambridge, 2003), pp. 158–76.

Diet in the Literary Sources

Perhaps because diet is one aspect of life over which — finances permitting — an individual can exercise some form of control, and has the potential to maximize quality of life as well as lifespan, texts on health and diet have been enduringly popular over the millennia: early medieval Northern Italy is no exception. As discussed in the Part I introduction on health and medicine, in classical and medieval medicine 'diet' signifies not just food but the correct nourishment and treatment in order to retain or restore health. The first-century writer Cornelius Celsus, in the preface on the history of Greek medicine states that: 'During the same times the Art of Medicine was divided into three parts: one being that which cures through diet, another through medicaments, and the third by hand.'[28]

Celsus devotes a substantial portion of his second book to the properties of foods. He describes which foods are good for heating or cooling the body, or promoting or hindering bowel movements.[29] Anthimus, a doctor who lived in Italy in the early sixth century at the court of the Ostrogothic king Theodoric after he was exiled from Constantinople, builds on this tradition in his work, *On the Observance of Foods*.[30] He wrote this treatise in the form of a letter for the Frankish king Theuderic. Anthimus was Ostrogothic ambassador to the Franks, and probably wrote his tract while posted in Gaul.[31] In his introduction he states that:

> I have taken care, to the best of my ability, following the directions of medical writers, of a plan of diet for Your Reverence which will be of benefit to you, because in men excellence of health corresponds to the suitability of food. By that I mean: if food has been prepared well, it helps towards good digestion, but if it has not been cooked properly, it causes a heaviness in the stomach and bowels.[32]

[28] 'Iisdemque temporibus in tres partes medicina diducta est, ut una esset quae victu, altera quae medicamentis, tertia quae manu mederetur.' Celsus, *De medicina*, Spencer, I, p. 6.

[29] Celsus, *De medicina*, Spencer, I, Book II.

[30] Anthimus, *De observatione ciborum* = *On the Observance of Foods*, ed. and trans. by M. Grant (Totnes, 1996).

[31] *Anthimus: De observatione ciborum*, Grant, pp. 27–28.

[32] 'Rationem observationis vestrae Pietati, secundum praecepta auctorum medicinalium, ut potui vobis exponere profuturam generaliter procuraui, quoniam prima sanitas homimum in cibis conguis constat. Id est, si bene adhibiti fuerint, bonam digestionem corporis faciunt, si autem non bene fuerint cocti, gravitatem stomacho et ventri faciunt.' *Anthimus*, Grant, pp. 46–47.

Throughout he emphasizes the importance of food being fresh and well cooked, and also notes the medicinal effects of dishes. In an acutely observed passage on asparagus, for example (as anyone who has eaten overcooked, unseasoned asparagus spears will tell you), he says:

> Both cultivated and wild asparagus are quite good. Asparagus is diuretic if it is boiled in water with the addition of celery or fennel root, and some coriander or mint is added just when the cooking liquor is drunk with wine. Do not boil asparagus for too long, for it will lose its power and flavour unless it is strong. Eat it with salt and oil.[33]

Did such exhortations from a royal physician, politician, and diet guru, however, have any relevance for the majority of inhabitants of early medieval Northern Italy? Anthimus's contemporary at the Ostrogothic court, Cassiodorus, says that 'we have had a winter without storms, spring without mildness, summer without heat, which is affecting crops'.[34] Paul the Deacon states that in the late sixth century that there was extensive flooding in Northern Italy, followed by famines the following summer. It has been suggested that this is essentially rhetoric employed for dramatic effect, but as with Cassiodorus, there well may be a kernel of truth among the hyperbole.[35] Christie argues that, although evidence of settlement abandonment and a shift in the rural economy in this period is usually ascribed to economic factors, there is convincing archaeobotanical evidence for the onset of cooler, wetter weather in the fifth and sixth centuries.[36] Further, Stathakopoulos's sweeping survey of incidents of famine and pestilence reported in late antique and early medieval literary sources in Western Europe and the Near East highlight an ongoing cycle of food short-

[33] 'Asparagi vero satis boni sunt, et domestici et agrestes, et urinas provocant, si in calda illorum apii radice admixta vel eniculi radice, coriandri modico ad horam misso vel mentae, cum vino ipsa calda bibatur. Et asparagi vero non debent nimium elixari, nam perdent virtutem et saporem, nisi fortiores sint et in sale et oleo comedantur.' *Anthimus*, Grant, ch. 54, pp. 68–69.

[34] Cassiodorus, *Variarum*, Fridh, XII, 25, cited in Christie, *From Constantine*, p. 486. 'Habuimus itaque sine procellis hiemem, sine temperie uernum, sine ardoribus aestatem.' Cassiodorus, *Variarum*, Fridh, p. 493.

[35] On this debate see Christie, *From Constantine*, pp. 488–89.

[36] Christie, *From Constantine*, p. 487. On the evidence from both tree rings and written sources, see K. Randsborg, *The First Millennium AD in Europe and the Mediterranean: An Archaeological Essay* (Cambridge, 1991), pp. 23–29, cited in Christie, *From Constantine*, p. 487.

ages and epidemics, although in Italy's case these were often linked to periods of warfare.[37]

At the other end of the spectrum, though, from failed harvests and the risk of famine, early medieval penance books circulating in Northern Italy focus on the sins of overeating and pollution of the body. This perhaps reflects the different preoccupations of the administrator and the monk or cleric, although as Ambrose of Milan and Cassiodorus himself show, the boundaries between the two in late antique and early medieval Italy are porous. (Both went from high secular office in the Roman and Ostrogothic regimes respectively to a high profile life in the ecclesiastical hierarchy, with Ambrose as a Bishop and Cassiodorus as monastic founder). A tenth-century manuscript preserved at the Vatican, containing a copy of a penance book called the Merseburg penitential, which was possibly designed for use by a bishop, states that if pain is felt in the stomach as a result of overeating, one day's penance should be given, but if culinary excess results in vomiting, a full week's penance should be undertaken.[38] Similar penances were handed out for inebriation.

In the same penance book, however, despite concerns about polluting material, based on the eleventh chapter of Leviticus in the Old Testament, it is accepted that sometimes less than perfect food is eaten. In the Merseberg penitential, where hens, for example, have fallen into wine, oil, and honey, these things should not be consumed, but 'the oil can be used for lighting or other necessities. Similarly honey can be used for medicines'.[39] Rather than being detached from everyday life, the compilers recognized the balance physical and spiritual purity with the need to 'make do and mend'. These provisions reflect both the range of potential sins and recipients of absolution, and the variable nature of the food supply. Some, however, were obviously more protected from food shortages than others, not least monasteries. Much archaeo-botantical data on diet in early medieval Northern Italy comes from monastic sites, and I therefore will consider this evidence separately from the cemetery material.

[37] Stathakopoulos, *Famine and Pestilence*: see for example, nos 95–101, pp. 271–77, concerning famine and epidemics during the course of the Gothic-Byzantine wars in the late 530s.

[38] 'Si quis autem per superfluitatem ventris distinctionem doloremque satietates sentit, I die peneteat, si autem ad vomitum, si infirmitatem VII die peneteat.' *Paenitentialia Minora*, Kottje, ME1, 54, lines 722–30, p. 142; V23, 56, lines 722–30, p. 142.

[39] 'De surice uel gallina aut alium aliquid, si ceciderit in uino uel in aqua, de hoc enim nemo bibat. Et si in oleo ceciderit uel in mel, oleo spendatur in lucerna vel in altera necessitatem. Similiter et mel ad medicina.' *Paenitentiale minora*, Kottje, 54, lines 590–94, p. 200.

The Monastic Diet? The Case of St Giulia, Brescia

> Everyone, apart from those who are very weak, should abstain completely from eating the meat of four-footed animals, *Rule of St Benedict*, ch. 39.[40]

St Benedict, writing in sixth-century Southern Italy, advocates moderation in diet, avoiding meat or excess in any form. On the other hand, the ninth-century monastic plan still preserved at St Gallen, over the Alps from Northern Italy in present day Switzerland looks more like the estate of a grand manor house or castle. Much debate has centred on whether any of this ambitious building project was ever carried out, or whether it was simply a vision of the ideal 'modern' Carolingian monastery.[41] At the very least, though, it indicates what a wealthy and well-connected monastery throughout the Carolingian Empire might aspire to. There is a house for the chicken and goose keeper, together with separate yards for geese and poultry.[42] Similarly, accommodation is marked for the keepers of the pigs, sheep, goats, and cows, respectively.[43] There are courts for drying fruit and grains, a medicinal garden, and an orchard in the cemetery.[44] For processing food there is a mill, bakery, and brewery, and cellars for storage.[45] It is obviously possible that the intention of keeping four footed animals was for the milk, leather, and so on, or for workers to consume rather than monks, but we cannot be sure. How, then, are we to make sense of these conflicting pictures of life and diet in a monastery? Given the large chronological and geographical range, not to mention the many different kinds of monastic institution, can we even talk of a monastic diet in the singular?

One unique excavation in Northern Italy that might shed some light on these issues is the monastic site of St Giulia in Brescia, almost halfway between

40 'Carnium vero quadripedum omnimodo ab omnibus abstineatur comestio praetor omnino devils egrotos.' B. Venande, *Rule of St. Benedict* (Cambridge, MA/London, 2011), ch 39, p. 138. For an up-to-date translation, see Benedict of Nursia, *Rule of Benedict*, trans. by C. White (London, 2008).

41 See the online resource on St Gallen <http://www.stgallplan.org/> accessed 19 January 2013, or in book form the three-volume classic, W. Horn and E. Born, *The Plan of St Gall: A Study of the Architecture and Economy of, and Life in a Paradigmatic Carolingian Monastery* (London, 1979).

42 P. Riché, *Daily Life in the World of Charlemagne*, trans. by J. A. McNamara (Philadelphia, 1978), pp. 36–37. Horn and Born, *Plan*, I, p. xxiv.

43 Riché, *Daily Life*, pp. 36–37.

44 Riché, *Daily Life*, pp. 36–37.

45 Riché, *Daily Life*, pp. 36–37.

Milan and Verona. This was a female Benedictine monastery built on the site of a Lombard settlement, and excavators have analysed layers for the whole of the early medieval period and beyond.[46] This allows us to compare both between monastic and secular diets on the site, and assess whether a recognizably monastic diet along the lines envisaged by St Benedict was being consumed in the monastic era on the site.

For both the Lombard and Carolingian monastic period on the site sheep, pigs, and cattle remains dominate, so it is certainly not a meat-free site at any point in its history.[47] What is particularly interesting, however, are the differences between the Lombard period and the ninth and tenth centuries in terms of food which supplemented this domesticated meat supply. In the Lombard period evidence of the hunting of wild animals, such as red deer, brown deer, hare, possibly wild boar, and even bear has been found.[48] In the later strata, however, the only wild animals for whom bone fragments have been recovered are hares.[49] Instead, in the post-Lombard period on the site more birds and fish appear to have been consumed.[50] Birds represent 7–8% of animal remains found in the Lombard strata on the site, but 30% in the later, monastic strata.[51] However, Pat Baker, who has analysed the osteo and archaeo-botanical finds in depth, points out that the differences may not be as dramatic as they appear since some areas were sieved and others not: sieving results in much better recovery of small fragile bones such as those belonging to birds.[52]

However, what is clear is that different species of birds were being consumed between the Lombard and Carolingian periods on this site. For example, only one goose bone was found in the earlier strata, but 17% of the recovered bones for the ninth- and tenth-century strata were geese bones, although it is not possible to say whether these were wild or domesticated.[53] Some domestic duck bones were found for both periods, but in the ninth and tenth centuries a range

[46] G. P. Brogiolo, ed., *S. Giulia di Brescia: gli scavi dal 1980 al 1992, reperti preromani, romani e alto medievali* (Firenze, 1999).

[47] P. Baker, 'The Vertebrate Remains from the Longobard and 9th–10thC Occupation of S. Guilia, Brescia', in *S. Giulia di Brescia: gli scavi dal 1980 al 1992, reperti preromani, romani e alto medievali*, ed. by G. P. Brogiolo (Firenze, 1999), pp. 425–49 (pp. 428 and 444).

[48] Baker, 'Vertebrate Remains', pp. 339–440.

[49] Baker, 'Vertebrate Remains', p. 440.

[50] Baker, 'Vertebrate Reamins', p. 428.

[51] Baker, 'Vertebrate Remains', p. 440.

[52] Baker, 'Vertebrate Remains', p. 440.

[53] Baker, 'Vertebrate Remains', p. 442.

of wild birds, such as heron, pigeon, grey partridge, and winter migratory birds such as the cormorant and grey heron.[54] Therefore, in both periods wild vertebrates were consumed, but for the Lombard period it was principally game, whereas by the ninth and tenth centuries, wild birds were more popular. This may well be a cultural difference rather than anything connected with a monastic or secular lifestyle. Further, the Lombard phase of the site would appear to have been home to a much less wealthy community than that of the nuns of St Giulia, although as I shall discuss below in the section on cemetery evidence, determining status through the number of grave goods (or lack of them) is a blunt instrument, particularly in an era of rapidly changing belief systems on the Italian peninsula.

In terms of fish consumption, for the Lombard period on this site only ten fish bones have been recovered.[55] In the ninth- and tenth-century strata, however, fish bones are much more numerous.[56] In both periods, as might be expected for an inland site, the types of fish eaten are from rivers and lakes: pike, tench, and trout. For the ninth and tenth centuries, migratory fish such as eels and sturgeons were also eaten.[57] It is tempting to suppose that, since, according to the Rule of St Benedict, the eating of meat was discouraged except for the sick, this explains the increased role of fish in the diet. Certainly fish played an important role in the diet at religious festivals and during Lent.[58]

It must be remembered though, that by no means all living on this site would have been professed monks: lay brothers and sisters, craftsmen, and so on also formed part of the monastic 'household' in its widest sense.[59] Also, Rules were not necessarily interpreted to the letter, and the large quantity of sheep, cow, and pig bones, showing butchery marks which indicates they were killed for meat, suggests that meat formed part of the diet for many if not all of the site's inhabitants in the ninth and tenth centuries. The bones of horses, donkeys, and mules have been found on the site for both periods, but show no cut marks to suggest they were used for meat.[60] The Lombard period bear remains do not

[54] Baker, 'Vertebrate Remains', p. 443.

[55] Baker, 'Vertebrate Remains', p. 443.

[56] Baker, 'Vertebrate Remains', p. 443.

[57] Baker, 'Vertebrate Remains', p. 443.

[58] Baker, 'Vertebrate Remains', p. 448.

[59] On monasticism in Italy see the ongoing series, Monasticon Italiae (Cesena, 1981–). A classic general introduction is still C. H. Lawrence, *Medieval Monasticism: Forms of Religious Life in Western Europe in the Middle Ages* (London, 1984).

[60] Baker, 'Vertebrate Remains', pp. 439–40.

necessarily prove that bear was eaten, as it could have been killed for its skin and teeth.[61]

One of the strengths of the analysis at the St Giulia site in Brescia, however, is that it also includes plant and seed remains. One of the perhaps more surprising findings is the range of cereals and grains present at the site. For example, barley (*hordeum vulgare*) was found in samples dating from before the fifth to the end of the seventh century, and it appears that they had been toasted and roasted, indicating processing for a specific culinary purpose.[62] It was found in greatest quantities for the period 450–569 AD. Indeed, it is in this period — during which time the last Western emperor was deposed, and the Ostrogoths ruled only to be toppled after a long conflict by the Byzantines from the East — that the widest range of grains appear at the St Guilia site.[63] Rye is found for both the phases 450–569 and 569–680, but in larger quantities in the earlier phase. Likewise two varieties of wheat (*Triticum aestivum/durum* and *Triticum dicoccum*) are more common in this early phase, although another type — *Triticum monococcum* — appears to be equally popular in both the 450–569 and 569–680 AD periods. The remains of two different types of millet (*Panicum miliacum* and *setaria*) are also more numerous for the period 450–569 AD. Sorghum (*sorghum bicolor*) and spelt (*triticum pipo spelta*), though, are found only in the 450–569 AD phase.[64] Oats (*avena*) are found in equal quantities on the site in both early medieval phases.[65]

The use of these grains in the period 450–569 AD and, in a more restricted way also up to 680 AD, represents a real break with the past as far as this particular site is concerned, as for the pre-fifth-century phase no samples at all of oats, rye, millet, sorghum, or two of the various varieties of wheat (*triticum monococcum* and *triticum diococcum*) were found.[66] Sorghum is perhaps the most surprising find to modern eyes, as even today it is a grain almost exclusively grown and consumed in its native home of the African continent.[67] It is

[61] Baker, 'Vertebrate Remains', p. 448.

[62] E. Castiglioni, M. Cottini, and M. Rottoli, 'I resti botanici di Santa Guilia a Brescia', in *S. Giulia di Brescia: gli scavi dal 1980 al 1992, reperti preromani, romani e alto medievali*, ed. by G. P. Brogiolo (Firenze, 1999), pp. 401–24 (p. 410).

[63] Castiglioni, 'I resti botanici', p. 410.

[64] Castiglioni, 'I resti botanici', p. 410.

[65] Castiglioni, 'I resti botanici', p. 410.

[66] Castiglioni, 'I resti botanici', p. 410.

[67] See for example <http://www.vurv.cz/altercrop/sorghum.html>, accessed 18 January 2013.

mentioned in Pliny's *Natural History* and was probably introduced into Italy in the first century AD but had not become particularly popular by the end of the Western Empire, although it would become more widely distributed in Northern Italy in later periods.[68]

This expansion in the range of grains found for the early medieval phases of this site can be interpreted in many ways. First of all, it can perhaps be seen as a response to political and economic uncertainty and upheaval, particularly during the bloody Gothic wars in the first half of the sixth century.[69] Livestock are relatively expensive to raise and are also vulnerable to raids since they can be either carried away or killed and eaten. There is obviously also a risk that crops will be destroyed as armies pass through or have battles in the region. However, crops still growing in the fields are less attractive as military provisions as they require harvesting and processing before they can be cooked. Grain stores are another matter, however, and there is evidence of an early communal grain store at the St Giulia site.[70] However, the crops grown may also represent the agricultural practices and consumption patterns of incomers — whether Ostrogothic or otherwise — who settled in Northern Italy as a result of the dramatic political change taking place on the Italian peninsula in the period 450–569 AD.[71]

We do not know, though, whether all these grains were for human and/or animal consumption. The toasted barley would almost certainly have been for human consumption, whether as food or alcoholic drink, and it is likely the wheat would have been used for bread. The other grains could be cooked to make gruel or porridge, but equally could have been used as fodder for animals.[72] We also need to consider the possibility, where the sample shows no evidence of processing and is found scattered rather than in a larger concentrated quantity, that it may even have been considered a weed. Certainly plants which grow as weeds in cereal crops, such as corn buttercup (*ranunculus arvensis*) and brome grass (*Bromus secalinus*), are found in the samples from St Giulia.[73]

[68] Castiglioni, 'I resti botanici', p. 419.

[69] W. Pohl, 'Invasions and Ethnic Identity', in *Italy in the Early Middle Ages, 476–1000*, ed. by C. La Rocca (Oxford, 2002), pp. 11–33 (p. 20) and Castiglioni, 'I resti botanici', p. 424.

[70] Castiglioni, 'I resti botanici', p. 424.

[71] So suggest the authors of the archeo-botanical report. See Castiglioni, 'I resti botanici', p. 418.

[72] On sorghum as food and fodder see 'Sorghum', in *Consultative Group on International Agricultural Research* <http://www.cgiar.org/impact/research/sorghum.html> accessed 18 January 2013.

[73] Castiglioni, 'I resti botanici', p. 422.

The same is true of the red/grass pea or red vetchling (*lathyrus cicera vel sativus*).[74] However, while it can indeed grow as a weed in other crops, ancient farming manuals also describe it as a crop in its own right.[75] It does not appear at the St Giulia site until the period 450–569 AD, with smaller quantities found for the period 569–680 AD. Arguably the systematic raising of crops is suggested by both the range and quantities of not just grains but also lentils. Lentils (*lens culinaris*) were found in the greatest quantities in the period 450–569 AD.[76] This is a source of protein but its dried foliage (straw) can also be used as fodder for animals.[77] The remains of peas (*pisum sativum*) and broad beans (*faba minor*) have also been found at the site, but only for the period 450–569 AD.[78] Peas can also be used for fodder as well as human consumption.[79] It may be that species suitable for both human and animal use were deliberately chosen.

More exotically, the edible berries from the cornelian cherry (*cornus mas*), the peach tree (*Prunus persica*) and even the black mulberry (*morus nigra*) are found in small quantities post-450 AD.[80] The mulberry was possibly introduced into Italy in the Roman period, but attestations are usually later than the St Giulia find, so this sample is significant. None of these are native to Northern Italy, and the quantities found suggest that they were specimen trees, luxuries, rather than being systematically grown as a crop, although fruit in general may have played a larger role than previously thought in the early medieval diet.[81] Hazel (*corylus avellana*) and sweet chestnut (*Castanea sativa*), however, are both endemic in Europe, but were also found only in small quantities for the periods post-450 AD and 569 AD respectively.[82] This suggests that the diet was possibly supplemented by foraging, but only on a small scale, or perhaps examples of both of these trees may have grown on or near to the site.

[74] M.-P. Ruas, 'Aspects of Early Medieval Farming from Sites in Mediterranean France', *Vegetation History and Archaeobotany*, 14.4 (2005), 400–15 (p. 409). See also Castiglioni, 'I resti botanici', p. 420.

[75] Ruas, 'Aspects of Early Medieval Farming', p. 409.

[76] Castiglioni, 'I resti botanici', p. 410.

[77] 'Lentils', in *Consultative Group on International Agricultural Research* <http://www.cgiar.org/impact/research/lentils.html>, accessed 18 January 2013.

[78] Castiglioni, 'I resti botanici', p. 410.

[79] 'Pisum sativum', in *Floridata* <http://www.floridata.com/ref/P/pisu_sat.cfm>, accessed 18 January 2013.

[80] Castiglioni, 'I resti botanici', p. 410.

[81] Castiglioni, 'I resti botanici', p. 420.

[82] Castiglioni, 'I resti botanici', p. 410.

Overall, however, the range of animal bones and plant remains found at St Giulia in its monastic phase reflect most closely those listed in the Carolingian monastic plan of St Gallen. It would be a mistake, however, to characterize this diet as uniquely Carolingian or monastic: the Carolingians were avid copiers of Roman and Merovingian treatises on diet, and Emperor Justinian's *Digest* of Roman law includes discussion of many of the foodstuffs found at St Giulia.[83] Book thirty-two on legacies states that herd animals include 'all four-footed creatures that feed gregariously', including pigs. Giulia in its monastic phase therefore, perhaps should be characterized as representative of a thriving, wealthy Carolingian estate that happened to include some nuns.[84] As on any large estate, secular or monastic, the owners and workers were likely to have had differing diets anyway.

Beyond the monastery, there is the diet of the clergy as well as the laity to consider. An episcopal capitulary issued at Pavia between 845–50 AD states that when bishops tour their dioceses, they should not oppress their own archpriests, and receive only fixed quantities of the following: bread, milk, wine, chicken, eggs, lamb, pork, feed for horses, hay, honey, oil, and wax.[85] This only states what is expected to be available, not necessarily what archpriests or others would eat or use everyday, although the items listed would appear to be the staples needed for both man and beast. Again, it would appear that wealth and social status (into which religious status was obviously interwoven) were the key factors determining the range and type of foodstuffs consumed. Is this confirmed by the cemetery evidence outside of monastic sites?

Diet and Disease Beyond the Monastery

Dental Evidence, Illness, and Vitamin Deficiency

One of the limits of archeo-botanical evidence is that, particularly in socially mixed households such as that found on monastic complexes or large estates,

[83] Riché, *Daily Life*, p. 169; Justinian, *Digest*, Book 32, 65.4–7 and 66.

[84] On this issue see also R. Fleming, 'Bones for Historians', p. 47.

[85] 'Statuimus etiam, ne episcope, quando pro confirmando populo parroechias circumeunt, archipresbyteros suos gravent, ut huiusmodi dispensa contenti sint: panes C, frischingas IV, vinum sextaria L, pullos X, ova L, agnum I, porcellum I, annonam ad caballos modios VI, foenum carradas III, mel, oleum, cera, quod sufficit.' Azzara and Moro, *I capitolari italici*, no. 36 (210), ch. 15, p. 172.

we cannot be sure who is eating what, or even if a plant was simply a weed growing in the courtyard! Human osteo-archaeological evidence, on the other hand, can provide more specific indicators as to an individual's overall diet and health, although interpretation of the data remains complex and often inconclusive.

Teeth can be analysed for caries and for the type of wear on the enamel. Caries can, as today, signal a fairly refined, sweet diet while visible wear on the teeth suggests a diet rich in rough, unrefined food.[86] However, as Ginatempo points out, elements of both can be found in the same set of teeth.[87] Where this occurs, however, this in itself is informative, as it indicates quite a varied diet. Teeth can also be analysed for their strontium and zinc levels, with high strontium levels suggesting a diet based mainly on cereals and legumes with little meat. In contrast, high zinc and low strontium levels point to a diet with far more meat in it: Ginatempo argues that this indicates a higher status individual.[88] A lower level of zinc can be seen as a marker of a more milk and cheese based, pastoral diet.[89] However, as he himself points out, vitamin deficiencies can also be hereditary or due to anaemia sideropenica rather than as a result of a poor diet.[90]

Two of the other principal dental markers used by archaeologists as evidence of nutritional deficiencies and disease are dental hypoplasia and *criba orbitalia*.[91] Dental hypoplasia is a line visible in the dental enamel, indicating some interruption in growth.[92] It can indeed be an indicator of deficiencies in diet, specifically a lack of sufficient quantities of Vitamins A or D.[93] However,

[86] Ginatempo, 'Corpi e uomini' 7–64 (pp. 24–25). For an example of such a study see B. Bonfiglioli, P. Brasili, and M. G. Belcastro, 'Dento-Alveolar Lesions and Nutritional Habits of a Roman Imperial Age Population (1st–4th C AD): Quadrella (Molise, Italy)', *Homo*, 54.1 (2003), 36–56. I am grateful to Brigitta Hoffmann for the reference and a copy of this article.

[87] Ginatempo, 'Corpi e uomini', p. 25.

[88] Ginatempo, 'Corpi e uomini', p. 27.

[89] Ginatempo, 'Corpi e uomini' p. 27.

[90] Ginatempo, 'Corpi e uomini', pp. 28–29.

[91] See, for example, E. Bedini and others, 'Paleobiologia del gruppo umano altomedievale della chiesa cimiteriale di Centallo (Cuneo)', in *L'italia centro-settentrionale in eta longobarda: atti del convegno, Ascoli Piceno, 6–7 ottobre 1995*, ed. by L. Paroli (Firenze, 1997), pp. 345–64 (p. 358). On hypoplasia and cribra orbitalia in general, see Fleming, 'Bones for Historians', pp. 31–34.

[92] S. Hillson, *Teeth* (Cambridge, 1990), p. 125. See also Ginatempo, 'Corpi e uomini', especially p. 30.

[93] Hillson, *Teeth*, p. 130.

it can also sometimes be caused by specific episodes of malnutrition or fever, or a combination of both.[94] Additionally, though, it can also signal low birth weight, diabetes or an inherited condition.[95] *Criba orbitalia* is similar to hypoplasia in that, being a developmental 'interruption' visible in the bones of the skull, it can indicate iron-deficiency anaemia.[96] It can also be caused by a form of *microcitemia* (*thalassaemia*, inherited/carried anaemia).[97]

The difficulty therefore lies in distinguishing between these multifarious causes, or identifying a specific episode of illness responsible for a hypoplasmic line running around the tooth enamel.[98] Further, even if a specific episode of malnutrition or fever is suggested for skeletons displaying signs of hypoplasia, it can be seen as a sign of a robust, fairly healthy community rather than a sickly, vitamin deprived one.[99] This is because for those who died immediately due to a febrile disease, for example, would not show signs of hypoplasia: dental hypoplasia is a sign that a child survived an illness or period of malnutrition.[100] In relation to the rates of hypoplasia found at the seventh-century central Italian site of La Selvicciola, near Viterbo, it has been suggested that the age at which a child is weaned and genetic susceptibility to changes in dental enamel may account for different values.[101]

[94] Hillson, *Teeth*, p. 130. See also Bonfiglioli, 'Dento-Alveolar Lesions', 36–56 (p. 52).

[95] Hillson, *Teeth*, pp. 127 and 130. See also Fleming, 'Bones for Historians', p. 32. On the complexity of interpreting signs of hypoplasia and other dental anomalies, see the recent article by K. C. Hoover and others, 'Exploring the Relationship Between Hypoplasia and Odontometric Asymmetry in Isola Sacra, an Imperial Roman Necropolis', *American Journal of Human Biology*, 17.6 (2005), 752–64. I am grateful to Brigitta Hoffmann for the reference and a copy of the article.

[96] Fleming, 'Bones for Historians', p. 31.

[97] Mallegni, 'Su alcuni gruppi', p. 250.

[98] Hillson, *Teeth*, pp. 129–30.

[99] See Roberts and Cox, *Health and Disease*, p. 220, and Fleming, 'Bones for Historians', p. 34. For the Anglo-Saxon evidence Fleming does argue that individuals showing signs of *cribra orbitalia* or hypoplasia do tend to have shorter lifespans overall than those without.

[100] I am grateful to Sally Crawford for discussion on this point: any errors and infelicities in my analysis of the archaeological evidence, remain, however, entirely my own.

[101] G. Manzi and others, 'Discontinuity of Life Conditions at the Transition from the Roman Imperial Age to the Early Middle Ages: Example from Central Italy Evaluated by Pathological Dento-Alveolar Lesions', *American Journal of Human Biology*, 11 (1999), 327–41 (p. 338). See also M. Blakey, T. E. Leslie, and J. Reidy, 'Frequency and Chronological Distribution of Dental Enamel Hypoplasia in Enslaved African Americans: A Test of the Weaning Hypothesis', *American Journal of Physical Anthropology*, 95 (1994), 371–83.

With Vitamin D deficiency, pseudofractures can occur, which can then develop into actual fractures, healing imperfectly, or the spine can twist (scoliosis/kyphosis).[102] However, as with hypoplasia or *cribia orbitalia*, for scoliosis and kyphosis there are several — usually developmental but also possibly genetic — causes of this condition.[103] Further, a vitamin deficiency — even where it causes a degree of spinal curvature for example — does not necessarily affect an individual to the extent that they cannot take part in normal social and economic activities within a community. Likewise a childhood illness, although serious at the time, might, over a lifetime, be of relatively short duration and significance in the context of a whole lifetime, yet still leave a record in the dental enamel.

What then, if anything, do either vitamin deficiencies (anaemia) or evidence in teeth of interrupted growth tell us? Iron deficiencies (anaemia) have been detected at both the high status rural cemetery at Centallo in North East Italy, and in the Lombard era cemetery at St Guilia, Brescia, dating from the sixth and seventh centuries, before the site became the prestigious nunnery.[104] The individuals buried there are described as a 'hybridized' local and Lombard population, with few grave goods.[105] Whether this automatically equates to a 'lower-status' cemetery however, is debatable. A low number of grave goods could be interpreted as a sign of lower status, but equally may reflect changing belief systems. Further, there is evidence that many of the graves had been broken into in preceding centuries, so they may have originally been richer.[106] In general in Northern Italy early Lombard graves were likely to be furnished while native Roman ones by the sixth century, when the Lombards invaded,

[102] On Vitamin D deficiencies in history, see M. Brickley, S. Mays, and R. Ives, 'Skeletal Manifestations of Vitamin D Deficiency Osteomalacia in Documented Historical Collections', *International Journal of Osteoarchaeology*, 15 (2005), 389–403 (pp. 392–95). See also M. Brickley, S. Mays, and R. Ives, 'An Investigation of Skeletal Indicators of Vitamin D Deficiency in Adults: Effective Markers for Interpreting Past Living Conditions and Pollution Levels in 18th and 19th Century Birmingham, England', *American Journal of Physical Anthropology*, 132 (2007), 67–79.

[103] Brickley, 'Skeletal Manifestations', pp. 395–96. On a possible genetic basis for some cases of scoliosis, see <http://www.iscoliosis.com/articles-gene.html>, accessed 18 January 2013.

[104] G. P. Brogiolo and C. Cuni, 'Le sepolture di età longobarda di S. Giulia in Brescia', *Rivista di Studi Liguri*, 54 (1988), 145–58; G. P. Brogiolo, *Brescia altomedievale: Urbanistica ed edilizia dal IV al IX secolo* (Mantua, 1993), pp. 90–96, cited in Christie, *From Constantine*, p. 252.

[105] Christie, *From Constantine*, p. 252.

[106] Brogiolo and Cuni, 'Le sepolture', p. 145.

generally were not.[107] Determining ethnic identity simply from grave goods is an uncertain business, though, and above ground rituals may have been used to distinguish pagan, Arian, and Catholic as much as the type of burial.[108] However, in the case of this Lombard era burial site at St Giulia, dating from the sixth to seventh century, the osteo-archaeological evidence is more convincing as to their precarious economic status, as the remains show evidence of widespread malnutrition.[109] In the most serious cases it may have caused the individual's death.[110] Of the twenty-two Lombard era skeletons at this site, nine are under sixteen, and of the adults, all but two are young adults between sixteen and twenty five.[111] It is therefore unclear whether this is a 'whole of population' burial site or not. It is possible, therefore, that the causes of iron deficiency, and its severity, not to mention its impact on the various age groups within a community, differed between the sites at Centallo and St Giulia. It also perhaps challenges the idea, however, that even higher status individuals necessarily had a balanced diet or one always high in red meat, one of the main sources of iron.

Conversely, even more humble communities, if they had access to a wider range of foodstuffs, could fare better than the young inhabitants of Lombard-era St Giulia. Just thirteen kilometres from that site at Brescia, the Villa Carcina, a contemporary burial site, reveals much better nutrition for the community there.[112] Brogiolo and Cuni argue that this reflects the contrasting microeconomies in the region: the community at Villa Carcina lived at a fairly high altitude, and had access to milk and milk products, while at the domus at St Giulia the inhabitants were instead reliant on a poor mixed economy, without the benefit of the wide range of provisions and distribution networks that could be available in cities.[113] The later nunnery of St Giulia on the same site, well connected and with estates to draw on, perhaps largely avoided many of the dietary problems faced by the earlier inhabitants.

[107] Christie, *From Constantine*, p. 150.

[108] Christie, *From Constantine*, pp. 149–50. See also A. Schülke, 'On Christianization and Grave-Finds', *European Journal of Archaeology*, 2.1 (1999), 77–106, cited in Christie, *From Constantine*, p. 150.

[109] Brogiolo and Cuni, 'Le sepulture', p. 155.

[110] Brogiolo and Cuni, 'Le sepulture', p. 155.

[111] Brogiolo and Cuni, 'Le sepulture', p. 155.

[112] Brogiolo and Cuni, 'Le sepulture', p. 156.

[113] Brogiolo and Cuni, 'Le sepulture', p. 156.

At Rivoli, just south east of Turin, thirty seven individuals, buried in thirty-three tombs datable to between the sixth and eighth centuries, have been excavated.[114] Only two of the thirty seven skeletons are of children or adolescents: of the adults nineteen are male, twelve female, and for three sex is not determinable.[115] The majority are in earth graves. One male and one female skeleton show signs of having had rickets (Vitamin D deficiency) in infancy.[116] This does not, however, on its own, necessarily indicate low status or a poor or very restricted diet: Sources of vitamin D are found in dairy products, eggs, liver, and oily fish, but only in small amounts: 90–100% of vitamin D needed in the human body is activated by exposing skin to sunlight.[117] It is therefore, even today in the age of fortified milk and cereals, possible to be Vitamin D deficient while eating a fairly varied and balanced diet if there is not sufficient exposure to sunlight. About a quarter of the adult skeletons from the Rivoli cemetery had *criba orbitalia*, however.[118] This would suggest frequent illness or an uncertain food supply, but which the individuals concerned were none the less hardy enough to survive.

Similar levels are found in the early medieval phase of the cemetery of Centallo, in the Cuneo region, about 60 km south of Turin.[119] Interestingly, though, it was almost absent from the samples from a cemetery near the Roman arena at Acqui terme, about 65 km south west from Alessandria in southern Piedmont, and Chieri, not far from Turin. Acqui terme is a cemetery excavation of equivalent size to Rivoli, and which also has a broadly similar mix of children, adults, males, and females as Rivoli.[120] It was used, however, over a longer and later time period, from the seventh to the eleventh century.[121] Chieri, however, is earlier than either Rivoli or Acqui, the skeletons dating to the fifth and sixth century. It is also a larger excavation, uncovering forty-eight skeletons, of which six were children or adolescents, twenty-five male, twelve female, and five where the sex

[114] Mallegni, 'Su alcuni gruppi', p. 234.

[115] Mallegni, 'Su alcuni gruppi', p. 234.

[116] Mallegni, 'Su alcuni gruppi', p. 251.

[117] Brickley, 'Skeletal Manifestations', p. 391.

[118] Mallegni, 'Su alcuni gruppi', pp. 250–51.

[119] Mallegni, 'Su alcuni gruppi', p. 251.

[120] Thirty-three skeletons, of which four were children and adolescents. Of the adult remains, nineteen were male, and ten female. Mallegni, 'Su alcuni gruppi', p. 234.

[121] Mallegni, 'Su alcuni gruppi', p. 234.

was not determinable from the remains.[122] The authors of the article conclude that such differences are attributable to differences in diet or hygiene between these communities.[123] This may be the case, or may even conceivably indicate an episode of disease or malnutrition. It is certainly true that at Centallo, the diet of those excavated from the early medieval phase appears from the strontium and calcium levels to have been rich in vegetables and cereals and low in animal proteins.[124] It is suggested the population as a result suffered from iron deficiencies.[125] In contrast, at Acqui the relative levels of strontium and calcium and zinc and calcium indicate a more balanced diet.[126] (Within this, there are gender differences as at Acqui women appear to have eaten less meat, but slightly more than men at Centallo, and the authors acknowledge that it is difficult to know whether this is statistically significant or causal or not.)[127]

Given the relatively small samples and large timescales involved, however, it is impossible to say to what extent differences in diet played a role in the prevalence of *cribra orbitalia* in the excavated skeletons. Further, although the balance of children, adults, males, and females is roughly similar between these cemeteries, that is relatively few children and adolescents and a consistently higher number of adult males than females, it is difficult to say with any precision if their status and role in the community is similar between the groups represented. It is certainly clear that none of these sites represent 'real' populations in the sense of a representative sample, given the relatively low numbers of child and female skeletons found at these cemeteries.[128]

Joint Conditions and Fractures in the Osteo-Archaeological Evidence

While the impact of vitamin deficiencies and fluctuating food supplies continues to be debated, there is no doubt that the early medieval population of Northern Italy, as elsewhere, suffered from many joint problems despite a life

[122] Mallegni, 'Su alcuni gruppi', pp. 234–35.

[123] Mallegni, 'Su alcuni gruppi', p. 251.

[124] Mallegni, 'Su alcuni gruppi', p. 253.

[125] E. Bedini and others, 'Paleobiologia del gruppo umano altomedievale della chiesa cimiteriale di Centallo (Cuneo)', in *L'italia centro-settentrionale in eta longobarda: atti del convegno, Ascoli Piceno, 6–7 ottobre 1995*, ed. by L. Paroli (Firenze, 1997), pp. 345–64 (p. 358).

[126] Mallegni, 'Su alcuni gruppi', p. 253.

[127] Mallegni, 'Su alcuni gruppi', p. 253.

[128] See, for example, the burial sites discussed by Christie, *From Constantine*, pp. 252–59.

expectancy much lower than that in the developed world today. In Latin pain in the hands can be termed *chiragra*, *arthritis*, or *articularis*, but these terms can also denote gout (*podagra*), a condition about which a tract was written by Alexander of Tralles.[129] Both conditions are discussed together in some detail by Cornelius Celsus. He states that:

> Joint troubles in the hands and feet are very frequent and persistent, such as occur in cases of podagra and cheiragra. These seldom attack eunuchs or boys before coition with a woman, or women except those in whom the menses have become suppressed.[130]

In modern medicine, arthritis is now divided into multifarious types and of these, forms such as gouty- and osteo-arthritis are visible in the archaeological record, although rheumatoid arthritis is considered a more recent disease.[131]

At the Lombard cemetery at Centallo, in North-East Italy, osteoarthritis was found most frequently in the vertebral column, but also in knees, and nearly 8% of the skeletons analysed had shin splints.[132] Arthritis was also found in the jaw of two males buried at Centallo, and a further two at another Lombard cemetery in Piedmont, Rivoli.[133] Osteoarthritis in the back and knees could be caused by repetitive movements, but is also associated with being overweight.[134] Shin splints (*periostitis*) could have been caused by lack of Vitamin C or extensive horse riding.[135] Also in Piedmont, at the cemetery of the castle of Monte de Croce, dating from the eleventh century, around two thirds of the skeletons

[129] See Notre Dame University online Latin dictionary at <www.nd.edu/~archives/latin.htm>, accessed 14 April 2014; Valerie Knight is preparing a PhD thesis at Manchester University in the Department of Classics and Ancient History on the gout treatise.

[130] 'In manibus pedibusque articulorum vitia frequentiora longioraque sunt, quae in podagris cheragrisve esse consuerunt. Ea raro vel castratos vel pueros ante femina coitum vel mulieres, nisi quibus menstrua suppressa sunt, temptant.' Celsus, *De medicina*, Spencer, I, Book IV, ch. 31, p. 455.

[131] See, for example <http://www.bbc.co.uk/health/conditions/arthritis>, accessed 18 January 2013. On forms of arthritis and in the archaeological record see P. Bridges, 'Review of *A Field Guide to Joint Disease in Archaeology*, by J. Rogers and T. Waldron', *American Antiquity*, 61.3 (1996), 630, and J. Rogers, I. Watt, and P. Dieppe, 'Arthritis in Saxon and Mediaeval Skeletons', *British Medical Journal*, 283.6307 (1981), 1668–70.

[132] Mallegni, 'Su alcuni gruppi', pp. 233–61 (p. 251).

[133] Mallegni, 'Su alcuni gruppi', p. 251.

[134] <http://www.bbc.co.uk/health/physical_health/conditions/in_depth/arthritis/aboutarthritis_osteoarthritis.shtml>, accessed 18 January 2013.

[135] Mallegni, 'Su alcuni gruppi', p. 251.

show arthritic changes in the breastbone, collar bone, shoulder blade, and arm, with around a third having arthritis in their elbows or knees.[136] As the authors of the report point out, the skeletons concerned are not of an advanced age, and therefore must have led a very physically active life.[137]

Many of the bones also show signs of microtraumas (small injuries that have not healed), caused by, the authors of the report argue, excessive lifting or other heavy work.[138] It is recognized, however, that arthritic changes can be caused by a combination of age and/or genetic factors as well as heavy work.[139] Like Centallo, this cemetery is of high status individuals, and therefore the physical activity witnessed in the bones is likely to been due to considerable riding, and presumably also training for warfare and so on.[140] A few individuals suffered from anaemia, one from a probably benign leg tumour, another possibly from leukaemia.[141] In the case of severe anaemia or leukaemia the affected individual would struggle to take a full part in the life of the community, and would almost certainly have required at least basic care.

There is therefore arguably something of a mismatch between the emphasis given in a large late antique medical text, such as Caelius Aurelianus's work, and at least some of the chronic ailments suffered by much of the population, as we can only presume that arthritic problems were no less of an issue for lower status members of a community doing manual labour. Mirroring this is the relative lack of attention paid by historians of medicine to arthritic conditions, in contrast to archaeologists for whom it has become a mainstay of palaeopathological analysis.[142]

The emphasis in the legal codes on accidental and occupational injuries discussed in chapter one does not accord the same attention by medical writers, but many herbal recipes, discussed in the following chapter, do seek to aid wounds and breaks. Further, the surviving archaeological evidence supports the prevalence of accidents and injuries in early medieval Northern Italian communities. In the Piedmontese cemeteries of Centallo, Rivoli, and Acqui, fractures of the

[136] Fornaciari, 'Paleopatologia', p. 718.

[137] Fornaciari, 'Paleopatologia', p. 718.

[138] Fornaciari, 'Paleopatologia', p. 717.

[139] Fornaciari, 'Paleopatologia', p. 718.

[140] Fornaciari, 'Paleopatologia', p. 718.

[141] Fornaciari, 'Paleopatologia', p. 719.

[142] For the brief mentions of arthritis in Classical medical surveys, see A. Cruse, *Roman Medicine* (Stroud, 2004), p. 137 and Nutton, *Ancient Medicine*, p. 23.

ulna (forearm) are fairly common: at Centallo, all three cases are male, but at Acqui one is female, and another female at Acqui had a broken femur (thigh bone).[143] Fractures of the tibia (shinbone) can also be found at all three sites. All these injuries could be acquired from falls, work-related accidents or fights.

Conclusion

Was life in early medieval Northern Italy, then, nasty, brutish, and short? On the whole, as elsewhere in early medieval Europe — certainly in comparison with modern Western standards of living and life expectancies — the answer must be yes. There were, however, particularly dangerous phases in the life cycle, such as early infancy, and for women, child-bearing years. That having been said, although, as seen above, individuals could be injured or killed in the course of warfare or disputes, a man living above the breadline might nevertheless hope to see his fortieth birthday.

What the evidence at the St Giulia site at Brescia shows, when comparing the data from the earlier Lombard era settlement phase and later monastic community, is that a good diet was not all about location, location, location, although it certainly could help. On this site the Lombard era inhabitants relied heavily on hunting for their meat, but the evidence from their cemetery suggests that their food supply was sometimes precarious. The later monastic community on the same site, with much greater economic resources at its disposal, could grow, raise, or buy in a wide range of meat, grains, and other foodstuffs. Nevertheless, choosing a good location for a settlement with access to dairy products as well as grains could ensure that less wealthy, non-monastic communities such as that at Villa Carcina could still enjoy a relatively balanced and healthy diet.

The majority of inhabitants of early medieval Northern Italy certainly led an active, physically demanding life, which would explain the number of osteo-arthritic changes seen in the osteo-archaeological evidence from cemeteries. The dental evidence, although difficult to interpret, would also appear to support Cassiodorus's and Paul the Deacon's accounts that food supplies remained uncertain and fluctuating, with surpluses one year, and famine the next. Those of high status, or connected with large, well run estates, whether monastic or secular, were to a degree at least protected from some of these vagaries of food supply. Diet manuals were popular with the wealthy, but presuppose a choice of

[143] Mallegni, 'Su alcuni gruppi', p. 252.

foodstuffs and physical activity, and therefore had little relevance for the bulk of the population.

What united the wide range of communities found in Northern Italy, however, whether big, small, monastic, secular, mountainous or urban, was an interest in preventing or curing disease or infection, principally with herbs, but also through medical — or divine — intervention, the subject of the following chapters.

Chapter 3

Treating Illness: Herbs, Scalpels, and Cupping Vessels

In the absence of any medical records, or the patient feedback forms and government statistics on treatment times and outcomes which are now so integral to the running of healthcare in modern Britain and the West, how do we know if anyone in the early Middle Ages actually received medical treatment? The short answer is, with great difficulty. Apart from passing references to the ministrations of doctors and others in chronicles or saints' lives, and scattered archaeological evidence on surgeon's tools and medical intervention such as trepanning (drilling a hole in the skull) and setting fractures, we are principally reliant on legal and medical texts and recipes for evidence of medical practice. However, just as I have only cooked a very small percentage of the recipes from the many cookery books I own, is the same true of medical recipe books, herbals, or manuals on bleeding patients with cupping vessels or other medical instruments (phlebotomy)? In order to address these issues this chapter is divided into three sections. I begin with the area on which we have the most evidence, medical recipes and *Herbals*, before turning to texts on bleeding and, finally, the area on which we have the least evidence, surgical procedures.

Lotions and Potions

There are two principal types of medical recipes. The first include several ingredients, and are often found in miscellanies or collections (some called *antidotaria*). Such collections are regularly organized in terms of types of problem or illness (e.g. childbirth, poisonous stings, and so on) or they might start with diseases of the head and work down the body to the feet. The second type of recipe is *simples*, that is, remedies based on one individual plant. These are often found in *Herbals*, which are arranged according to plant, usually with a brief discussion of habitat and other names by which it is known before listing remedies.[1] Both of these types of medical recipes and collections are to be found in early medieval Northern Italian manuscripts. Some of these codices appear either to have been intended for export or were part of personal manuscript collections, as two arrived north of the Alps at the imperially favoured monastery of St Gallen, possibly fairly soon after they were produced: they are St Gallen, Stiftsbibliothek, MSS 217 (from page 252 onwards as the manuscript is currently paginated) and 751.[2] In contrast, Modena, Archivio Capitolare, MS O.I.11 is an early ninth-century medical miscellany which almost certainly has remained for over a thousand years in the region in which it was originally copied.[3] I discuss all three manuscripts below as representative case studies of the variety of medical collections circulating in early medieval Northern Italy. However, individual recipes could also be scribbled into blank pages or flyleaves of existing manuscripts. These have received far less attention from scholars, but, I shall argue, are a key part of the argument in favour of the practical use of medical and herb based recipes, since they demonstrate a process of active selection on the part of the anonymous copyists who squeezed them into pre-existing manuscripts.

Mind the Gap: Theory and Practice in Recipes and Remedies

The type of source to have received the most attention in terms of the relationship between text and practice, though, is the *Herbal*. As far back as 1927 Singer's study of herbal compendiums warned against assuming a practical use for these manuscripts.[4] Henry Sigerist's study of early medieval herbal literature five years before Singer's focused on the ancient heritage of these texts and on

[1] See, for example, M. Collins, *Medieval Herbals: The Illustrative Traditions* (London, 2000), p. 156.

[2] Collins, *Medieval Herbals*, p. 183.

[3] Lowe, *CLA* III, no. 368, p. 30.

[4] C. Singer, 'The Herbal in Antiquity and its Transmission to Later Ages', *Journal of Hellenic Studies*, 47 (1927), 1–52.

transcriptions of early medieval recipe collections.[5] As recently as 1982 Jakob Büchi outlined the principal ancient and medieval herbal recipe collections, emphasizing their academic and monastic nature rather than any 'folk' origins.[6] However, Linda Voigts has forcefully argued for the practical utility of herbal remedies. Voigts points to evidence of the substitution of hard-to-obtain ingredients with those more readily available in the region where a particular recipe or set of recipes was copied.[7] In response to the criticism that antique and medieval plant illustrations are often imprecise, Voigts counters that a plant does not need to be drawn with botanical accuracy in order to be recognized. After all, modern road signs do not aspire to realism, yet are clearly recognizable and understood.

John Riddle also places great emphasis on the practical use of herbs, specifically to limit female fertility and as abortifacients. His methodology is to examine both the frequency with which a specific herb is mentioned in ancient and medieval medical texts and anthropological and clinical studies which suggest a degree of efficacy for the plant in question, in order to assess their use in the medieval and post-medieval world.[8] He also stresses the importance of oral transmission of medical knowledge about herbs and their uses.[9] While he is undoubtedly right to highlight the role of orality, and point to the practical applications of many of these herbs, there are obvious difficulties in using modern data, plants, growing conditions, and anthropological studies to try and replicate or evoke the sometimes vague descriptions or illustrations of plants and recipes from ancient and medieval manuscripts. These problems were acknowledged in a series of experiments testing the antibacterial properties of Anglo-Saxon eye salve recipes: the results showed that while individual ingredients used did inhibit bacteria, the mixtures advocated in the recipes practically cancelled out any antibacterial effect.[10] This chapter focuses on the practi-

[5] Sigerist, *Studien und Texte*.

[6] J. Büchi, *Die Entwicklung der Rezept-und Arzneibuchliteratur*, 3 vols (Zürich, 1982–86), I (1982), 68.

[7] L. Voigts, 'Anglo-Saxon Plant Remedies and the Anglo-Saxons', *Isis*, 70 (1979), 250–68.

[8] See J. M. Riddle, *Contraception and Abortion from the Ancient World to the Renaissance* (Cambridge, MA, 1992), pp. 74–107; J. M. Riddle, *Eve's Herbs: A History of Contraception and Abortion in the West* (Cambridge, MA, 1997), pp. 44–52.

[9] Riddle, *Eve's Herbs*, p. 51.

[10] B. Brennessel, M. Drout, and R. Gravel, 'A Reassessment of the Efficacy of Anglo-Saxon Medicine', *Anglo-Saxon England*, 34 (2005), 183–95 (p. 184).

cal use of medical recipes by individuals who presumably believed they worked, whether or not they were actually bio-medically efficacious.

Similarly, rather than attempting to pass judgement on the efficacy or otherwise of medical recipes, Minta Collins has undertaken the task of a holistic study of late antique and medieval copies of the *Herbals*, considering them not just as members of a particular branch of a textual tradition, but in their original context of production.[11] She therefore considers aspects such as the materials used, page layout, types and extent of illustrations, and possible exemplars in order to assess the intended audience and use.[12] She concludes that while luxury herbal compendiums were probably designed as a cornerstone to a grand learned library, more modest copies could be used by learned medical practitioners.[13] Following on from this, I shall argue that the historiographical emphasis on large scale medical manuals and recipe collections has overshadowed manuscripts containing either individual recipes or smaller, more focused collections or miscellanies that may provide clues as the actual use and adaptation of recipes. Clearly, as Eliza Glaze has shown, some texts, such as those focusing on anatomy, were probably copied primarily for intellectual or teaching purposes rather than practical use.[14] What is needed, as Faith Wallis has argued, is a greater emphasis on the individual characteristics, aims, and possible audiences of each codex.

An additional way to attempt to assess the degree to which such recipes, modest or costly, were at least commonly known if not used is to explore references to recipes and remedies in other genres of texts. In Charlemagne's capitulary *De Villis*, issued in or just before 800 AD, herbs which he expects to be grown on his estates include many to be found in the recipes discussed above, such as roses or fenugreek (*fenicrecum*).[15] Of course, this essentially constitutes a wish list for the ideal royal estate, and may have only been executed either partially or on selected estates. The capitulary also does not state precisely for what purpose these herbs and vegetables were to be grown, or who was to use them. What it does show, however, is that these herbs were both known and thought

[11] Wallis, 'The Experience of the Book', pp. 101–26.

[12] Collins, *Medieval Herbals*.

[13] Collins, *Medieval Herbals*, p. 302.

[14] Glaze, 'The Perforated Wall'.

[15] 'Volumus quod in horto omnes herbas habeant: lilium, rosas, fenicrecum, costum, salviam, rutam, abrotanum, cucumeres, pepones, cucurbitas, faiolum [...].' *Capitularia regum Francorum*, I, no. 32, p. 90 no. 70.

to be necessary, and a combined culinary and medicinal purpose is therefore likely. Further, contemporary lists exist of herbs to be bought by monks at the market or fair.[16] St Gallen, Stiftsbibliothek, MS 751 includes remedies added in a contemporary hand at the end of a large medical compendium, demonstrating at the very least an active process of seeking out and copying herbal recipes.[17] In Justinian's sixth-century *Digest*, the compendium of Roman law, it is assumed that lay individuals also had stocks of ingredients at hand for medicinal, culinary, and cosmetic purposes. In book thirty-four of the *Digest*, on legacies of gold, Pomponius is quoted concerning the nature of unguents:

> Where ungent has been left as a legacy, the legacy is regarded as comprising not only those perfumes which are used for pleasure but also items for medicinal purposes, such as commagenum, glaucium, crinum, rose, muracolu, pure nard oil; in fact, women use this too to make themselves more decorative and attractive.[18]

The fact this passage is included in a book on legacies of gold indicates how valuable these items were, but also suggests that they played a key role in the wealthy late Roman household. However, did the range of ingredients available in Western Europe reduce from the sixth century onwards?[19] Certainly *negotiatores* (merchants) were numerous enough in the Lombard kingdom for King Aistulf to legislate on them in 750 AD, and the will of an early ninth-century doge of Venice includes legacies of imported spices, much as envisaged by Justinian's legal compilation discussed above.[20] We do also have a manuscript possibly commissioned or owned by a travelling doctor that shows evidence of local adaptations of ingredients for medical recipes, St Gallen, Stiftsbibliothek, MS 217, to which I now turn.

[16] See B. Guérard, *Polyptique de l'abbé Irminon*, 2 vols (Paris, 1844), II, 336 and A. Schulte, *Geschichte des mittelalterlichen Handels und Verkehrs zwischen Westdeutschland und Italien mit ausschluss von Venedig*, 2 vols (Leipzig, 1900), I, 73, cited in MacKinney, *Early Medieval Medicine*, p. 169, n. 99.

[17] Beccaria, *I codici*, p. 380, no. 35b.

[18] 'Unguentis legatis non tantum ea legata uidentur, quibus unguimur uoluptatis causa, sed et ualetudinis, qualia sunt commagena glaucina crina rosa muracolum nardum purum: hoc quidem etiam quo elegantiores sint et mundiores, unguuntur feminae.' Justinian, *Digest*, Book 34, 2, 21.1.

[19] R. Lopez and I. Raymond, *Medieval Trade in the Mediterranean World* (London, 1955); P. Horden and N. Purcell, *The Corrupting Sea: A Study of Mediterranean History* (Oxford, 2000), pp. 153–70.

[20] See Lopez, *Trade*, documents 9 and 10, pp. 37–41. See also M. McCormick, *Origins of the European Economy: Communications and Commerce AD 300–900* (Cambridge, 2002).

The Manuscript of a Travelling Doctor? The Case of St Gallen, MS 217

St Gallen, Stiftsbibliothek, MS 217 was once believed to actually have been copied at St Gallen but was judged by the palaeographer Bernhard Bischoff to have a Northern Italian origin, possibly from the monastery of Bobbio.[21] It was reorganized before the fourteenth century, and according to Beccaria is comprised of two parts, albeit with similar handwriting. The first section contains a treatise on bleeding, gynaecological recipes, a *Liber fisicum*, and the *Liber Vettonicus*.[22] The second includes a *Bestiarum*, recipes and a *Herbal*.[23] Both are written in a minuscule dating from the first half of ninth century, with the pages divided into two columns. In the first, some titles and numbers are in red with some large decorated initials. The second has rubrics and spaces for plant and animal illustrations, most unfilled.[24] It was used by Voigts — before Bischoff's judgement on its origin — as an example of the inclusion of regional (alpine) plants alongside those included in Classical and late antique herbals.[25] Bobbio, founded in the seventh century, although set in a valley at about 270 m above sea level, is situated in the heart of the Ligurian Appennine mountain range.[26] Some alpine plants therefore could have been cultivated by the monks themselves and others obtained from higher altitudes.[27]

[21] P. Köpp, *Vademecum eines frühmittelalterlichen Arztes: Die gefaltete lateinische Handschrift medizinischen Inhalts im Codex 217 und in der Fragmentensammlung 1396 der Stiftsbibliothek in St. Gallen* (Aarau, 1980). Köpp combines folios from St Gallen, MSS 217 and 1396 into what he believes to be the original order of the manuscript — see p. 15 of his study for a table detailing this. See also the earlier study by E. Landgraf, 'Ein frühmittelalterlicher Botanicus', *Kyklos*, 1 (1928), 114–46.

[22] Beccaria, *I codici*, p. 369.

[23] The medical manuscript is the second in St Gallen, Stiftsbibliothek, 217, pp. 251–342. Within this Beccaria outlines two sections: the first pp. 251–74 and pp. 335–42 and the second pp. 275–334. Page 251 was used as a cover and is decorated with saints and animals. See Beccaria, *I codici*, p. 369.

[24] Beccaria, *I codici*, p. 370.

[25] Voigts, 'Anglo-Saxon Plant Remedies', p. 256. She follows Landgraf, 'Botanicus', p. 120.

[26] G. Cantino Wataghin, E. Destefanis, and S. Uggé, 'Monasteri e territorio: l'Italia settentrionale nell'alto medieovo', in *Sepolture e luoghi di culto in età longobarda: il modello regio: il Congresso Nazionale di Archeologia Medievale*, ed. by G. P. Brogiolo (Firenze, 2000), pp. 311–16 (p. 313).

[27] J. Jermyn, *Alpine Plants of Europe: A Gardener's Guide* (Portland, OR, 2005), p. 21. See also pp. 21–29 on Alpine zones in Italy and Europe.

It is certainly true that twenty-six plants in this manuscript do not appear in other major herbals such as Pseudo-Apuleius or Pseudo-Dioscorides, but of these twenty-six, half are not identifiable.[28] This may of course indicate local names for particular plants, strengthening Voigt (and Riddle's) argument, despite the original misattribution of the manuscript, but some textual corruption cannot be excluded either. Minta Collins argues that this manuscript was probably copied in a hurry, as spaces for illustrations were not filled in, and there were many spelling errors.[29] This is persuasive, as the scribes may have been working to a tight deadline if the commissioner wanted to take it with them on a journey: Bischoff argues that it was originally carried unbound and folded. However, spelling and other errors can creep in for many reasons, not least if the exemplar is in a script unfamiliar to the scribe or scribes copying it.

It has been speculated that it was for use by a travelling doctor, but the fact that it is largely unillustrated arguably may have limited its practical use.[30] Spaces had been left for illustrations, but only two were ever filled, and then only roughly.[31] Equally, however, the lack of botanical drawings surely would also have reduced its value as a natural history reference volume? It was certainly a substantial collection, since it runs to three hundred and forty-two pages, although not a deluxe display copy.[32] It is organized into clear sections, and as it currently stands (there is evidence of reorganization), it begins with a chapter on bloodletting, followed by one on recipes to help childbirth, an *antidotarium* (in this case selected recipes for different ailments) and a recipe collection organized from head to foot.[33] The *antidotarium* section (labelled *Antidotus Atrianus*, that is, 'Hadrian's Antidotary'), includes recipes with quite precise instructions, not least proportions of ingredients, which is not standard in many early medieval recipes. For example, to make 'an ungent for a headache [which] is not cold or a migraine (*emigrania*): mix one ounce of Spurge (*euphorbia*) in a mortar with three ounces of wax and one pound of best oil'.[34]

[28] Collins, *Medieval Herbals*, p. 184.

[29] Collins, *Medieval Herbals*, p. 184.

[30] Büchi, *Die Entwicklung*, p. 105; *contra*, see Collins, *Medieval Herbals*, p. 184.

[31] Beccaria, *I codici*, p. 370.

[32] See Büchi, *Die Entwicklung*, p. 105, and Beccari, *I codici*, no. 131, pp. 369–71.

[33] Büchi, *Die Entwicklung*, p. 105. Another Northern Italian example with an antidotary is Karlsruhe, Badische Landesbibliothek, Cod. Reichenau 120 (CXX) — see Beccaria, *I codici*, pp. 214–17. This manuscript includes extracts from Soranus Democritus and Caelius Aurelianus, placing the remedies in a learned context.

[34] 'Confectio unctionis ad capitis dolorem eine ad emigrania vel ad frigdorem: Euforbii –I

Another for earache, however, gives no quantities: it advises one to heat myrrh, aloe, opium, water, and honey in a chalice, place the mixture in hot water and then put it into the ear using a cloth.[35] While many of the recipes use vegetables and locally available ingredients, it is clear that ingredients such as euphorbium, myrhh, aloe, and opium, for example, would have had to have been imported from much further afield than Italy, from Africa, the Middle East, and perhaps even China.[36] Another remedy in St Gallen, MS 217 to cure all sorts of ailments, from stomachache and epilepsy to pain in the breast or side, includes the spices white and black pepper, cinnamon, mastic, ginger, and cassia bark.[37] Alongside these expensive ingredients, however, are the more prosaic rhubarb and honey.[38]

The final three sections of St Gallen, MS 217 (not included in Köpp's reconstruction) are: a table of synonyms for plants and ingredients (*Interpretatio erbarum siue pigmentorum*), a *Liber botanicus* (Pseudo-Apuleius's *Herbarius* with additions), and a *Liber bestiarum* (attributed in this manuscript to Sextus Placitus) which lists remedies obtained from animals.[39] This codex has a complex history: folios 275–334 are in a different hand and decoration, while small parts of the manuscript are also to be found in St Gallen, Stiftsbibliothek, MS

teres in mortario, caere-III, oleo optimi libram I, facis cerotum.' St Gallen, Stiftsbibliothek, MS 217, p. 258, transcribed and translated into German by Köpp, *Vademecum*, p. 41 and p. 110. See also Büchi, *Die Entwicklung*, p. 109.

[35] 'Ad aurem dolorem: murra, aloae, opiu cum aqua et melle spissum sit calefactum in calice, deponas in aquae calida, sic in aure panno imponis et mittis colando, fis(icum).' p. 267, transcribed and translated into German by Köpp, *Vademecum*, p. 55 and p. 114. See also Büchi, *Die Entwicklung*, p. 109.

[36] Büchi, *Die Entwicklung*, p. 112. See also Lopez, *Medieval Trade* and S. Loseby, 'The Mediterranean Economy', in *The New Cambridge Medieval History*, I: *c. 500–c. 700*, ed. by P. Fouracre (2005), pp. 605–38; Horden and Purcell, *The Corrupting Sea*, especially pp. 267–70; McCormick, *Origins of the European Economy*, p. 689 and pp. 708–16.

[37] See Kopp, p. 27, trans. p. 106. See also: 'Antidotum theodosion faciens ad multas passiones: accipitur vernum et autumnum qui facit ad dolorem [...] et epilemticis [...] et ad pectoris suiue laterum dolorum [...] ad dolorem ventris suiue stomaci.' cited in Buchi, p. 109. K. Krützfeld, 'Pfeffer als Gewürz und Arzneimittel: Eine Geschichte mit Höhen und Tiefen', *Deutsche Apotheker Zeitung*, 141.51–52 (2001), 42–48.

[38] 'reuponticu XII [...] mel dispumatum sufficit'.

[39] Büchi, *Die Entwicklung*, p. 105; Collins, *Medieval Herbals*, p. 166 and p. 183. E. Howald and H. E. Sigerist, eds, *Antonii Musae de herba vettonica, liber. Pseudoapulei herbarius. Anonymi De taxone liber. Sexti placiti Liber medicinae ex animalibus* (Berlin, 1927), although some of their conclusions are no longer valid — see Collins, *Medieval Herbals*, pp. 166–67 for discussion of the edition.

1396, a collection of recipe fragments, which Köpp has used in his 'reconstruction'.[40] Whichever elements of the manuscript as it now stands you include, or in whatever order, overall the manuscript obviously has a practical emphasis, since it includes two of three principal forms of early medieval treatment, namely herbal (and animal) remedies, and bloodletting, without any theoretical sections.

What is absent however, is that other key early medieval tool, prognostical calendars (such as the so-called Egyptian book of days): these determined whether a patient was to recover or not, and when they should be treated.[41] Further, there is no text dedicated to diet in this compilation: two differences with this manuscript's more glamorous cousin, also produced in Northern Italy in the ninth century, Karlsruhe, Badische Landesbibliothek, cod. Reichenau 120.[42] However, these *lacunae* do not necessarily preclude its practical use, since while it perhaps aspires to encyclopaedic proportions, it is principally focused on remedies. It could be argued, therefore, that rather than a general volume it was designed to reflect the particular expertise, interests, or needs of its original owner. Whether it was ever used, or intended to be used, in medical practice, we cannot say for certain: the range of ingredients, not to mention the sheer size of this collection mitigate against this being an everyday 'home remedies' aide-memoire, and the very practical orientation and simple decoration argue for some sort of practical use by a medical practitioner. This argument also presupposes, however, that it was only ever designed for one use or purpose, and that a learned interest in herbs and their origins could not be combined with their practical application.

A Medical Recipe Miscellany: Modena, Archivio Capitolare, MS O.I.11

The same could be said for Modena, Archivio Capitolare, MS O.I.11, folios 22–103, dating from the early ninth century. This squat, unshowy, and almost pocket-sized manuscript, however, is an unusually narrowly focused medical miscellany, particularly in comparison with other contemporary medical man-

[40] Beccaria, *I codici*, no. 131, pp. 369–70 and no. 140, pp. 393–94. See Köpp, *Vademecum*.

[41] On calendars see F. D. Gröenke, *Die frühmittelalterlichen lateinischen Monatskalendarien: Text, Übersetzung, Kommentar* (Berlin, 1986); C. Weißer, *Studien zum mittelalterlichen Krankheitslunar* (Pattensen, 1982).

[42] Beccaria, *I codici*, pp. 214–17. My impression of Karlsruhe, Badische Landesbibliothek, Cod. Reichenau 120, having viewed it, is that it was very carefully copied on creamy parchment and is decidedly a step-up from 'workhorse' manuscripts.

uscripts from Northern Italy. It contains no treatise of bloodletting or calendar of prognostication, and contains virtually nothing on surgery. Instead it focuses almost entirely on medical recipes, interspersed with part of the Hippocratic *Aphorisms*, which are a series of pithy observations on factors affecting the health of patients and the probable course of illnesses. It could easily have been used by an educated layperson as much as a medical practitioner. The choice and organization of these texts within this manuscript, therefore, deserve closer attention.

Modena, MS O.I.11 is composed of two distinct but related codicological units.[43] To date, most of the discussion concerning this manuscript has focused on its palaeographical characteristics, the presence of Anglo-Saxon runes on folio 72, and its significance as an early manuscript witness for the Latin version of Hippocrates' *Aphorisms*.[44] All parts of this manuscript are relevant to our discussion, however, even though the first does not contain medical material. This first section, folios 1^{v}–21^{v}, is a somewhat battered portion of Isidore of Seville's *Chronicle*, covering in this manuscript world history from Adam to Emperor Heraclius.[45] It is written in what Bischoff describes as an 'unregulated half-cursive' script, and is certainly rich in ligatures (two or more letters joined together into one character).[46] It was helpfully dated and signed by the scribe Iohannes in 801.[47] Unfortunately, however, Iohannes gives no clue as to his status — was he a cleric or a monk? It is also a mystery as to the location of the scriptorium where Iohannes worked. The manuscript in its entirety was recorded for the first time in Modena's library catalogue in 1818.

The second section was probably written slightly later than the first: Bischoff characterizes the script as an early Carolingian minuscule, although Lowe considered the whole manuscript to be written in pre-Carolingian minuscule.[48]

[43] E. A. Lowe treats them as one codicological unit (see *CLA*, III, no. 368, p. 30) but Bernhard Bischoff and Loretta Piccinini both consider them as codicologically and palaeographically distinct, but probably from the same scriptorium. See Bischoff, *Katalog*, II, 191–92 and L. Piccinini, 'Rune anglosassoni in un codice latino (Archivio Capitolare di Modena, O.I.11)', *Romanobarbarica*, 12 (1992–93), 173–88 (p. 173).

[44] Piccinini, 'Rune anglosassoni'; M. Canedi, *Runica manuscripta: un nuovo alfabeto runico* (Verona, 1983), K.-D. Fischer, 'Neues zur Überlieferung der lateinischen "Aphorismen" im Frühmittelalter', *Latomus*, 62.1 (2003), 156–64.

[45] Piccinini, 'Rune anglosassoni', p. 174.

[46] Bischoff, *Katalog*, II, 191.

[47] fol. 21^{v}.

[48] Bischoff, *Katalog*, II, p. 192; Lowe, *CLA* III, p. 30.

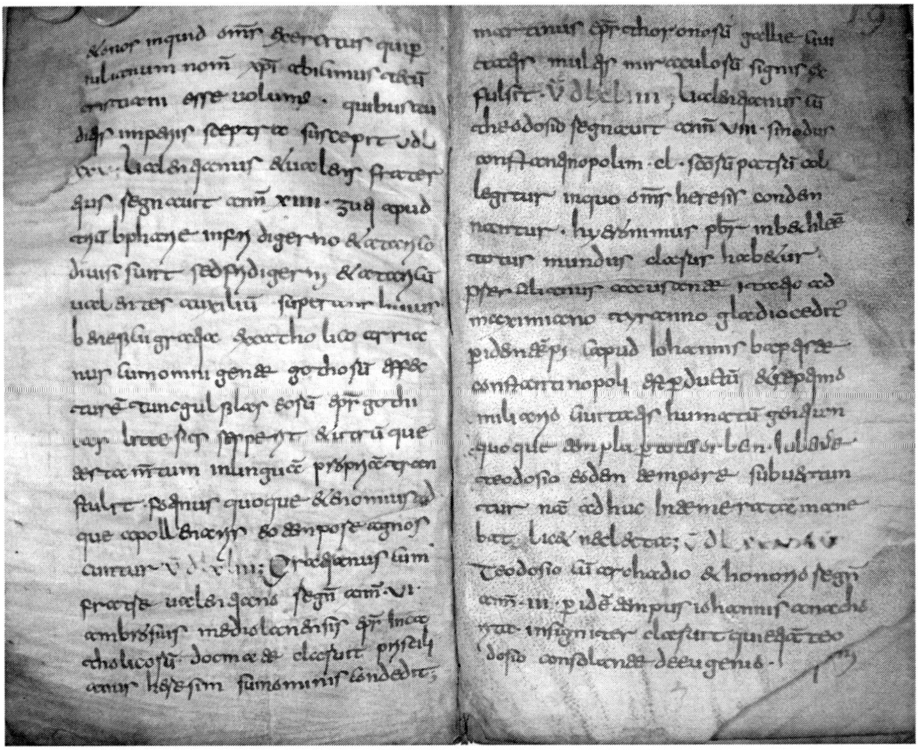

Figure 1. Modena, MS O.I.11, Scribe 1 (folios 1–21), Isidore of Seville's *Chronicle*. Photo taken and reproduced by kind permission of Lorenzo Pongiluppi.

What is important, however, is not how the scripts are categorized according to modern definitions, but how they, together with page layout and decoration, relate to each other. The scribe of Isidore's *Chronicle* writes in a mid-brown ink, with chapter numbers copied in what is now an orange colour[49] (see Figure 1). The second scribe, the copyist of the remedies on folios 22–24 and 37–103, writes in a small, neat hand, in a pale brown ink, with tall ascenders reminiscent

[49] The scribe's hand is quite rounded, with tall, quite thick ascenders. He uses d with a curved ascender, two forms of g, one with a closed bowl, the other, more rarely, with a flat top. There is a double height c with a broken back, and oc=a. It is also a ligature-rich script, using ri, te, ti, and ru ligatures. It is written on twenty-one lines, with some word separation. I am very grateful to Chief Archivist Monsignor Guido Vagarani, and Vice-archivist Lorenzo Pongiluppi for their generous assistance while I was consulting this manuscript in the original at the Archivio Capitolare, Modena. All figures for this manuscript given below are from photos taken by Lorenzo Pongiluppi.

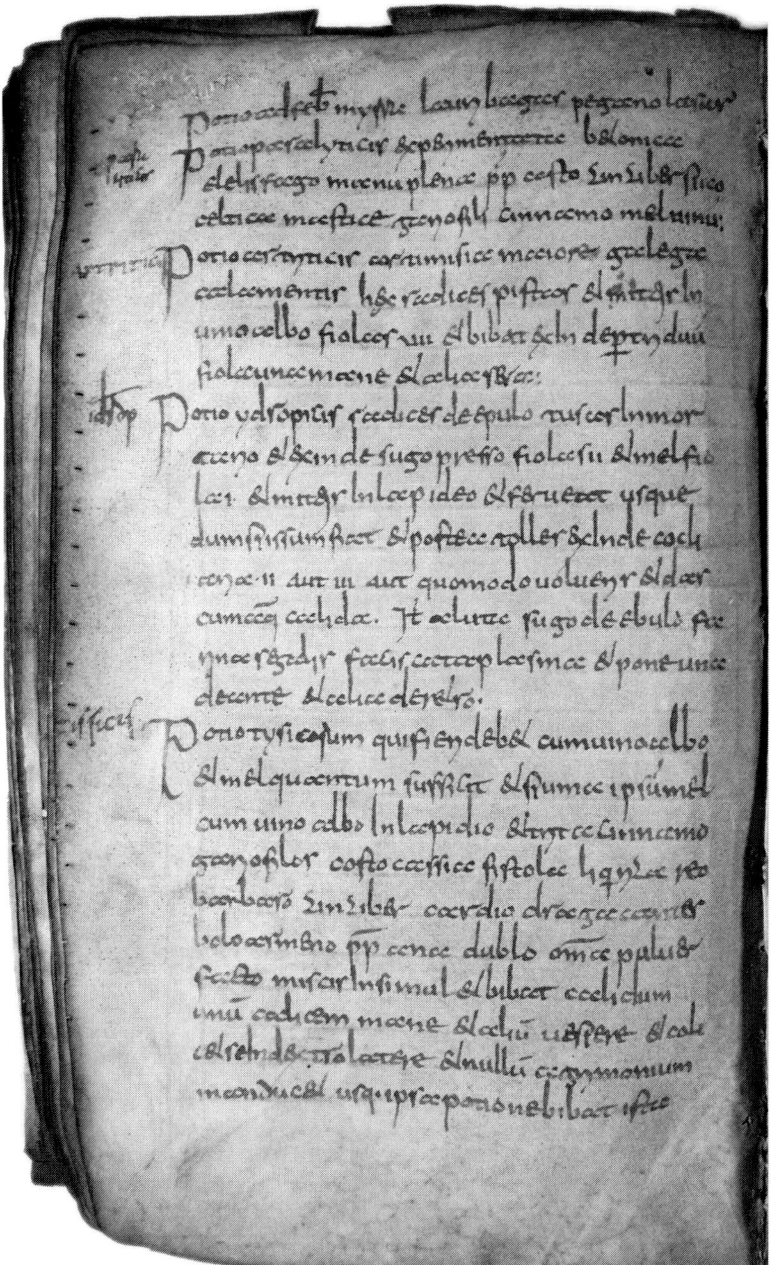

Figure 2. Modena, MS O.I.11, Scribe 2 (folios 22–24 and 37–103), Medical remedies. Photo taken and reproduced by kind permission of Lorenzo Pongiluppi.

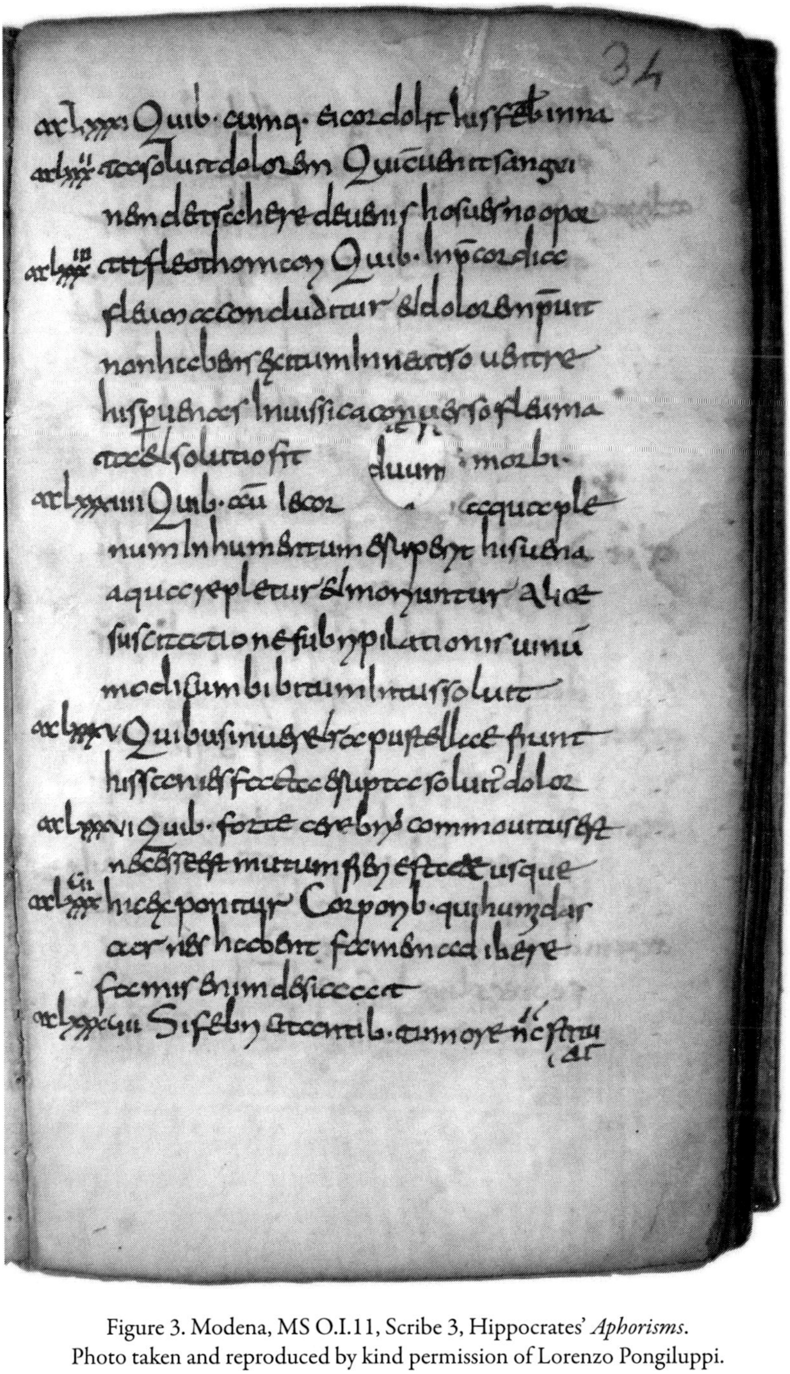

Figure 3. Modena, MS O.I.11, Scribe 3, Hippocrates' *Aphorisms*.
Photo taken and reproduced by kind permission of Lorenzo Pongiluppi.

of scribe one (see Figure 2).[50] Scribe 3, the copyist for the *Aphorisms*, writes 21 lines per page in a larger hand with much darker ink, almost black. He uses the same form of the letter g and curved d to scribe 2, but also has palaeographical links with scribe 1 in the tall, sometimes broken-backed c (see Figure 3).

Given the great similarities in script it therefore makes sense to see Modena, MS O.I.11 as a snapshot of a scriptorium at two key points in its development in the first quarter of the ninth century. Based principally on the characteristics of the handwriting, this manuscript has been attributed to Northern Italy, and the monastery of Nonantola has been suggested as a possible location.[51] However, Loretta Piccinini argues, following Mirella Morelli and Marco Palma, that this manuscript does not fit with other known Nonantola codies.[52] Piccinini, however, goes one step further and suggests the monastery of Bobbio.[53] Neither Lowe nor Bischoff though, would be drawn beyond saying that it was written in Northern Italy, despite being very familiar with manuscripts ascribed to Bobbio.[54] Ultimately, there is nothing to say that it this manuscript is not the last surviving product of a scriptorium with access to or links with Insular learning which we unfortunately simply cannot any longer identify.

This manuscript certainly did not remain untouched at the bottom of a book box or cupboard, as several folios have been annotated at various stages in its history. At the base of 24 verso an alphabet, in a later form of Carolingian minuscule than that which this manuscript is written in, is added in black ink. On 36 verso, Hippocrates' *Aphorisms* ends on line 14 with a handful of Greek letters, to which an anonymous reader has added, in a very pale ink, further Greek characters, the meaning of which is obscure. On several pages between 61 and 71, though, are added glosses or running titles which help the reader find remedies for particular ailments, such as coughs, arthritis, quartan fevers, deaf-

[50] The exception is the d, which is sometimes curved, but with a short ascender. The bowl of the g is closed, but with a connective line at the top of the bowl reaching right. The form of the letter a is the same however, as is the spiky r. Ligatures are still frequent: ri, et, and te in particular. The number of lines fluctuates between 22 and 26 lines.

[51] G. Cencetti, 'Scriptoria e scrittura nel Monachesimo benedettino', in *Il monachesimo nell'Alto medioevo e la formazione della civiltà occidentale* (Spoleto, 1957), pp. 187–219 (pp. 200–02); Beccaria, *I codici*, no. 93, p. 291.

[52] Piccinini, 'Rune anglosassoni', p. 187; M. Morelli and M. Palma, 'Indagine su alcuni aspetti materiali della produzione libraria a Nonantola nel secolo IX', *Scrittura e civilta*, 6 (1982), 23–98 (p. 28).

[53] Piccinini, 'Rune anglosassoni', p. 187.

[54] Lowe, *CLA* III, no. 368, p. 30; Bischoff, *Katalog*, II, 191–92.

ness or gout.[55] Some of these appear to have been added by the original scribe: for example, on folio 62 verso, lines 12–13, 'quartaniis' is added in apparently the same ink as the main text, and with the same form of a, cc=a. The same is true for the running title for a remedy for paralysis on folio 66 verso, line 2.[56]

It is possible, however, that a slightly later annotator added further marginal titles. These are in paler ink than that of the main text: on line 13 of folio 61 verso, the marginal title for *podraga* (gout) uses, unlike the scribe of the main text, a different form of the letter a, the one which would, in the course of the ninth century, became standard in Carolingian minuscule, and which we still use today.[57] Similarly, on folio 61 verso line 7, the marginal addition for deafness is also in the same pale ink with a rounded 'a'. A few folios on, line 2 of folio 66 verso has 'artritia' added in the margin, again using the later Carolingian minuscule form of the letter 'a'.[58] It would therefore appear that a reader sought to improve what might be termed the navigational tools of the manuscript by adding additional marginal titles. Only certain remedies, however, were selected: those for some of medicine's more intractable conditions, such as arthritis or gout, seem to have been privileged. Further, only folios 61 verso to 71 appear to have been annotated in this way, whether by the original scribe or a possibly later annotator.

Whenever the marginal titles between folios 61–71 were added to the main body of the text, it still demonstrates a concern that key recipes could be found easily by readers, whether for practical use and/or study. Further, there is evidence on the final folios that this manuscript was indeed being read and used, in all likelihood for practical medicinal purposes, in the centuries following its production. At the base of folios 102 verso and 103 recto was added, in a similarly diminutive script to the main body of the text, but with a very thin nib, instructions for the making of tinctures.[59] On folio 103 verso are further anno-

[55] Fols 61^{v}, 62^{r-v}, 63^{r}, 64^{r}, 66^{v}, 67^{v}, 68^{v}, 69^{v}, 70^{v}, 71^{r}.

[56] See also fols 63^{r} line 19 and 66^{v} line 9.

[57] B. Bischoff, *Latin Palaeography: Antiquity and the Middle Ages*, trans. by D. Ó Cróinín and D. Ganz (Cambridge, 1990), p. 112.

[58] See also fol. 66^{r}, lines 13–14.

[59] Fol. 102^{v}, 'Ad maculas de panno tollendas siue da oleo aut de qualicumque alia tinctura: accipis caseum vetus et albument eguali pondere et pista in simul fortiter et cum bene pistatum fuerit ungues ipsas maculas et fricas multum et mitte in lexivas quod bugada dicitur, et dum ibi iacuerit postea quando lavaberis purgabitur.' Simonini's transcription, 'Formulario in "Medicinae Varia" codice Mss. dell'VIII secolo conservato nella Metropolitana di Modena', *Atti e Memorie dell'Accademia di Storia dell'Arte Sanitaria*, 39.6 (1940), p. 68. An alternative reading by Loretta

tations in black ink, the clearest of which reads 'Cassa mu(m) id(em) sem(en) cassiae q(uo)d dicitur'.

There is nothing in any of the marginalia to suggest that either section of this manuscript ever left the region in which it was produced. In particular, the regional gloss 'quod bugada' in the additions on folios 102 and 103 prove that it was in Northern Italy in the eleventh century at least.[60] It is also possible that the two sections of this manuscript were placed together at an early date, in the scriptorium at which they were produced. At the very least they travelled together to their current home, the Archivio Capitolare in Modena. Although the first section concerns world history, and the second medical advice and recipes, both can be seen as works of knowledge and learning about the universe and ancient world. This is underlined by the presence of Greek letters, and a runic alphabet, on folio 72^{r}. We have no way of knowing, however, at precisely what stage in the manuscripts' history they were bound together.

In order to attempt to answer the fundamental question, as to how folios 22–103 of Modena, MS O.I.11 were intended to be used, we need to look at the contents and organization of this part of the manuscript. Folios 22^{r}–24^{v} are, in all probability, an incomplete series of recipes. These include several unguents to soothe itching, a powder (*pulver*) to deal with black teeth (*dentes nigros*) and remedies to rid the body of lice.[61]

Pinccinini is: 'Ad maricas depanno tollenda siue de oleo [...] ut de qualicumque alia tincura accipis caseum vetis et aull [...] dere et pista in simul facttem et cum bene [...] fuerit ungues ipsas maculas et fricas multum et [...] tre. In lex [...] asquid bugada dicitur et dum ibi iacuerit posteri quando lavaberis purgabitur.' transcription by L. Piccinini, 'Scheda codicologica di Archivio Capitolare di Modena Ms O.I.11' (unpublished transcription), by kind permission of Modena, Archivio Capitolare, p. 15. Some of the differences may be explained by the fact that some of the lettering could have been clearer seventy years ago when Simonini was studying Modena, Archivio Capitolare, O.I.11. For this reason, I have given Simonini's reading first, rather than my own attempt or Piccinini's. I am very grateful to Mons. Vigarani and Lorenzo Pongiluppi of the Archivio Capitolare, Modena, for making available to me hard-to-find and unpublished work connected to Modena, Archivio Capitolare, O.I.11. See also fol. 103^{r}, 'Item ad idem. Si tinctura fuerit ex arbore aut herba. Mitte illu(m) in folio vascul(um) et ex ipse herba aut arbore mitte aliquid int(er) circhu(m) et [dona?] ubi ipse pann(um) in bugada steterit. Altera die lava multu(m) bene et ipsas maculas non parebunt. P(ro)batissimum est.' transcription by myself, combined with Simonini's transcription, 'Formulario in "Medicinae Varia", p. 68.

60 Beccaria, *I codici*, p. 292.

61 See fols 22^{r}, 23^{r-v}. These folios, Piccinini notes, form an incomplete quire: see Piccinini, 'Rune anglosassoni', p. 174.

A second scribe copies folios 25r–36v, chapters from Hippocrates' *Aphorisms*.[62] Scribe 1, who copied folios 22–24, continues his work from folio 37 to the end of the manuscript.[63] There has obviously, therefore, been a division of labour between the scribe working on the *Herbarius* and herbal recipe sections of the manuscript, and the copyist of Hippocrates' *Aphorisms*. The *Aphorisms* begins on a new quire and the rest of the page is left blank where the *Aphorisms* ends, half way through the second quire used for this text.[64] The positioning of the *Aphorisms* is therefore somewhat curious, interjecting as it does between herbal recipe collections. It could be that this organization reflects the diverse exemplars used for the various elements of this second section of Modena, MS O.I.11, or that scribe 1 decided or was instructed to add further recipes to the blank folios of the Aphorisms quires, and continued from there.

The *Aphorisms* begin midway through with a chapter on the effects of cold.[65] It is therefore likely that this was originally a complete copy, since it reproduces almost in its entirety the final sections of the *Aphorisms*. Although, given the colophon for the Isidorian section of the manuscript, this composite codex was almost certainly intended for a male community, whether clerical or monastic, sections on pregnancy and problems of the womb have not been omitted. This is probably in the name of textual completeness and reverence for ancient Hippocratic knowledge, although it could possibly also have had relevance for female relatives and servants. Further, some chapters of the *Aphorisms* included in this manuscript, such as those on *podraga*, gout, accord well with the surrounding herbal remedies.

The recipes from folios 37r–72r include remedies for a wide range of problems identified by the copyist as weariness, tiredness, or faintness (*lassitudo*), coughs, fevers, and melancholy to paralysis, rabies, arthritis, or a lack of menstruation.[66] This recipe section is organized, unlike many recipe collections, not by body part from head to foot, but by the type of remedy used, i.e. *potio*

62 Piccinini, 'Rune anglosassoni', p. 175.

63 Piccinini, 'Rune anglosassoni', p. 175.

64 Piccinini, 'Rune anglosassoni', p. 174.

65 See Beccaria, *I codici*, p. 292.

66 See for example: *Potio ad lassitudine(m)* fol. 65v (tiredness/weakness); *Pessariae ad menstruam provocandam* fol. 39r (for periods); *Antidotum qui dicitur maurentius faciens ad stomachi dolorem* fol. 37r (stomach pains); *Potio ad rabia* fol. 65r (rabies); *Catarticum melancolicum* fol. 55v (melancholy); *Electarium ad tussem* (coughs); *Trociscus ad capitis dolorem* fol. 42v (pains in the head); *Potio ad plagas* fol. 66r (wounds); *Potio paralyticis* fol. 66v (paralysis); *potio artriticis* fol. 66v (arthritis).

(liquid), *unguentum* (unguent, ointment), or *pulvis* (powder). Some categories, such as unguents, appear more than once, perhaps suggesting multiple exemplars, and that this system of organization is not particularly rigorous.

This way of organizing the recipes potentially does make it a little bit trickier for the reader looking for a particular remedy, for example for a stomach ache, as they may have to look under several categories to compare remedies and pick the one best suited to their requirements. Since the opening folio of this section of Modena, MS O.I.11, folio 22, may once have been preceded by one or perhaps many previous pages, it is possible that an index or chapter headings helped the reader navigate through the hundreds of recipes listed. Further, the two scribes of this section of Modena, MS O.I.11 do include what might be termed basic 'visual signposting' to aid the reader in distinguishing between different remedies. Although no colour is used in these sections, and new lines are not necessarily used for each remedy, the initial letters of recipes, sections, or sentences, depending on the text, are enlarged and often indented. There is also some word spacing and punctuation employed.

One element of Modena, MS O.I.11 which has long been remarked on, but little studied until the work of Marisa Canedi and, more recently, Loretta Piccinini, is the presence of runic and Greek alphabets on folio 72 recto.[67] The same scribe who copied the herbal remedies added a Greek-Latin and a runic alphabet. Piccinini has suggested, given the alphabet's juxtaposition with herbal remedies, that its function may have been magico-medical, although she acknowledges that the link between runes and magical practices are contentious.[68] Such a use certainly cannot be discounted, but it is equally possible that the runes, particularly as they appear alongside the Greek alphabet, were copied by the scribe to complete the page, and that they represent another aspect of ancient knowledge and learning. Certainly the overwhelming emphasis in the recipes themselves is on using a combination of herbs, spices, and minerals, mixed with honey or wine, to heal, rather than incantations or other magico-medical rituals.

Folios 72–87, the Pseudo-Apuleius's *Herbarius*, include the treatise on the uses of betony, and unlike any of the previous recipe collections, has both an incipit and explicit. The *Herbarius* is a Latin compilation, probably dating from the fourth century, which owes much to Pliny and the anonymous late

[67] Canedi, *Runica manuscripta*; Piccinini, 'Rune anglosassoni', pp. 173–88.

[68] Piccinini, 'Rune anglosassoni', p. 186.

antique compilation, the *Medicina Plinii*.[69] It is a simple, that is, a herbal where remedies from a single plant are described. Seventy-eight out of a total of one hundred and thirty or one hundred and thirty-one chapters are included in this manuscript.[70] What is unusual about this copy of the *Herbarius* is that it is not illustrated, because pictures of the plants described were an integral part of the original text.[71] Illustrations were obviously important since they could help the user correctly identify the leaf, root, or flower of the plant they required. However, Modena, MS O.I.11 is by no means unique in containing unillustrated chapters from a herbal. St Gallen, Stiftsbibliothek, MS 217, as we have seen, is another example of this, although it was originally planned to be illustrated.[72]

In the case of Modena, MS O.I.11, were illustrations omitted to reduce the cost of the manuscript or because the necessary expertise for such drawings was not available in the scriptorium where the manuscript was copied? Certainly neither section of Modena, MS O.I.11 could be considered deluxe, with the first part in a space saving semicursive script, and the second with no coloured initials, just enlarged ink letters. Further, folio 26 has four holes in the parchment which have been written around, demonstrating that every scrap of available parchment was used for this compilation. However, whether considered together or in separate sections, Modena, MS O.I.11 still represents, at hundred and three folios in total, of which eighty two folios make up the medical section, a considerable investment in parchment (and hence sheep).

It could be argued that the lack of illustrations means that it was not designed for practical use. However, lavishly illustrated herbals equally could be prestige, luxury items, certainly not designed to be carried about, or risk being damaged by frequent thumbing. At 203mm × 119mm Modena, MS O.I.11 is a manuscript of quite modest proportions, about the size of a modern paperback. This contrasts starkly with the surviving folios of what must once have been monumental copies of the *Herbarius* like Ivrea, Biblioteca Capitolare, MS 94 (XCII), at 335 × 245mm.[73] Further, the *Herbarius* in Modena, MS O.I.11 is organized according to remedies for specific body parts or medical problems,

[69] Collins, *Medieval Herbals*, p. 165.

[70] Collins, *Medieval Herbals*, p. 165, and Beccaria, *I codici*, p. 292.

[71] Collins, *Medieval Herbals*, p. 165.

[72] Collins, *Medieval Herbals*, p. 184.

[73] Collins, *Medieval Herbals*, p. 229, n. 126, and *CLA* III, no. 301.

such as a fractured skull, not by plant.[74] This fits in well with the other sections on remedies in the manuscript: although the recipes in the other sections are organized according to the type of preparation used, the remedies all begin by listing the body parts or illnesses they were designed to treat. Between folios 85^{v}, when the *Herbarius* ends, and 88^{r} is a short section on when and how to collect some of the plants discussed in the preceding work.[75] The inclusion of this, and its positioning, is the strongest evidence yet that this was indeed designed as a practical manual.

Finally, on a new quire the scribe returns again, on folios 88^{r} to 103^{v}, to medical recipes entitled *Anditu(m) Theodotion*. It begins with a remedy for various ailments from a headache to indigestion and stomach ache. Remedies for coughs and stomach problems are prominent in this section, along with remedies for fever and vomiting. Therefore, while this is a relatively tightly defined collection of medical material, the compiler(s) have not reorganized the material from their exemplars radically — if they had, different recipe collections would have been combined together, and the *Aphorisms* placed either at the beginning or the end of the collection. The organization of the manuscript perhaps reflects in turn the way in which the scriptorium was run.

Whatever the factors affecting the order in which texts were copied into this manuscript, however, the juxtaposition of the *Aphorisms* with medical recipes was deliberate, providing a broader medical context for the remedies. Both the remedies and the *Aphorisms* would have required some basic knowledge of the body, humoral theory and diseases: specific terms for illnesses such as *podraga* (gout) or *melancholia* (melancholy) were employed in both sets of texts, and as discussed above, archaic terms for unguents and potions were used to organize the remedies sections. If this manuscript was for teaching or purely academic purposes, however, it certainly could not have served as a general guide or overview to ancient medicine. Theoretical and practical use, as I suggested above, are not necessarily exclusive, and one can lead to the other. Most likely, however, I argue, the principal aim of this compilation was to be a primer for the art of treating patients. Firstly, the age, sex, and complexion/balance of humours could be assessed, and perhaps also, following the *Aphorisms*, by the examination of stools and urine. Hundreds of medical recipes could then be scanned to find the most appropriate remedy.

[74] R. Simonini, *'Apulei Liber', Medicinae Varia in codice dell'VIII secolo conservato nell'archivio capitolare della metropolitana di Modena* (Modena, 1929), p. 28.

[75] On this see Simonini, *'Apulei Liber'*, p. 26.

Although a substantial compilation, as discussed above, its relatively small size and plain appearance, with a complete lack of illustrations, preclude any use simply as a 'display' manuscript. Unfortunately we know nothing about the individuals or communities who used the manuscript other than from the annotations, particularly on the final folios: in its long history clerical, lay, and monastic contexts are all possible. What this manuscript arguably represents, ultimately, however, is the backbone of early medieval medicine: practical advice and medical recipes, sometimes using expensive ingredients, but which could be concocted by any able and experienced individual, whether in the home, monastery or clerical community.

Vile Scraps: Recipe Fragments

However, ingredients for medical recipes were not just copied into legal compendiums or large medical collections, miscellanies, or *Herbals*. They could also be scribbled into the margins of medical manuscripts or added onto non-medical material. Unlike the expensive *Herbals* or grandiose medical compilations, these recipes were, particularly from the eighth-century onwards, not written in a laborious, time-consuming (and therefore expensive) bookhand where the pen is raised from the page for each letter, but in rapid cursive 'joined up' scripts. Many of these sorts of manuscripts containing medical recipes survive only as fragments, often written over, which highlights their more ephemeral nature. It is perhaps because of this that they have received relatively little attention from historians of medicine. Yet, if we accept that this type of low-cost, small-scale manuscript would have had a very high rate of attrition, originally it could have been one of the most popular methods for the copying of herbal recipes.

Fragments of recipes that have been attributed to Northern Italy before *c.* 1000 AD include Città del Vaticano, Biblioteca Apostolica Vaticana, MS Vat. Pal. lat. 187 (fol. 7) and MS Vat. Urb. lat. 293 (fols 95–96), St Gallen, Stiftsbibliothek, MS 912, London, British Library, MS Harley 5792, Milan, Biblioteca Ambrosiana, MS C.105 inf., and Sélestat, Bibliothèque municipale, MS 1 (A).[76] Of these, the Sélestat fragment, dating from the second half of the seventh century and written in uncial, may have once been part of a larger collec-

[76] C. Stornajolo, *Codices Urbinates Latini* (Roma, 1942), p. 264; G. Carbonelli, *Frammento medico del secolo VII: Cod Vat urb lat 293* (Roma, 1921); Lowe, *CLA* I, no. 80b, p. 24; *CLA* I, no. 116; *CLA* II, no. *203; *CLA* III, no. 2489a; *CLA* VI, no. 830, p. 38.

tion, since it includes a medical fragment as well as medical recipes.[77] St Gallen, Stiftsbibliothek, MS 912 is a fragment of gynaecological recipes, copied at the end of the fifth century or beginning of the sixth century in Northern Italy, and then some two hundred years later erased and reused for a glossary.[78] Milan, Biblioteca Ambrosiana, MS C.105 inf., is another palimpsest of medical recipes.[79] It was originally copied in the sixth century in a cursive script, together with a fragment of the *Carmen de VII fratribus Machabaeis*.[80] Apart from the unusual combination of texts, both the choice of script — cursive is relatively rapid and therefore makes copying quicker and cheaper — and the fact that the manuscript was reused for a new text in the eighth century, emphasizes its utilitarian origins and, ultimately, disposability. This also appears to be reflected in the London Harley fragment, copied in the eighth century, which contains a Latin-Greek glossary as well as recipes.[81] Several remedies for common complaints such as fevers, coughs, and stomach pains are included, along with cures for snakebites and growths (tumores).[82] The glossary is divided into two columns, but the recipes (folios 273–76) are written as continuous lines.[83] The two types of text are therefore clearly divided visually. The use of uncial script in this manuscript, however, sets it apart from Modena, MS O I 11. Whereas the Modena codex is written in a local, North Italian minuscule script, the compiler of the Harley manuscript consciously decided to employ an ancient and statuesque script, presumably to evoke the glories of antiquity.

Vat. Pal. lat. 187 (folio 7) dating from the eighth century, also contains non-medical material, and links with the Greek speaking East. It contains just two

[77] Lowe, *CLA* VI, no. 830, p. 38.

[78] Lowe, *CLA* VII, no. 973, p. 38. See also M. Elsakkers, '*Procicit, purgat et sanat*: Early Medieval Gynaecology: Recipes for Emmenagogues and Prugatives' (unpublished paper delivered at the Conference of the Classical Association of South Africa, July 2007). I am grateful to Marianne for supplying me with a copy, now reprinted in her unpublished PhD thesis. See also L. Totelin, 'Old Recipes, New Practice? The Latin Adaptations of the Hippocratic Gynaecological Treatises', *Social History of Medicine*, 24.1 (2011), 74–91. See also the survey article by M. Green, 'Women's Medical Practice and Health Care in Medieval Europe', *Signs*, 14.2 (1989), 434–73.

[79] Lowe, *CLA* III, p. 16.

[80] Lowe, *CLA* II, no. 324, p. 16.

[81] Lowe, *CLA* II, no. *203, p. 25.

[82] London, British Library, MS Harley 5792, fol. 275^{r-v}.

[83] Lowe, *CLA* II, no. *203. The origin of this manuscript is unclear: it has links with both Northern Italy and France, according to E. A. Lowe.

recipes, added onto the last — originally blank — folio of part of a psalter. The psalter fragment, consisting only of the first two psalms and the opening lines of psalm three, is written in a fairly large, eighth-century individualistic minuscule script with some uncial elements.[84] There are headings and enlarged initials in black and red.[85] It is by no means a deluxe manuscript, but is clearly laid out for practical use. In contrast, the recipes are scribbled in an eighth-century Northern Italian cursive script, and the scribe has not bothered to rule the folio, or use colour.[86] The headings for the two recipes are in uncial, but they are not on a separate line, and follow on immediately from each other, obviously to squeeze them into the available space.[87] Of the two recipes, the first is an unguent to cure stomach ache: ingredients include aloe, rose, a cypress leaf (*foliu cypera*), '*galbanum*' (the resin of a plant originating from Syria), and crocus. (It is not clear whether it is the stamens of a particular variety of crocus (i.e. saffron) or other part of crocus in general which should be used.) The types of ingredients suggest a Near Eastern origin, perhaps Byzantine, and therefore translated from the Greek. Whatever the exemplar, it is an expensive method for curing stomach ache, and the ingredients are highly specialized.

The second recipe, however, labelled as a physic potion (*potio ad physicos*), provides a complete contrast. The principal ingredients for this recipe are a heavy or large chicken (*pullum grassum*), lard (*lardu*) and bone marrow (*medulla*). Other ingredients include radishes, oil, and honey. Should we see this as an early version of chicken soup?![88] Unlike the first recipe, many of the ingredients would be to hand in a well-stocked domestic household. Further, the use of lard as well as oil suggests a Northern Italian or Northern European rather than a Mediterranean or Near Eastern origin.

[84] Lowe, *CLA* I, no. 80a, p. 24.

[85] Lowe, *CLA* I, no. 80a, p. 24.

[86] Lowe, *CLA* I, no. 80b, p. 24.

[87] Città del Vaticano, Biblioteca Apostolica Vaticana, MS Palatini latini 187, fol. 7. I am grateful to the library for supplying me with a digital copy of this manuscript. Unfortunately due to the closure of the archive for renovation at the time of writing this book, I was unable to consult the original.

[88] In Exeter, Cathedral Library, MS 3519, dating from the fifteenth century, the eating of a young chicken (with pepper, anise, and dill) is recommended as part of an elaborate aid to conceive. I am grateful to Teresa Tyers for alerting me to this parallel. See T. L. Tyers, 'Manuscript 3519 Revisited in the Cathedral Library, Exeter: An Analysis of a Medieval Medical Compendium' (unpublished master's thesis, University of Nottingham, 2006), p. 30.

These recipes are followed, on the same folio, in half-uncial, a list of plants and herbs. There are no illustrations however, apart from an ink sketch of a bird on folio 38 verso. On folio 54 recto the subject matter appears to switch from the natural world to Emperor Maximus and his exploits in Spain. Yet another new hand is employed here. It would therefore seem that while the herbal recipes were deliberately inserted to link in with the herbal treatise, the manuscript has also been added to by different scribes with a variety of subject matter presumably of interest to the community or individual who owned it.

For whom, therefore, were these two recipes intended? The fact that they were copied into the back of a psalter might suggest a clerical owner: as I shall show from the charter material in chapter six, several clerics also describe themselves as a *medicus*. However, library catalogues and wills show that in the early Middle Ages the well-educated laity (male and female) also owned psalters.[89] The recipes themselves fail to resolve the issue of the type of owner for this manuscript. The first recipe, with its exotic (for Northern Italy, at least!) ingredients, and lack of exact quantities for many of those listed, may argue for a medical practitioner.

However, there is long tradition, from the Roman writer Celsus to Isidore of Seville and beyond, of educated men who were not themselves necessarily trained medical practitioners writing about medicine.[90] Further, many works which were by medical practitioners, such as Galen's popular letter *Ad Glauconem*, were written as 'self-help' manuals for the educated public.[91] There is evidence of lay ownership of medical books, and it is reasonable to assume that heads of households (including women, if the example of early modern England is anything to go by) practised 'self-help' medicine for themselves and their dependents whenever possible, and had some medical knowledge, however basic or practically orientated.[92] This is assuming however, that the first

[89] See R. McKitterick, *The Carolingians and the Written Word* (Cambridge, 1989), ch. 6. On literacy in Italy under Lombard rule see N. Everett, *Literacy in Lombard Italy* (Cambridge, 2003).

[90] Nutton, *Ancient Medicine*, p. 5.

[91] D. W. Peterson, '"*Ad Glauconem*" as a Text for an Amateur Practitioner', in his 'Galen's Therapeutics to Glaucon and Its Early Commentaries' (unpublished doctoral thesis, John Hopkins University, 1974), ch. 2, pp. 25–46. See also K.-D. Fischer, 'Anweisungen zur selbstmedikation von Laien in der Spätantike', *xxx Internationaler Kongress für Geschichte der Medizin* (Düsseldorf, 1988) pp. 867–74.

[92] On women and 'self-help' medicine in early modern England see L. M. Beier, 'In Sickness and in Health: A Seventeenth-Century Family's Experience', in *Patients and Practitioners:*

recipe was indeed intended for practical use in the first place rather than being an exotic curiosity. The second recipe, however, is definitely far more achievable and accessible on a fairly modest domestic scale, without extensive medical knowledge. The texts on plants, and Roman history, again suggest either an erudite layman or clerical or monastic owners with broad interests in history and the natural world.

Città del Vaticano, Biblioteca Apostolica Vaticana, MS Vat. Urb. lat. 293, fols 95–96 also dates from the eighth century — Lowe thought it probably was written in Italy, but its precise origin is uncertain. Unlike Vat. Pal. lat 187 it is copied in uncial, but apparently as rapidly as the scribe could: Lowe describes it as 'careless': it has been systematically corrected in a minuscule hand.[93] The corrector may even be 'Bernrat', whose name is scribbled into the margin around a hole in the parchment at fol. 96.[94] It was probably corrected from the exemplars immediately after copying, although a later reader cross-referencing cannot be ruled out.[95] It was almost certainly part of a larger compendium of recipes: roman numerals are given in the margins for the majority of the recipes but there are no gaps between recipes.[96] However, they are not sequential even in this short fragment — the numbering appears to have been imported wholesale from the original exemplars.[97] Carbonelli deplored what he termed the grammatical and orthographical errors, arguing that the scribe had no comprehension of what they were copying.[98] It is true that he (or she) may not have had medical knowledge, and that errors can creep into any copying, but at least some of the orthographical and grammatical 'errors' point towards contemporary usage and pronunciation rather than simple carelessness or ignorance.

Lay Perceptions of Medicine in Pre-Industrial Society, ed. by R. Porter (Cambridge, 1985), pp. 101–28; L. Hunter, 'Women and Domestic Medicine: Lady Experimenters, 1570–1620', in *Women, Science and Medicine 1500–1700*, ed. by L. Hunter and S. Hutton (Stroud, 1997), pp. 89–107; L. W. Smith, 'Reassessing the Role of the Family: Women's Medical Care in Eighteenth-Century England', *Social History of Medicine*, 16.3 (2003), 327–42.

[93] Lowe, *CLA* I, no. 116. On overall discussion of the fragment, Carbonelli, *Frammento medico*, pp. 3–5.

[94] Lowe, *CLA* I, no. 116.

[95] Carbonelli argues that this correction was undertaken in the eleventh or twelfth century: see Carbonelli, *Frammento medico*, p. 4.

[96] Città del Vaticano, Biblioteca Apostolica Vaticana, MS Urbinates latini 293. I am grateful to the library for supplying me with a digital copy. Due to the closure of the archive I was unable to consult the original.

[97] Carbonelli, *Frammento medico*, p. 5.

[98] Carbonelli, *Frammento medico*, p. 4.

The fact that the recipes were corrected by another hand indicate also that the text was being read and verified, not simply copied unthinkingly — parchment was too expensive for that. The choice of script is curious, however. This is obviously not a deluxe manuscript in any way, and with no single numbering system, titles or line separation between recipes, it is not particularly user-friendly either. Why, then, choose to write in an uncial script, which takes up more space than minuscule, and takes much longer to write than heavily abbreviated cursive scripts? It could be that the idea was to make the text look late antique, to lend gravitas and the authority of age to the recipes.

Certainly the way the recipes are organized is very traditional, starting from the top of the body and working down. It begins with various remedies for problems with the head, distinguishing between pains in the head with heat or fever and those without.[99] One contains, among other things, dried rose (petals?) and cypress leaf, sesame, and fenugreek, which were to be placed on the head with water.[100] Another directs rose oil to be placed on the back of the head.[101] For a feverish headache, however, the unknown compiler advises abstinence from wine as well as the application of the ubiquitous rose oil.[102]

Between the first two recipes for headaches, however, is one for the 'flow of women' which involves heating pitch, making it into a powder, and then placing it in leather (a pouch?) with sesame, on the navel.[103] It would appear

[99] 'Ad caput calidum lavandum [...] Ad capitis diversis doloribus quod si capitis dolor nimio per calore obveneret [...] Si autem superveniet febrientibus capitis dolor [...].' Carbonelli, *Frammento medico*, p. 7 and p. 9.

[100] 'Ad caput calidum lavandum. Nitri assi et triti uncia una, melcoctum, vitella ovorum tria. Haec teres in unum, et ante pridie infundes in aquae congium unum cum sesamo, rosa sicca, cypero, foeno graeco ad tertias; et lava cum supradicto medicamine et cum ipsa aqua caput.' Carbonelli, *Frammento medico*, p. 7.

[101] 'Ad capitis diversos dolores. Quod si capitis dolor nimius propter calorem obvenerit, convenit sine sale oleo roseo et non vetere infundere cutem capitis: et parcius erunt unguenda posteriora capitis loca, id est in initio: neque enim hoc sine causa praecipimus: quia in initio medullae spinalis haec passio accidit. Non invento oleo, de omphacio ungues oleo: si nec hoc fuerit, camilino. Infantis pueris vel mulieribus, et quibus molles sunt vel solute carnes, quibus espediunt infrigidare loca nimis, hoc modo offerenda sunt adiutoria. Necesse est ut in aqua nimis.' Carbonelli, *Frammento medico*, p. 7.

[102] 'A vino autem absteneant qui dolores capitis patiuntur [...] roseum oleum ei sufficiet [...].' Carbonelli, *Frammento medico*, p. 9.

[103] 'Item ad profluvium mulieris; picem mundam mittes in caccabum [...] Et mox si remiserit, mittes super spongiam [...] Et mox ut exarxerit pix e spongia tota, tolles de foco, et cum refriguerit facies pulverem et sparges in aluta super tabula calentem, et cum sesamo pones

to be for irregular or abnormally heavy bleeding.[104] It certainly interrupts the flow of the general organization of this fragment, as it appears between recipes for problems of the head and ocular disorders, including remedies for injured as well as painful eyes.[105] This inclusion of this recipe does not, unfortunately, necessarily narrow down the possible context or intended audience for this fragment: such a recipe could have been copied by monks or clerics for the care of female servants, nuns for their own use, or could even have been intended for a lay household.

MSS Vat. Pal. lat 187, fol. 7 and Vat. Urb. lat 293 therefore demonstrate that the interpretation of medical recipes and their use is complex and context dependent, and that any discussion cannot exclude either individual recipe additions or the possibility of lay as well as clerical and monastic owners. Nor can a simple binary division be made between large collections and herbals containing recipes and individual recipes added to non-medical material such as those in MS Vat. Pal. lat. 187, folio 7. Karlsruhe, Badische Landesbibliothek, MS Cod. Reichenau 120, copied in Northern Italy in the ninth century, is an impressively large and carefully copied medical compendium. Yet, it includes a simple recipe for stimulating a woman's period: ingredients include parsley, hartwart, rue, black pepper, lovage, thyme, and celery seeds.[106] All of the herbs listed (excluding pepper) would have grown in a reasonably well-appointed herb garden in Northern Italy: thyme, rue, and lovage are all Mediterranean in origin but were grown in Northern Europe from an early date.[107] The Latin name for lovage, *ligusticum*, may even derive from the region Liguria, in Northern Italy.[108]

unum in umbilico usque ad pectionem, et alium ad renes.' Carbonelli, *Frammento medico*, p. 7. On menstruation, see M. Green, 'Flowers, Poisons and Men: Menstruation in Medieval Western Europe', in *Menstruation: A Cultural History*, ed. by A. Shail and G. Howie (Basingstoke, 2005), pp. 51–64.

[104] M. Elsakkers, 'Procicit'; Riddle, *Eve's Herbs*; Riddle, *Contraception*.

[105] Carbonelli, *Frammento medico*, pp. 10–13.

[106] Riddle, *Contraception*, p. 104 and n. 93.

[107] J. McVicar, *Jekka's Complete Herb Book* (London, 1994), pp. 108–09, pp. 166–67, and pp. 200–03. S. Malcolm, *The Encyclopaedia of Herbs and Herbalism* (London, 1979), p. 272, pp. 256–67, and pp. 214–15. J. Riddle, 'Pseudo-Dioscorides' *Ex herbis femininis* and Early Medieval Medical Botany', *Journal of the History of Biology*, 14 (1981), 43–81.

[108] McVicar, *Complete Herb*, p. 108 and Malcolm, *Encyclopaedia*, p. 214.

Conclusion

What unites the compilers and copyists of early medieval Northern Italy's medical and herbal recipes is a keen interest in some exotic ingredients and learned Classical medicine, but carefully selected, and where necessary, adapted for practical use. As in Vat. Pal. lat 187, recipes including rose petals and saffron rub shoulders with those the main ingredients of which are lard and chicken. Even larger compilations such as Modena, MS O.I.11 were copied into easily portable manuscripts that were never going to win any beauty prizes, but ensured the maximum amount of content was squeezed into the minimum amount of parchment. The end user could therefore equally have been an educated layperson, cleric, and/or medical practitioner. These collections, I have shown, were highly focused, selecting the parts of Classical Medicine, such as Hippocrates' *Aphorisms* in Modena, MS O.I.11, which could help diagnose and predict the course of an illness, and then treat it using the plethora of available medical recipes. One aspect of medical practice where a skilled specialist was considered essential, though, was phlebotomy, bleeding, the importance of which to early medieval medicine is demonstrated through the number of texts copied on this subject in Northern Italy.

Phlebotomy

Bleeding patients in order to rebalance the humours is the most iconic (and despised) of early medieval medical treatments. Despite the modern popular association between leeches and medieval medicine, in early medieval Western Europe bleeding appears to have been carried out principally by the cutting of a vein with a special tool called a *phlebotamus*, that is, a lancet or knife.[109] In the *iatrosophista* Agnellus of Ravenna's commentary on Galen's *De Sectis*, he describes how a doctor will show his pupil the instruments of his trade: 'Look, this is a lancet (*phlebotamus*) for cutting veins.'[110] This is not, however, a word found only in medical texts. Gregory the Great relates the story of an unauthorized preacher who had a dream in which he saw his words filling a *phlebotamus* in his mouth.[111] The correct time and manner of bleeding was a central

[109] Niederhellmann, *Arzt*, p. 71.

[110] 'Ecce hic est flebothomus ad incidendam venam.' *Agnellus of Ravenna*, Westerink, p. 10.

[111] Gregory, *Dialogues*, I, 4. 8, cited in S. Cosentino, 'La figura del medicus in italia tra tardoantico e altomedioevo: Tipologie sociali e forme di rappresentazione', *Medicina nei secoli, arte e scienze*, 9.3 (1997), 361–89 (p. 377).

concern, as witnessed both by the many prognostical calendars and treatises and also by scattered references in the legal codes and other literary sources.[112] The medical teacher Agnellus of Ravenna, discussed in the introduction to Part I, elucidates Galen's humoral framework, teaching that:

> We do not open the veins in winter because the weather is cold; if we open the veins we make the patient colder, and in taking away the heat of the blood we do more harm than we give help. We do not open the veins in summer because the body is dried out by too much heat.[113]

Bleeding is therefore best carried out in spring and autumn. Instructions on the timing of bleeding are also to be found in medical writers' discussions of specific illnesses. Aurelianus states that when a patient has phrenitis (a frenzy, combining physical and psychological symptoms), bleeding should always take place by the third day at the latest.[114] Despite the reputation of medieval doctors and barber-surgeons to bleed at the drop of a hat, according to the late antique reception of Galenic lore, a decision about whether to bleed or not should also take into account the patient's age, temperament, occupation, and strength:

> We do not draw blood from children, because not only does it help as nutrition, but also makes them grow [...] We do not open the veins of old men because watery and moist phlegm abounds in them [...] warm and dry temperaments are not to be subjected to blood-letting, because if their veins are opened they are harmed by the extraction of moisture from the blood [...] if they lead leisurely lives and are found at the tables of the mighty we open their veins; but if their place is in manual work, and worry, their veins are not opened [...] if strength is good we open the veins, if it is not good we do not open the veins.[115]

[112] F. Ageno, 'I giorni egiziaci', *Lingua Nostra*, 13.3 (1951), 69–70; Groenke, *Monatskalendarien*.

[113] 'In hieme non fleuotomamus quia tempus est frigidus, si fleuotomamus plus infrigdamus, subtractum calorem sanguinis plus ledimus quam iuuamus; in estatem non fleuotomamus quia desiccatum est corpus a nimio calorem.' *Agnellus of Ravenna*, Westerink, pp. 66–67.

[114] 'At si sola atque vehemens strictura aegros in phreniticam extemplo passionem perduxerit, designat adhibendam esse phlebotomiam permittentibus viribus, atque, si passio cogit, intra diatriton, si minus, in ipsa prima diatrito, ultra numquam, vexantur enim in eiusmodi aegritudinibus corporis vires.' *Caelius Aurelianus*, Bendz and Pape, *Celeres Passiones*, I, ch. X, pp. 63–63.

[115] 'Infantes non fleuotomamus quia non solum in nutrimentum eos iuuat in melius, sed et crescere eos facit [...] temperantia calida et sicca non sunt fleuotomandi, quia si fleuotomati fuerint, subtractam humectationem sanguinis leduntur [...] si sunt in otiositatem et in mensas potentum inueniuntur, fleuotomamus; si autem in labore sunt positi et in cogitationibus, isti non

Similarly, the first-century Roman writer Cornelius Celsus also considered the particular nature of children in relation not just to phlebotomy, but treatment in general:

> But if a child is the sufferer (of the pestilence), and not robust enough for blood-letting to be possible, thirst is to be used in his case, the bowels are to be moved by a clyster whether of water or of pearl-barley gruel; then and not before he is to be sustained by light food. Indeed in general children ought not to be treated like adults. Therefore, as in any other sort of disease, we must set to work with more caution in these cases; not let blood readily, not readily clyster, not torment by wakefulness and by hunger or excess of thirst, nor is a wine treatment very suitable. After the remission of the fever a vomit is to be elicited, then food of the lightest nature is given, after which let the child sleep; next day, if the fever persists, let the child be kept without food, and on the third day return to food as above. Our aim should be, as far as possible to sustain the child, by food when suitable, with abstinence in between when suitable, omitting all else.[116]

As MacKinney argued as early as 1937 — and the early medieval Italian evidence supports this — bleeding was apparently done by *medici* rather than, as in later periods, by barber-surgeons.[117]

Less attention has been paid, however, to the exact contexts in which texts on the art of phlebotomy are copied. For example, there are two very different Northern Italian manuscripts, now preserved at St Gallen, in present day Switzerland, which contain texts on the art of bleeding. The first, dating from the first half of the ninth century, is St Gallen, Stiftsbibliothek, MS 217, discussed above in relation to medical recipes. The importance of bleeding in early medieval therapeutics is arguably signalled by the fact that the first text in the first manuscript of the medical section of St Gallen, Stiftsbibliothek, MS 217 as

fleuotomantur [...] virtus si bona fuerit fleuotomamus, si non fuerit bona non fleuotomamus.' *Agnellus of Ravenna*, Westerink, pp. 68–69.

[116] 'Quod si puer est qui laborat, neque tantum robur eius est, ut ei sanguis mitti possit, siti ei utendum est, ducenda alvus vel aqua vel tisanae cremore, tum denique is levibus cibis nutriendus. Et ex toto non sic pueri ut viri curari debent. Ergo, ut in alio quoque genere morborum, parcius in his agendum est: non facile sanguinem mittere, non facile ducere alvum, non cruciare vigilia fameque aut nimia siti, non vino curare satis convenit. Vomitus post febrem eliciendus est, deinde dandus cibus ex levissimis, tum is dormiat; posteroque die, si febris manet, abstineatur; tertio ad similem cibum redeat. Dandaque opera est, quantum fieri potest, ut inter oportunam abstinentiam cibosque oportunos, omissis ceteris, nutriatur.' Celsus, *De medicina*, Spencer, I, Book III, ch. 7, pp. 262–65.

[117] MacKinney, *Early Medieval Medicine*, p. 39.

it now stands is an *Epistula de phlebotomia*. This details which vein to cut, how to bleed, and when bleeding should be avoided.[118]

In contrast, St Gallen, Stiftsbibliothek, MS 751 is a massive medical compilation of some five hundred pages, and contains no less than three texts on bloodletting. The first, an *epistula de fleutomia Gallieni*, is sandwiched between a letter on what is required of a *medicus* and a letter which is supposedly a debate between Plato and Aristotle.[119] The second and third are grouped together towards the end of the codex, after a dietetic calendar. The only material that comes after them are some recipes added in a contemporary hand. The manuscript is divided into distinct sections — and has a second index at folios 424^r–428^r. It therefore appears that the treatises were retained in the original order of the exemplars used rather than being reorganized into a separate section on phlebotomy. Between the three texts there is some overlap: both the *Epistulae de fleotomia Gallieni* and the final *Epistula de phlebotomia* begin with an instruction to cut the right hand vein.[120]

The compendium overall might be characterized as a learned medical arts handbook: as well as Pliny's *De medicina*, the Pseudo-Galenic *Liber tertius*, and Galen's treatise on urine and Vindicianus's *Gynaecia*, several of the texts consciously display their Greek (and hence by implication learned) origin by stating that they were translated from Greek into Latin.[121] Yet there are also several prognostical works, essential for any medieval medical therapeutics to predict the course of a patient's illness and whether they will recover or die, and a dietetic calendar as well as herbal recipes.[122] The number of texts on phlebotomy arguably also shows that this compendium at least in part was intended to aid medical practice as well as enhance learning and Classical knowledge.

No clean divide between 'therapeutic' and 'learned' texts could or should be made, however, nor can these terms necessarily be equated in an uncomplicated way with 'practice' and 'theory'. For example, as I showed above, many of the

[118] Beccaria, *I codici*, p. 370. Köpp, *Vademecum*.

[119] Beccaria, *I codici*, p. 377, no. 23a.

[120] Beccaria, *I codici*, p. 377, no. 23a and p. 380, no. 23b.

[121] See for example, Beccaria, *I codici*, p. 373 no. 373. On the Pliny extract see K.-D. Fischer, 'Quelques réflexions sur la structure et deux nouveaux témoins de la Physica Plinii' (C-St. Gallen 217 and 751), in *Pline L'ancien: temoin de son temps*, ed. by J. Pigeaud and I. Orozius (Nantes, 1987), pp. 53–65. On the *Liber tertius*, see K.-D. Fischer, 'Der Pseudogalenische Liber tertius', in *Galenismo e medicina tardoantica: fonti greche, latine e arabe*, ed. by I. Garofolo and A. Roselli (Napoli, 2003), pp. 101–32, and edited text, pp. 285–346.

[122] Beccaria, *I codici*, p. 373, no. 3. See also Köpp, *Vademecum*.

ingredients in herbal remedies originate from the East and therefore evoke Greek (and learned) antecedents. In any case, it is unlikely that either the compilers or users of this manuscript were troubled by such distinctions. The addition of recipes on a spare folio suggests that this manuscript was designed to be a 'one-stop shop' for medical knowledge, but that this was an ongoing process in which the monks actively engaged rather than simply preserving Classical learning.

This compilation, St Gallen, MS 751, has been attributed to the monastery of Nonantola and it is from monasteries that much of our evidence for bleeding comes from. A Carolingian monastic capitulary dated 10 July 817, over forty years after the invasion of Northern and Central Italy, states that set times for bleeding are not observed, but each person is permitted as the necessity of their condition dictates.[123] Special food and drink is also to be supplied.[124] An earlier capitulary is concerned about over-frequent bleeding in monasteries.[125] On the St Gallen monastic plan a special room for bleeding was envisaged.[126] In how many monasteries, if any, this idea was ever actually carried out, we do not know. However, the fact that it is specified on the plan at all demonstrates its perceived centrality to monastic therapeutic practice, whether or not it was carried out in a special room. In his account of John of Beverley, Bede stresses the importance of correct bleeding procedure to avoid any complications.[127]

Bleeding, therefore — by whatever means — was a key part of early medieval medical practice, but was by no means indiscriminate, and was one option among several. Based on the manuscript evidence from early medieval Northern Italy, however, it enjoyed much greater prominence than surgery.

Surgical Procedures

The much scarcer and more scattered evidence for surgery than for other medical interventions reflects the limited range and use of surgery in early medieval

[123] 'Ut certum flebotomiae tempus non observant, sed unicuique secundum quod necessitas expostulate concedatur', *Capitularia regum Francorum*, I, no. 170, ch. 11, p. 344.

[124] 'Et specialis in cibo et in potu tunc consolatio praebeatur', *Capitularia regum Francorum*, I, no. 170, ch. 11, p. 344.

[125] Cited in Riché, *Daily Life*, p. 168. Capitulary of 789, *Capitularia regum Francorum*, I, p. 63.

[126] For a facsimile of the plan see Horn and Born, *The Plan of St Gall*, I, xxiv.

[127] Cited in V. Nutton, 'Medicine in Late Antiquity and the Early Middle Ages', in *The Western Medical Tradition 800 BC to AD 1800*, ed. by L. Conrad and others (Cambridge, 1995), pp. 71–88 (p. 85).

medical practice. This should not necessarily be viewed as a complete break with the past, however. In Greek and Roman medicine too, the emphasis was very much on using diet and drugs to prevent and treat ailments, and only resorting to surgery when absolutely necessary.[128] This does not mean that surgery was not discussed in Classical medical texts. Cornelius Celsus, whose work was known and copied in early medieval Northern Italy, devotes the whole of Book VII of his massive compendium on health and treatment to surgery.[129] The dangers, though, are recognized:

> There is no bone in the abdomen, but all the same fistulae there are so dangerous that Sostratus thought them incurable. Experience, however, shows that this is not always the case. Indeed — and this may seem very remarkable — a fistula which forms over the liver, spleen, or stomach, is safer than one right over the intestine, not because a fistula there is more harmful, but because it opens the way to another danger.[130]

This is perhaps why virtually all early medieval copyists and compilers in Northern Italy largely bypassed what work there was in the ancient and late antique world, in the Hippocratic corpus and elsewhere, on surgery, instead focusing on the medical recipes and treatises on bleeding discussed above, together with works on about the impact of environment on health, and aids to predict the course of an illness, or analyse urine.[131] Having said that, up to the late Roman period there have been many finds, scattered across the Roman Empire, of doctors' and surgeons' instruments. In Rimini, in North-East Italy, for example, a

[128] V. Nutton, 'Roman Medicine 250 BC to AD 200', *The Western Medical Tradition 800 BC to AD 1800*, ed. by L. Conrad and others (Cambridge, 1995), pp. 39–70 (p. 54).

[129] Contemporary manuscripts including parts of Celsus's works include; Firenze, Biblioteca Medicea Laurenziana, Plutei LXXIII codex 1, Beccaria, *I codici*, no. 88, p. 278; Città del Vaticano, Biblioteca Apostolica Vaticana, MS Vaticani latini 5951, Beccaria, *I codici*, no. 102, p. 312.

[130] 'Ventri nullum os subest, sed ibi perniciosae admodum fistulae fiunt, adeo ut Sostratus insanabiles esse crediderit. Id non ex toto ita se habere usus ostendit. Et quidem, quod maxime mirum videri potest, tutior fistula est contra iecur et lienem et ventriculum quam contra intestina, non quo perniciosior ibi sit, sed quo alteri periculo locum faciat.' Celsus, *De medicina*, Spencer, III, Book VII, ch. 3, pp. 308–11.

[131] On surgery in the Hippocratic corpus see Jouanna, *Hippocrates*, pp. 87–91 and pp. 395–96. The large medical compilation Uppsala, K. Universitetsbiblioteket, MS Med. 6, copied in Northern Italy in the first half of the ninth century, is a typical early medieval compilation, with texts on bleeding, environmental factors and herbs. See Beccaria, *I Codici*, pp. 344–50.

set of one hundred and fifty surgeon's tools, dated to 257–58, was found in the excavation of a Roman house.[132] It has been argued that since the differences between these instruments within the set are often subtle, that this suggests a high degree of specialization.[133] This is very true, but we do not know how many tools the set's owner actually used on a regular basis: so large a collection surely also functioned as a status symbol and professional identifier as well as having a practical use.[134] It has been assumed that similar tools remained in use in the early medieval period, although our evidence for this is less rich due to changing burial practices, for example. The fact remains, however, that a dateable set from the early Middle Ages for this region has yet to be uncovered.[135] Similarly, early medieval evidence for trepanning (drilling a hole in the skull) is strongest for Anglo-Saxon England.[136]

Legal sources do discuss surgery, although their interpretation is not always straightforward. It is unlikely, for example, that castration was common in late antique or early medieval Italy. Nevertheless, a statute on it is retained in Justinian's law code:

> Should anyone act in defiance of my edict, the doctor performing the operation shall suffer a capital penalty, as shall anyone who voluntarily offered himself for surgery.[137]

The punishment for the doctor as well as the patient is severe, and was presumably designed as a deterrent. It is interesting that it is envisaged that a doctor, rather than a surgeon or any other form of medical practitioner, would carry

[132] J. Ortalli, 'Rimini: la Domus 'del chirurgo', in *Aemilia: La cultura romana in Emilia Romagna dal III secolo a.C. all'eta costantiniana*, ed. by M. Marini Calvani, R. Curina, and E. Leppolis (Bologna, 2000), pp. 512–26; R. Jackson, 'A Roman Doctor's House in Rimini', *British Museum Magazine*, 44 (2002), 20–23. See also R. Jackson, 'Roman Doctors and their Instruments: Recent Research into Ancient Practice', *Journal of Roman Archaeology*, 3 (1990), 5–27; Niederhellmann, *Arzt*, p. 79, and R. Watermann, *Medizinisches und Hygienisches aus Germania inferior* (Neuss, 1974), p. 128ff, cited in Niederhellmann, *Arzt*, p. 79.

[133] Nutton, *Ancient Medicine*, p. 185.

[134] See P. Baker, 'Roman Medical Instruments: Archaeological Interpretations of their Possible "Non-functional" Uses', *Social History of Medicine*, 17.1 (2004), 3–21.

[135] On Roman surgical tools see Cruse, *Roman Medicine*, ch. 6.

[136] See, for example, S. A. Mays, 'A Possible Case of Surgical Treatment of Cranial Blunt Force Injury from Medieval England', *International Journal of Osteoarchaeology*, 16 (2006), 95–103.

[137] 'At si quis aduersus edictum meum fecerit, medico quidem, qui exciderit, capitale erit, item ipsi qui se sponte excidendum praebuit.' Justinian, *Digest*, Book 48, 8, 4.2.

out the procedure. In early medieval Italy the practice of castration is certainly known and understood. In the *Vita* of an eighth-century Tuscan abbot called Walafred he is castrated in his dreams to prevent any more lustful thoughts or acts.[138] This idea of 'spiritual' castration, however, has a long Christian tradition, and does not prove that it was ever carried out in early medieval Italy, whether in the North or the South.[139]

In the Alamannian law codes, however, in force for Alamans living in Northern Italy in the early Middle Ages, deliberate castration by another as a form of assault is mentioned.[140] The earliest version of this code, the *Pactus Alamannorum* dates to the first half of the seventh century, and therefore is probably slightly more ancient than Rothari's edict.[141] This is followed by the early eighth-century *Lex Alammanorum*, from which the clauses on castration are drawn:[142]

> If someone completely cuts off another's genitalia, [the attacker] should pay 40 solidi in compensation. If [the attacker] castrates him, so that he loses his virility, he should pay 20 solidi in compensation.[143]

The compilers of the code remain silent on the possible motivation for such an act. Presumably more than one person would have to be involved unless the victim was unconscious. Perhaps there were cases where castration was carried out in revenge as a vigilante punishment for sexual crimes (Walafred's 'spiritual' castration was in response to an unspecified sexual misdemeanour) or alternatively specifically to prevent another member of the family producing rival

[138] C. Pilsworth, 'Sanctity, Crime and Punishment in the *Vita Walfredi*', *Hagiographica*, 7 (2000), 181–99; K. Schmid, ed., *Vita Walfredi und Kloster Monteverdi: Toskanisches Mönchtum zwischen langobardischer und fränkischer Herrschaft* (Tübingen, 1991), and C. Leyser, 'Masculinity in Flux: Nocturnal Emission and the Limits of Celibacy in the Early Middle Ages', in *Masculinity in Medieval Europe*, ed. by D. M. Hadley (Harlow, 1999).

[139] See Pilsworth, 'Sanctity'.

[140] Hlawitschka, *Franken*, and H. Beumann and W. Schröder, eds, *Die Transalpinen Verbindungen der Bayern, Alemannen und Franken bis zum 10. Jahrhundert* (Sigmaringen, 1987).

[141] Niederhellmann, *Arzt*, p. 12. *Pactus Alamannorum*, ed. by Merkel, *Leges Alamannorum*, ed. by G. Pertz, MGH Leges, 3 (Hannover, 1863).

[142] Niederhellmann, *Arzt*, p. 13. *Lex Alamannorum*, Merkel; *Leges Alamannorum*, Pertz.

[143] Cod A, 'Si aliquis alium genetalia ab totum absciderit, 40 solidos conponat. Si autem castraverit, ita ut virilia non tollat, cum 20 solidis conponat.' *Lex Alamannorum*, Merkel, LVII, chs 58–59, p. 127; Cod B 'Si aliquis alio genitalia tota absciderit, 40 solidos conponat. Si autem castraverit, ita ut virilia non tollat, cum 20 solidis conponat.' *Lex Alamannorum*, Merkel, LXV, chs 30 and 31, p. 127. See Pactus, XL, for the castration of horses.

heirs. How common such crimes were is unclear, but the fact that it is included at all in Alamannian law is notable: no such law exists in either the Lombard law codes or Justinian Roman law compilations.

The Alamannian law codes also describe injuries — sometimes using vernacular terms — and name specific medical instruments with a level of detail not found in other contemporary codes. This suggests, I argue, a direct engagement with contemporary medical practice and that knowledge of basic medical terms and injuries was assumed for readers of the code by those compiling it. The very first clause of the earliest Alamannian law code, the *Pactus*, opens with a statement on head injuries.

> If anyone breaks another's head so that the brain (*cervella*) appears, let him pay twelve solidi. And if a claim that the blow was not a major one arises between them over this altercation, yet a physician still inquires about this injury, let the physician take a solemn oath with his iron tools or find three witnesses who affirm this.[144]

The phrase concerning the doctor inquiring about the injury 'ut medicum ille querat' is opaque: unlike Lombard law, where a doctor should be called in for certain types of injuries, the phrasing here would indicate that the *medicus* has heard about the injury and seeks out the victim. In Alamannian law this is a legal or court doctor who specifically treats wounds, although no special term is used to denote this.[145] In the event of a dispute this doctor is also called as a witness, something that is not part of Lombard or Justinian law at all. As Niederhellmann has pointed out, the fact that, in Alamannian law the word of one doctor is worth that of three other witnesses indicates his high status. It also acknowledges his privileged role to determine the nature of a wound: a forerunner of the modern 'expert witness'.

Head injuries appear to have been a particular concern of Alamannian law makers into the eighth century as well, since the *Leges Alamannorum* repeats clauses from the *Pactus* concerning the scratching of the skull and the throwing

[144] 'Si quis alte[ri] caput frigerit, sic ut cervella pareat, solvat sol 12. Et si inter se de hoc intencione habe[an]t, ut non sit sic granda plaga, ut medicum ille querat, fort[e] medicus fuerit, in ferramenta sua previat sacramentum aut tres testes invenian[tur] [qui] dicant.' *Pactus legis Alamannorum* I, *Leges Alammanorum*, Merkel, chs 1 and 2, p. 34. Cited in Niederhellmann, *Arzt*, p. 66. Translated as *Laws of the Alamans and Bavarians*, trans. by T. J. Rivers (Philadelphia, 1977), p. 47. See also *Lex Alamannorum* 57.5: 'si autem ipsum ossum perdit medicus et non potest eum praesentare, tunc duce testes adhibeat, qui hoc vidissent, quod de illa plaga ossus tullisset, aut ille medicus hoc conprobet, quod verum fuisset, quod de ipsa plaga ossus tullisset.' cited in Niederhellmann, *Arzt*, p. 67.

[145] Niederhellmann, *Arzt*, p. 67.

of a bone against a shield. The eighth-century version, however, then adds three further clauses concerning treatment:

> If, however, a physician loses that bone and cannot present it, then let him call two witnesses who have seen that the bone broke away by that blow, or let that physician prove that the bone broke away by that blow. If, however, the skull is cut through so that the brain appears and a physician can touch it with a *pinna* or a cloth, let him compensate with twelve solidi. If, however, the brain protrudes from the wound, as often happens, so that the physician mends [the skull] with medication or silk and afterwards [the patient] recovers, and this is proved to be true, let him [the giver of the blow] compensate with forty solidi.[146]

It is clear from this that the doctor was expected to collect evidence (in this case a bone, or bone fragment) for presentation in court: one can only guess at the circumstances in which a *medicus* might mislay it! Perhaps the opposing side could even sometimes persuade the doctor to 'lose' the evidence. The 'medicamento' which could be used to heal the wound was presumably some sort of plaster, poultice, or unguent. 'Fanonus' (silk) obviously refers to the sewing up of the wound. Both types of treatment are carried out, the lawcode assumes, by a *medicus* rather than a barber-surgeon, for example. The language used to describe these injuries and their treatment is also interesting: in one version of the code, 'skull' is glossed by the vernacular term 'kebal'.[147] 'Pinna' is translated as 'feather' by Rivers but as a specific medical instrument by Niederhellmann.[148] 'Feather' does make sense in the context, however, since the alternative is a

[146] 'Si autem ipsum ossum perdit medicus et non potest eum presentare, tunc duos testes abhibeat, qui hoc vidissent, quod de illa plaga ossus tullisset, aut ille medicus hoc conprobet, quod verum fuisset, quod de ipsa plaga ossus tullisset. Si autem testa trescapollata fuerit, ita ut cervella appareat, ut medicus cum pinna aut cum fanone cervella tetigit, cum 12 solidis conponat. Si autem ex ipsa plaga cervella exierunt, sicut solet contingere, ut medicus cum medicamentum aut cum sirico stupavit, et postea sanavit, et hoc probatum est, quod verum sit, cum 40 solidis conponat.' *Lex Alamannorum*, Merkel, Cod. A, LVII, 5–7; Cod. B, LIX, 5–7, pp. 64–65; Rivers, *Laws*, LVII, chs 5–7, p. 86.

[147] *Lex Alamannorum*, Merkel, Cod. A, LVII, 6–7; Cod. B, LIX, 6. See Niederhellmann, *Arzt*, p. 77.

[148] *Lex Alamannorum*, Merkel, Cod. B, LIX, 6–7: 'Si autem testa (B9 id est kebal), transcapulata fuerit, ita ut cervella appareat, ut medicus cum pinna aut cum fanone cervella tetigit, cum 18 solidi conponat. 7. Si autem ex ipsa plaga cervella exierit, sicut solet contingere, ut medicus cum medicamento aut sirico stupavit (B9 id est virscoppot), et postea sanavit, et hoc probatum fuerit, quod verum ist, cum 40 solidis conponat.' Cited in Niederhellmann, *Arzt*, p. 78. Niederhellmann suggests that a 'pinna' is a cylindrical pointed instrument.

cloth, which is also light and relatively non-invasive (at least compared to a metal instrument such as that envisaged by Niederhellmann).

The question which has not been asked, however, is why this detailed treatment of head injuries which is so conspicuously lacking in other contemporary lawcodes? On a practical level, cranial injuries — and attempts at treatment such as possible trepanning — can be found in contemporary skeletons. In Anglo-Saxon England Bede refers to a head injury being cured by a doctor resetting the bones.[149]

Men in particular could have suffered head injuries in the course of fighting on campaign or in more localized disputes. Certainly axes or swords could cause at least some of the types of wounds being described. Work injuries, in construction, mining, or estate management, such as being hit by a falling branch or tree as envisaged in Justinian's *Digest*, must also have occurred relatively frequently. However, this must have been a feature of life for all citizens of Northern Italy as everywhere else, not just for Alamans.

Is this emphasis on the brain therefore related to the compiler or compilers' concept of the role of the brain in the functioning of the body? For Aristotle, the heart was the seat of the organic soul, while the brain functioned as a cooling system for the heart.[150] However, the philosopher Plato and the Greek anatomist Herophilus both located intellect in the brain.[151] Galen followed Plato's view that the rational soul was to be found in the brain.[152] Certainly Alamannic law, as discussed above, demonstrates a particularly active engagement with contemporary medical practice and theory, so it is possible that a Platonic or Galenic understanding of the brain informed the treatment of the different parts of the body in the Alamannic legal codes. One wound is when the attacker 'pierces the hand so that a cauterizing iron is not applied to the veins, and stops the bleeding'.[153] Double the compensation, however, three *solidi*, is given when it is necessary to apply 'a cauterizing iron [...] to stop the

[149] In Anglo-Saxon England Herebald is represented as being cured of a skull fracture by a combination of prayers, blessings and a doctor. Cited in Nutton, 'Medicine in Late Antiquity', p. 86.

[150] Nutton, *Ancient Medicine*, p. 118.

[151] Nutton, *Ancient Medicine*, pp. 116–17 and M. Grmek, ed., *Western Medical Thought from Antiquity to the Middle Ages* (Cambridge, MA, 1999), p. 87.

[152] Grmek, *Western Medical Thought*, p. 166.

[153] 'Si manum transpunxerit, ita ut focus non intret ad coquendum venas vel sanguinem stagnandu, conponat solidum unum et semis.' *Lex Alamannorum*, Merkel, Cod. A, LVII, 33 pp. 122–23; Cod B LXV 5, pp. 122–23.

bleeding'.[154] Cauterization as a treatment is also mentioned in the 813 Council of Châlons.[155] It can also be used to treat putrefied flesh, and is obviously also a common metaphor for the curing of sins.[156]

Since we are so reliant on Alamannic law for evidence of surgery, which in any case was not applicable to the vast majority of the population in early medieval Northern Italy, the prevalence of the use of surgical procedures in the region is very hard to assess. It is likely that some surgery did take place where absolutely necessary, perhaps most often in the context of accidents or warfare. It does not, however, appear to have been an everyday occurrence. If surgical procedures were performed, there is no evidence in this period of specialist surgeons. As I discuss in chapter six, in this period the *medicus*, the doctor, truly was a general practitioner, prescribing, bleeding and cutting as needed.

Conclusion

The weight of the surviving manuscript evidence is overwhelmingly tipped towards medical recipes and bleeding, alongside dietary and lifestyle advice, as the preferred treatment options for the inhabitants of early medieval Northern Italy. Parchment was simply too expensive (and time consuming to make) for copyists and compilers to waste their time on texts they could not use. As we have seen, every available page was used to add particular recipes to. None of the manuscripts discussed in this chapter could be described as deluxe or display copies: they had a job to do, and aesthetics were of secondary importance. Far from blindly copying the prestigious medical tomes of a lost, Classical civilization, the early medieval medical compilers and copyists of Northern Italy were highly selective and focused in their text choice and organization. How often, though, did people turn to higher powers than Hippocrates, Galen, or anonymous recipe authors, for cures? In the next chapter I re-examine the evidence for healing at holy places.

[154] 'Si autem ferrun calidum intraverit ad stagnandum sanguinem, cum 3 solidos conponat.' *Lex Alamannorum*, Merkel, Cod. A, LVII, 34 p. 123; Cod.B LXV, 6, p. 123.

[155] Cauterio aut ferro, *Concilium Cabillonense*, ed. by A. Werminghof, MGH Concilia, 2,1 (Hannover, 1906), p. 280, cited in Niederhellmann, *Arzt*, p. 82 and McKinney, *Early Medieval Medicine*, p. 41, n. 66. See also MGH Leges, Section 3, III, 283.

[156] McKinney, *Early Medieval Medicine*, nn. 110 and 111.

Part II

Healing: People and Places

Chapter 4

Shrines and Healing

When Europe fell apart, the Church remained as the only fixed point [...] the result was a return to religious medicine.[1]

This quote could easily be dismissed as the view of a modern medical professional without detailed knowledge of the early Middle Ages. However, Haegar is by no means a lone voice. Cosentino has argued that between the fifth and seventh centuries people turned more to healing saints such as Cosmas and Damian and the figure of the holy man, and that this is why our evidence for *medici* in Italy is more slight than in the preceding centuries.[2] However, the seventh century in particular is relatively poorly attested in general for Italy. The key factor here, surely, is that as communities adapted and altered to the new political, religious, and economic post-Roman climate, so too do the types of surviving source material alter: the number of inscriptions decrease, and the number of charters, for example, as the eighth century progresses, increase. Legendary accounts of the heroic lives of Northern Italy's many saints and martyrs also proliferate in this period. This shift in source material, as I shall argue also in chapters five and six on unsanctioned healers and doctors, respectively, can drastically affect which medical practitioners and methods of healing are most visible to us.

More specifically, the hagiographical literature can also potentially 'skew' our view of secular and religious healers, secular doctors in particular. Is this

[1] K. Haegar, *The Illustrated History of Surgery*, 2nd edn (London, 2000), p. 69.

[2] S. Cosentino, 'La figura del medicus', pp. 380–81.

true of Northern Italian saints' lives, though? For this chapter, I have chosen a representative cross section of four very different urban and two rural cult sites across Northern Italy. Two of the urban sites, Ravenna and Genoa, are ports or close to ports, while Pavia and Milan are inland, and Lombard and Roman capitals respectively. Pedona and Bobbio are the two selected rural cult sites as they both have contemporary hagiography associated with them, as well as being known cult sites. I shall focus on the principal early medieval saints' lives which contain episodes of healing for each location. I begin, though, by looking at how secular doctors are portrayed in this literature, and whether this indicates competition between secular and ecclesiastical forms of healing or not. I shall argue that healing at a saint's shrine in early medieval Northern Italy was not necessarily as ubiquitous as might be assumed.

The Failed Doctor

One 'marker' that historians have identified as indicating that a text may have been written in order to demonstrate the efficacy of saintly healing is the presence of the motif of the failed doctor. Typically in this motif the saint and his (or her) relics succeed with holy healing where the secular *medicus* has failed. Behind this motif historians such as Flint and Kazhdan have seen hostility and/or competition between different types of healers.[3] Skinner argues that, for medieval Southern Italy at least, the issue is not so much competition over choice of healer as a struggle for the assets which can accumulate from successful healing, secular or otherwise.[4]

In Northern Italian saints' lives written before *c.* 900 AD, however, the motif of the failed doctor is much rarer than in their Southern Italian or Byzantine counterparts: it is only present in two pre-eighth-century texts, the *Vita Epiphani*, from Pavia, and the Ravennate *Passio Apollinaris*. Apollinaris is styled in his *Passio*, probably composed in the sixth or seventh centuries, as the proto-bishop of Ravenna.[5] The *Vita Epiphani* was written by the sixth-century

[3] A. Kazhdan, 'The Image of the Medical Doctor in Byzantine Literature of the Tenth to Twelfth Centuries', *Dumbarton Oaks Papers*, 38 (1984), 43–51 (p. 48), and V. Flint, 'The Early Medieval Medicus, the Saint — and the Enchanter', *Social History of Medicine*, 2.2 (1989), 127–45.

[4] Skinner, 'A Cure for a Sinner', p. 305. See also C. Pilsworth, 'Medicine and Hagiography in Italy *c.* 800–1000', *Social History of Medicine*, 13.2 (2000), 253–64 (pp. 258–59).

[5] *Passio Apollinaris*, AASS, July V, 344–50. See also G. Zattoni, 'La data della Passio S. Apollinaris di Ravenna', *Atti delle R. Accademia delle scienze di Torino*, 32 (1904), 364–78 (repr. in G. Zattoni, *Scritti storici e ravennati* (Ravenna, 1975), pp. 115–28).

Bishop Ennodius of Pavia to honour his predecessor, Epiphanus.[6] Of the two, the *Passio Apollinaris* appears to follow the traditional *topos* of the failed doctor more closely.

After hearing of a soldier friend's son's miraculous healing by Apollinaris, a tribune asks for Apollinaris to be brought secretly to his house. The tribune's wife has been ill for several years, and is lying in bed. She has consulted doctors, but they have been unable to help her. Apollinaris takes her hand, telling her to rise in the name of Jesus Christ and to believe in him. The woman gets down from her bed, healthy, shouting the praises of the Lord.[7] This is a carefully crafted scene by the anonymous author of the *Passio*, with every element designed for maximum dramatic impact. Gesture, touch, and words are all combined in the figure of Apollinaris and the location is not just the woman's home, but her actual sick bed. It is the presence of Apollinaris which sanctifies the humble location, and no link is implied to a later cultic site.

It is in this context that the mention of *medici* in the text should be seen. There is no indication that the doctors consulted were inept, it is simply that this woman was considered beyond human medical aid. The emphasis by the author on the intractability of her unnamed condition and the considerable length of time she has been ill all contribute to a sense of the magnitude of Apollinaris's achievement in healing her so easily and rapidly. There are also obvious biblical echoes to this miracle to which the audience of this text is likely to have been attuned.[8]

Therefore the doctors in this narrative, I would argue, are simply the 'straight men' or foils for Apollinaris's sanctity and achievements. The doctors are not depicted as competing with Apollinaris in this narrative. Rather, the implication is that they have already given up and are happy to leave what they

[6] *The Life of Saint Epiphanius by Ennodius: A Translation with an Introduction and Commentary*, ed. and trans. by G. M. Cook (Washington, DC, 1942). There is now a critical edition and translation in Italian: *Ennodio. Vita del beatissimo Epifanio*, ed. and trans. by M. Cesa (Pavia, 1988). On Ennodius, see also the study by S. Kennell, *Magnus Felix Ennodius: A Gentleman of the Church* (Ann Arbor, 2000).

[7] *Passio Apollinaris*, in *Sanctuarium sue vitae sanctorum*, ed. by B. Mombritius (Paris, 1910; repr. New York, 1978), I, 116–22. In the version printed in AASS, July V, 244–50, ch. 4, p. 245, it is (presumably secular) medicine in general which has failed, not *medici* specifically: 'cui omnis medicina contraria extitit'.

[8] See J. Helm, 'Sickness in Early Christian Healing Narratives — Medical, Religious and Social Aspects', in *From Athens to Jerusalem: Medicine in Hellenized Jewish Lore and in Early Christian Literature*, ed. by S. Kottek and M. Horstmanshoff (Rotterdam, 2000), pp. 241–58.

consider hopeless cases to other methods of healing, since unhealed patients do nothing for a *medicus*'s reputation.

Crucially, I would also argue that the model underlying this vignette is not a straightforward one of pluralistic healing, with or without the 'medical market place' where patients more or less concurrently can seek help from many types of healer.[9] The picture painted is that of having consulted more than one doctor, but the focus then having shifted towards living with the condition rather than actively seeking to heal it. The implication in this text is that *medici* were the first, and possibly, except in extreme cases, only port of call for those that could afford it.[10] This might therefore perhaps be termed more accurately a 'hierarchy of resort'.[11]

It would also appear that *medici* (note again that this is in the plural) were automatically presumed to be the healer of choice for those of status in the *Vita Epiphani*: there is no suggestion by Ennodius that Epiphanus consulted anyone *but* doctors when 'congealed fluid flowed into his vital organs (an ailment which the doctors call catarrh), and, penetrating into the innermost parts, vent its fury upon the whole body'.[12]

Unlike the anonymous author of the *Passio Apollinaris*, though, Ennodius does explicitly accuse *medici* of having given inadequate care to Epiphanus during his final illness: he decries the lack of the skill of the doctors involved (*inperitia medicorum*). It is not clear if a 'panel' of doctors examined Epiphanus

[9] This term was first used in H. Cook, *The Decline of the Old Medical Regime in Stuart London* (Ithaca, 1986) but has been much discussed and critiqued since, not least on the basis that it focuses on consumers rather than the possible social and cultural factors determining behaviour. See D. Harley, 'Rhetoric', pp. 407–35. For an alternative view of medical pluralism, based on overlapping spheres of influence rather than the marketplace model, see D. Gentilcore, *Healers and Healing in Early Modern Italy* (Manchester, 1998), pp. 2–3.

[10] The order in which patients are depicted in hagiography as consulting medical practitioners and/or supernatural aid can obviously vary between regions and periods: for Byzantine examples, see P. Horden, 'Sickness and Healing', in *The Cambridge History of Christianity*, 9 vols (Cambridge, 2005–2009), III: *Early Medieval Christianities, c. 600–c. 1100*, ed. by T. F. X. Noble and J. M. H. Smith (2008), pp. 416–32 (p. 416).

[11] See L. Romanucci-Ross and others, eds, *The Anthropology of Medicine: From Culture to Method* (South Hadley, MA, 1983), part I, alluded to in M. Pelling, *Medical Conflicts in Early Modern London: Patronage, Physicians, and Irregular Practitioners 1550–1640* (Oxford, 2003), p. 230.

[12] 'Continuo eum coagulatus in vitalibus umor infudit, quem catarrhum medici vocant, qui se medullitus inserens in ruinam publicam saevibat.' *Vita Epiphani*, Cesa, *Ennodio*, p. 76. For translation see Cook, *Saint Epiphanius*.

together or whether second (and third?) opinions were sought after the initial *medicus* failed to heal the Bishop. Whatever the case, this vignette could clearly be seen as a version of the *topos* of the failed doctor. What is particularly striking about this text, however, is that no saint or their relics come to the rescue to effect a last minute miraculous cure for Epiphanus: the doctors fail, and he simply dies. It is also important to note that Ennodius's hostility is not towards doctors in general: the problem was that the doctors were inept (*inperitia medicorum*), not that they were secular healers. Why then include this incident at all, since it is hardly an advertisement for divine healing power?

The *Passio Epiphani* is obviously a very different text from the *Passio Apollinaris*, which was composed in simple language, centuries after Apollinaris was supposed to have lived, and with little material for the unknown author to go on. In contrast, the *Vita Epiphani* is written in complex, elegant Latin by someone who knew Epiphanus personally. Ennodius was writing about his predecessor inside living memory with a presumably educated and knowledgeable local audience primarily in mind. It has been argued, notably by Peregrine Horden, Paul Fouracre, and Valerie Flint, that in order for miracles to be credible hagiographers need to provide broadly reliable details about illness and treatment.[13]

Certainly it would appear that this is borne out in the *Vita Epiphani*: Ennodius uses the medical term 'catarrhus', and describes how this congealed fluid destroyed Epiphanus's internal organs. Was this what the doctors who treated Epiphanus had diagnosed, or is this Ennodius's own explanation? In Isidore's *Etymologies*, written around a century later but based on Classical learning, he describes catarrh as 'in Greek r<h>eumais [is] called eruptio, discharge, or fluor, flux. In Latin catarrhus, catarrh, is a continual flow of rheum from the nostrils'. He acknowledges, though, that it can also reach the throat and lungs.[14] The fifth-century medical writer Caelius Aurelianus also discusses catarrh in the context of both acute and chronic illnesses.[15]

[13] Horden, 'Sickness and Healing', p. 416; P. Fouracre and R. A. Gerberding, eds, *Late Merovingian France: History and Hagiography 640–720* (Manchester, 1996), pp. 45–46; Flint, 'The Early Medieval Medicus', pp. 130–31. It obviously very much depends on the hagiographical text in question, as Skinner has pointed out in her article, 'A Cure for a Sinner', p. 303.

[14] Isidore of Seville, *The Etymologies of Isidore of Seville*, trans. by S. Barney and others (Cambridge, 2006), IV.7.11. 'Reuma Graeca, Latine eruptio sive fluor appellatur. Catarrhus est fluor reumae iugis ex naribus quae dum ad fauces venerit, catarrh vocatur; dum ad thoracem vel pulmonem rheum dicitur.' Isidore of Seville, *Etymologiae*, ed. by W. M. Lindsay (Oxford, 1985).

[15] Caelius Aurelianus, *Akute Krankheiten: Buch I–III; Chronische Krankheiten: Buch IV–V*, ed. by G. Bendz, trans. by I. Pape, 2 vols (Berlin, 1990), I, p. 88 line 3; p. 198 line 7; p. 226, line 18; p. 294 line 16; p. 451 line 18; p. 542 line 12; p. 616 line 4; p. 664 line 5.

In Ennodius's account, however, no specific illness is named. Arguably, then, Ennodius is adding the patina of medical knowledge to his description, without necessarily telling us very much, or basing it on specific medical study. This would fit, though, if we assume an educated audience who were not medical specialists. The lack of a miraculous cure can also be attributed to this anonymous, and possibly select, intended audience: if they knew Epiphanus, they were well aware that he had not been healed. By laying the blame on unskilled doctors, Ennodius also neatly sidesteps the issue of Divine Will in Epiphanus's death, or indeed the relationship between illness and sin.

The 'marker' of competition between secular and holy healing is therefore almost completely absent in early medieval Northern Italian hagiography. Instead the only approach remaining is to analyse key saints' lives individually to see what type of healing miracles they depict and whether they are linked to a particular cultic location or not. I begin with the North Western sea port of Genoa and its patron saint, Syrus.

Genoa and the Cult of St Syrus

The only other *vita* I have come across in early medieval Northern Italian hagiography which rivals Ennodius's detailed description of Epiphanus's last illness, and which does not follow obvious biblical models, is that of Bishop Syrus of Genoa. It was probably written at the end of the eighth century or beginning of the ninth and appears in the Bobbio manuscript Città del Vaticano, Biblioteca Apostolica Vaticana, MS Vat. Lat. 5771, copied in the second half of the ninth century.[16] We are therefore in the unusual position of knowing that this text was definitely circulating in early medieval Northern Italy, possibly fairly soon after it was written. It is also atypical in that the miracle in question is post-mortem. The anonymous author does not however, unlike Ennodius, give any details about Syrus's final illness. It is simply stated that Syrus knew the date he would die. Syrus's body was then carried on a bier (*lectum*) towards the *Basilica Apostolorum*, surrounded, according to the hagiographer, by grieving crowds. The bier was set down, allowing the crowd, attempting to collect relics, to approach.

> Among them a skipper from the Province of Libya, acting in the fullest faith, when he had approached that sacred body, immediately saw blood flowing out of his

[16] J.-C. Picard, *Le Souvenir des évêques: sépultures, listes épiscopales et culte des évêques en Italie du Nord des origins au xe siècle* (Roma, 1988), pp. 600–02. The text, BHL 7973, is in AASS, June V, pp. 481–82.

> [Syrus's] nostrils. And swiftly taking a handkerchief, which he had on top of his head, he wiped up the flow of blood. [...] The skipper then returned to his ship, and stored (it) with diligent care [...] and when he approached his own country, after he had been dropped off there, many sick people, troubled by unclean spirits, ran from the distance to meet him, saying 'Behold, St Syrus comes, who has us to cleanse'.[17]

On landing, the bloodied handkerchief was accidentally dropped onto the shore, where people were healed. A basilica was built there and, claims the author, healing miracles continue to occur 'up to this day'.[18] As Picard has noted, the fact that the Libya described in this text is obviously pre-Islamic, points to a pre-seventh-century date, but the vagueness of the location — we are given no name for the port or the basilica in Libya — suggest that the author was probably writing about events in the distant past.[19]

The specificity of the moment at which the North African sailor obtained a contact relic of St Syrus seems to be at odds in this narrative with the singular lack of detail on the supposed Libyan healing shrine dedicated to the Genoese bishop. It is also notable that although the post-mortem nosebleed is implicitly miraculous, it is not until the sailor has left Genoa that healing miracles occur. If the *vita* was written to develop and promote a cultic site in Genoa, at which people could hope to be healed, surely it would have rated a mention (or three) in the text?

One explanation is that the author has found an ingenious way to attempt to kick-start Syrus's cult in Genoa and establish his healing credentials without actually claiming that healing miracles had already taken place there. Although Syrus is mentioned 'by-the by' in Pope Gregory the Great's sixth-century *Dialogues*, his feast day does not appear in any early martyrologies.[20] We therefore have no evidence of a cult before the appearance of the *vita* in Vat. lat. 5771, and even this only proves that the text was being read and copied, not that

[17] 'Inter quos etiam nauclerus Libyae Provinciae, plenissimam fidem agens, cum appropinquasset ad sanctum illud corpus; illico vidit de naribus eius sanguinem effluentem. Que festinus tollens sudarium, quod habebat super caput, sanguinem emanantem detersit. [...] nauclerus ad navem regressus [...] et diligenti cura reposuit [sudarium] [...] Cumque appropinquaret propriae patriae, adhuc procul posito occurrerunt ei obviam multitudo infirmorum, qui a spiritibus immundis vexabantur, dicentes: Ecce S. Syrus venit, qui nos habet mundare.' *Vita Syri*, ch. 7.

[18] *Vita Syri*, ch. 9.

[19] Picard, *Le Souvenir*, pp. 600–01.

[20] Picard, *Le Souvenir*, pp. 601–02. Gregory the Great, *Dialogues*, ed. by A. de Vogüé, 3 vols (Paris, 1978–80), III, Book 4, Chapter 55.2, p. 180, cited in Picard, *Le Souvenir*, p. 601.

there was cultic activity in Genoa centred on St Syrus. It is possible, therefore, returning to the idea of the knowledgeable local audience discussed above in relation to Epiphanus of Pavia, that the author of the *Vita Syri* was reworking an ancient legend or story attached to St Syrus, rather than attempting to make something up closer to home that would be unlikely to be believed.

There are several elements in this narrative that point to it being based on an existing story or tradition, whether written or oral. Firstly, the story does not follow biblical or even common hagiographical models, and involves a foreign sailor, which is entirely plausible and relates directly to Genoa's history as a port. Secondly, there is the close attention to odd details (reminiscent, as noted above, of Ennodius's specificity in relation to Epiphanus's last illness) such as the bleeding nose and the taking off of the handkerchief from the sailor's head. Of course, these could simply be the mark of a skilful storyteller, but in the context of early medieval Italian hagiography, these are extremely unusual *minutiae* and there are far more everyday post-mortem miracles that could have been inserted if the author was making it up from scratch.

Equally, the vagueness as to the location of the Libyan basilica is convincing if it is based on an ancient tradition where all the details have long since been lost, particularly unsurprising given the seventh-century Muslim invasion of the region. More cynically, of course, the generality of the location, and, in eighth-century terms, its inaccessibility to most Genoese, handily prevent any verification of the author's claims. At the same time, though, the author is emphasizing the power of Syrus's relics to heal, even far from his native Genoa.

Syrus is represented as performing a lone exorcism of a boy during his lifetime in the Genoa area, interestingly while still a priest.[21] The principal service he performs for the citizens of Genoa, however, is what perhaps could be termed snake exorcism: he cleanses a well near the *Basilica Apostolorum* in Genoa of a 'serpens' so that the water can be used again.[22] In terms of location, the *Basilica Apostolorum* is the key structure in Genoese topography in this text: it is also where Syrus is buried. All the miraculous events in the narrative, however, actually occur outside of the building. Its naming is also curious — the basilica, albeit virtually completely rebuilt, is known up to this day as San Siro, and there is evidence from Gregory the Great's *Dialogues* that it was known as such in the late sixth century, long before the eighth- or ninth-century supposed redaction of the *Vita Syri*.[23]

[21] *Vita Syri*, ch. 2.

[22] *Vita Syri*, ch. 5.

[23] Picard, *Le Souvenir*, p. 76.

The author may have been emphasizing Syrus's apostolic connections, as it is stressed that he dies on the day of the Feast of the apostles Peter and Paul.[24] Still, such coyness about the naming of a cultic site is highly unusual among hagiographic writers. The *Basilica Apostolorum*/San Siro is therefore both simultaneously present and absent in the narrative, the elephant in the room. Either, as I have suggested above, the author is somewhat cautiously advancing claims for the efficacy of Syrus's relics, or his aims in writing were not primarily to promote the basilica of San Siro as a healing shrine. Indeed, what Nick Everett has convincingly argued is that the *raison d'être* of much — above all episcopal — early medieval Northern and Central Italian hagiography is the promotion of apostolic roots, episcopal primacy, and boundary claims between sees.[25] This would certainly explain the number of healing miracles involving 'biblical' diseases and conditions such as blindness, demonic possession, and leprosy, and the close connection made in the texts between healing and evangelization of a region. If this is the case though, such texts would have little to tell us about healing shrines. One way to test this theory is to look more closely at the *Passio Apollinaris*, discussed above in relation to the *topos* of the failed doctor. Although Everett did not discuss it because it was composed in Byzantine rather than Lombard territory, the *Passio Apollinaris* has been seen by other scholars as epitomizing the type of apostolic, episcopally centred hagiographic writing he highlights.[26]

Ravenna and its Legendary First Bishop, Apollinaris

The dating of the *Passio Apollinaris* is disputed, but most commentators see it as a tool in the Ravennate see's struggle for independence and primacy, whether from Milan in the fifth century or Rome in the seventh.[27] In the *passio* of

[24] *Vita Syri*, ch. 7.

[25] N. Everett, 'The Hagiography of Lombard Italy', *Hagiographica*, 7 (2000), 49–126 (pp. 97 and 99).

[26] Picard, *Le Souvenir*, p. 694.

[27] See F. W. Deichmann, *Ravenna: Hauptstadt des spätantiken Abendlandes*, 5 vols (Wiesbaden, 1958–89), II: *Kommentar* (1976), p. 165; G. Zattoni, 'La data della Passio S. Apollinaris di Ravenna', *Atti delle R. Accademia delle scienze di Torino*, 32 (1904), 364–78 (repr. in G. Zattoni, *Scritti storici e ravennati* (Ravenna, 1975), pp. 115–28); F. Lanzoni, *Le fonti della leggenda di Sant'Apollinare di Ravenna* (Bologna, 1915), p. 4; E. Will, *Saint Apollinare de Ravenna* (Paris, 1936), p. 11. On the early history of the See of Ravenna, see A. Simonini, *La chiesa Ravennate: splendore e tramonto di una metropole* (Faenza, 1964), pp. 8–18.

Apollinaris his first healing miracle occurs before he has even reached Ravenna city centre. He is approaching Ravenna, having been ordered by the apostle Peter to convert the inhabitants of the city, when he meets a soldier with a blind son.[28] Apollinaris makes the sign of the cross over the boy's eyes. Just in case the reader might miss the symbolism of this miracle, as Apollinaris gestures over the eyes of the boy, he prays that both the boy's 'exterior and interior' eyes be opened.[29] The boy regains his sight, and he and his family are baptized in the river, in a scene presumably deliberately reminiscent of the ministry of John the Baptist.

Just as with the episode of the tribune's wife and the 'failed' doctor discussed above, Apollinaris's other healing miracles take place predominantly in domestic settings: he is sought out in the house of a widow where he has been recovering from wounds by a noble man, Bonefacius, who has lost the power of speech.[30] He also raises from the dead the daughter of Rufus the patrician upon entering their house: the daughter is subsequently consecrated to God.[31] Apollinaris's final healing miracles, however, take place not in a home but neither in a church: the sick meet him at night in secret outside of the city.[32] No post-mortem miracles are included which would seem to support the idea that the principal aim of the text is to present Apollinaris as a proto-apostle, of which healing miracles are part of the model in order to establish his credentials rather than as an advertisement for any specific cultic site. The domestic and outdoor settings for his miracles echo biblical accounts of Jesus's healing ministry: in the gospel of Matthew, for example, Jesus heals Peter's mother-in-law in her bed, where she had been suffering from a fever, and John relates how a long-time invalid at the pool of Bethesda picked up his mat and walked at Jesus's instruction.[33]

However, Apollinaris had two basilicas dedicated to him in early medieval Ravenna: the massive sixth-century structure of Sant' Apollinare in Classe

[28] *Passio Apollinaris*, Mombritius, *Sanctuarium*, 1, p. 117; AASS, July V, ch. 3, p. 345.

[29] *Passio Apollinaris*, Mombritius, *Sanctuarium*, line 43, p. 117, line 5, p. 118; AASS, July V, ch. 3, p. 345.

[30] *Passio Apollinaris*, Mombritius, *Sanctuarium*, line 56, p. 118, line 13, p. 119; AASS, July V, ch. 10, p. 346.

[31] *Passio Apollinaris*, Mombritius, *Sanctuarium*, lines 21–53, p. 119; AASS, July V, ch. 14, p. 345.

[32] *Passio Apollinaris*, Mombritius, *Sanctuarium*, lines 3–30, p. 122; AASS, July V, ch. 34, p. 350.

[33] Matthew 8. 14–15; John 5. 1–15.

and Sant' Apollinare Nuovo. The latter dedication, however, only dates from the ninth century when Apollinaris's relics were transferred from the outlying basilica at Classe to the safety of Ravenna city centre.[34] Arian Christian bishops during the reign of Theodoric may also have had a chapel dedicated to Apollinaris in the episcopal palace.[35] Did the *passio* really have no connection with any of these churches or chapels and their possible cultic activities?

The strongest candidate among these locations for a connection between text and the physical location of a saint's relics is Sant' Apollinare in Classe. This vast basilica was constructed in the sixth century a few miles from Ravenna itself by a banker, but the then Archbishop of Ravenna Maximinius ensured that it also housed Apollinaris's relics.[36] The theme of the connection between Apollinaris and the apostles which is so prominent in the *passio* is also emphasized in the apse mosaics in the basilica of Sant' Apollinare in Classe. Twelve sheep, representing the apostles and echoing also the story of the Good Shepherd, surround the figure of Apollinaris, hands aloft, praying.[37] It is as close as an artist could come to depicting Apollinaris as Christ-like. In the triumphal arch this symbolism is employed again in a seventh-century mosaic, with the sheep depicted as leaving Jerusalem and Bethlehem, representing the Gentile and Jewish nations.[38] Given the problems in dating the *passio*, however, it is unclear which came first, basilica or text. The only thing which is certain is that it dates to not later than the seventh century, because a small fragment of a manuscript containing the text survives.[39] Unfortunately it is not large enough to give us

[34] Deichmann, *Ravenna*, III, 307.

[35] Picard, *Le Souvenir*, p. 659.

[36] There is debate on the exact nature of the translation and the original placement of the inscription which records it; see F. Patini, 'I luoghi di sepoltura dei vescovi Ravennati nel "Liber pontificalis" di Andrea Agnello', *Felix Ravenna*, 98 (1968), 6–12, and G. Lucchesi, *Note agiografiche sui primi vescovi di Ravenna* (Faenza, 1941), pp. 63–73, cited in C. Pilsworth, 'Representations of Sanctity in Milan and Ravenna, *c.* 400–*c.* 900 AD' (unpublished doctoral thesis, University of Cambridge, 1999), p. 142, n. 20.

[37] Deichmann, *Ravenna*, III, 383, 385. See also online images and commentary by Mary Sullivan at <http://www.bluffton.edu/~sullivanm/italy/classe/santapollinare/santapollinare2.html>, accessed 18 January 2013.

[38] Deichmann, *Ravenna*, III, 385. See also online images and commentary by Mary Sullivan at <http://www.blufton.edu/~sullivanm/italy/classe/santapollinare/santapollinare2.html>, accessed 18 January 2013.

[39] St Petersburg (formerly Leningrad), Saltykov-Scredrin Public Library, MS F.v.I.12, written in uncial. See G. Cavallo, 'La cultura scritta tra antichità tarda e alto medioevo', in *Storia di Ravenna, 2.2 Dall'età bizantina all'età ottoniana: ecclesiologia, cultura e arte*, ed. by A. Carile

any idea of a context for the manuscript, nor do we know the exact location where it was copied.

There is a ninth-century crypt in the basilica which again suggests this was a possible pilgrimage site, but whether it had a particular reputation from an early date as a healing shrine is impossible to say. Whether the text pre or post dates the basilica, perhaps we should see Apollinaris's depiction in his *passio* as a healer rather than just a proto-bishop, but of the 'better sort', apostolic, in the mould of biblical New Testament heroes. It could also be argued that the fact that none of Apollinaris's healing miracles are explicitly enacted in Ravenna city centre, but instead take place in homes or on the outskirts, suggest that the author is themselves writing from outside the city walls. If this were the case though, it is odd that Classe, the port where the basilica was built, does not receive more prominence in the text. We should therefore be extremely careful about attempting to 'match' a text with a physical structure or healing cult.

We should, however, also look beyond hagiographical evidence: there are two 'doctor saints' with links to Ravenna. Cosmas and Damian are both the most obvious — and famous — saints to whom particularly potent healing powers were ascribed due to their status in their legend as doctors. A church was already dedicated to them in fourth-century Constantinople, but it was rebuilt in the sixth century by Emperor Justinian — Procopius relates that Justinian was rescued from death by the saints who appeared to him in a dream.[40] Deichmann has argued that the presence of Cosmas and Damian in the Byzantine era decoration at St Michele in Africisco in Ravenna can be attributed to the influence of Justinian's patronage of their cult, and that relics may have been brought from Constantinople.[41] However, Pope Felix IV (526–30) dedicated a basilica in the Forum of Vespasian to Sts Cosmas and Damien, so Rome may have provided another possible model.[42] Another factor for their inclusion is that church itself was built in fulfilment of a promise, *votum*, for a healing through the intercession of the Archangel Michael.[43]

(Ravenna, 1992), pp. 79–126 (p. 106), cited in Pilsworth, 'Sanctity', p. 142 n. 18. Lowe, *CLA* XI, no. 1608, p. 8.

[40] Cited in M. Maas, ed., *The Cambridge Companion to the Age of Justinian* (Cambridge, 2005), p. 307.

[41] Deichmann, *Ravenna*, II: *Kommentar*, 2, p. 43.

[42] R. Krautheimer, *Corpus Basilicarum Christianarum Romae*, 5 vols (Città del Vaticano, 1937–77), I (1937), 139 and 143.

[43] Deichmann, *Ravenna*, II: *Kommentar*, 2, p. 7.

Ravenna was also the setting for the healing of the late antique poet Venantius Fortunatus, who settled in Francia and was a confidant of the queen and subsequently nun Radegund, but who was originally from Italy. He relates how, in front of a picture of Martin at the Ravennate church of the Roman martyrs Sts Iohannes and Paulus, his sight was restored to him.[44] Much attention has centred on the relationship between the cure and the picture of Martin, since it goes to the heart of the impact of the Eastern debate about the use of images in Christianity (iconoclasm) in the West in late antiquity and the early Middle Ages.[45] However, the role of light, oil, and flame is arguably equally significant in the healing process in this narrative. Gregory of Tours and Paul the Deacon both give slightly abbreviated versions of this same healing miracle.[46] Deichmann argues that this incident must have occurred in Venantius's late youth, before he left for Francia.[47]

[44] 'Expete Martini loculum, quo iure sacelli iam desperatum lumen mihi reddidit auctor: munera qui tribuit, saltim, rogo, verba repende, est ubi basilicae culmen Pauli atque Iohannis, hic paries retinet sancti sub imagine formam: amplectenda ipso dulci pictura colore. sub pedibus iusti paries habet arte fenestram; lychnus adest, cuius vitrea natat ignis in urna. huc ego dum propero, valido torquente dolore, diffugiente gemens oculorum luce fenestris, quo procul ut tetigi benedicto lumen olivo, igneus ille vapor marcenti fronte recessit et praesens medicus blando fugat unguine morbos.' Venantius Fortunatus, *Vita S. Martini*, Liber IV, ed. by F. Leo, MGH AA, 4 (Berlin, 1881), pp. 369–70.

[45] Deichmann, *Ravenna*, II, 2, 334. J. W. George, *Venantius Fortunatus: A Latin Poet in Merovingian Gaul* (Oxford, 1992); R. Van Dam, *Saints and their Miracles in Late Antique Gaul* (Princeton, 1993), pp. 11–13 on the cult of St Martin, and also L. Brubaker, *Vision and Meaning in Ninth-Century Byzantium: Image as Exegesis in the Homilies of Gregory of Nazianzus of Paris* (Cambridge, 1999), pp. 27–33 on the debate on images. See also J. Pizarro, *Writing Ravenna: The Liber Pontificalis of Andreas Agnellus* (Ann Arbor, 1995), pp. 92–99, about the ninth-century Ravennate writer's own discussion of the power of images.

[46] Gregory of Tours, *S. Georgii Florentini Gregorii turonensis episcopi Opera omnia*, in *Patrologiae cursus completus: series latina*, ed. by J.-P. Migne, LXXI (1879), col. 927: 'Sibi quoque in Ravenna atque in rhetorica socio suo Felici, ex oleo, quod sub imagine picturae beati Martini in cicendili ardebat, dum tetigerunt oculos, lumen reddi(d)isse confessus est.' Paul the Deacon, *Historia Langobardorum*, 79: '[Venantius Fortunatus] sed tamen Ravennae nutritus et doctus, [...] Hic cum oculorum dolorem vehementissimum pateretur, et nihilominus Felix iste ipsius socius pari modo oculos doleret, utrique ad basilicam beatorum Pauli atque Iohannis quae intra eadem urbem sita est, perrexere. In qua etiam altarium in honore beati Martini confessoris constructum propinquam habet fenestram, in qua lucerna ad exibendum lumen est constituta. De cuius oleo mox sibi isti, Fortunatus scilicet et Felix, dolentia lumina tetigerunt.' Cited in Deichmann, *Ravenna*, II: *Kommentar*, 2, p. 333.

[47] Deichmann, *Ravenna*, II: *Kommentar*, 2, p. 334.

The emphasis in this account, however, is on the personal and unique aspects of this healing: there is no indication that Venantius was jostling with other sick petitioners in front of the picture. Rather, healing flowed from quiet personal devotion and pictures of saints could hang in any church or indeed home. To try and find evidence of healing at specific cultic sites we need to look at one of the secular and ecclesiastical powerhouses of late antique and early medieval Italy, Milan.

Milan

As Ravenna gradually slipped into relative obscurity by the end of the early Middle Ages, the city of Milan in North West Italy retained its importance in both secular and ecclesiastical circles. This can be attributed to its status as a late Roman Western capital, but also the Europe-wide fame of its bishop Ambrose. Perhaps it is also no coincidence that this is one Northern Italian episcopal *vita*, at least, where healing miracles are prominent.[48] There is also a clear focus on the veneration of Ambrose in Milan in the shape of the basilica and subsequently monastery of Sant'Ambrogio (originally the *Basilica martyrum*, commissioned by Ambrose and constructed between 379 and 382 in a burial zone near the Porta Vercelliana in Milan).[49] In chapter twenty-one of the *Vita*, Paulinus, writing in North Africa but having known Ambrose personally, relates how a secretary was tormented by an unclean spirit:[50]

> The devil abandoned him (the secretary) as he left Rome, fearing to be brought to the holy man (Ambrose). And so, as long as the servant was in Milan with the bishop, the devil appeared to exercise no power over him. But, when he left Milan

[48] Edited in M. Pellegrino, *Paolino di Milano: introduzione, testo critico e note a cura di Michele Pellegrino* (Roma, 1961). For a translation of Pellegrino's edition, see *Ambrose*, ed. and trans. by B. Ramsey (New York, 1997), pp. 195–218.

[49] C. Bertelli, ed., *Milano, una capitale da Ambrogio ai Carolingi* (Milano, 1987), p. 127. On the basilica see also F. Reggiori, *La basilica di Sant'Ambrogio* (Milano, 1966). On the cult of Ambrose see, for example, P. Courcelle, *Recherches sur Saint Ambroise: 'Vies' anciennes, culture, iconographie* (Paris, 1973). On the manuscript tradition of the *vita* see A. Paredi, 'Paulinus of Milan', *Sacris Erudiri*, 14 (1963), 206–30 (p. 221). See also L. Ruggini, 'Sulla fortuna della Vita Ambrosii', *Athenaeum*, n.s., 41 (1963), 98–110. M. Ferrari, 'Manoscritti e cultura', in *Milano e i Milanesi prima del mille: X Congresso internazionale di studi sull'alto medioevo* (Spoleto, 1986), pp. 270–73, identifies four main 'families' of manuscript, the earliest being Paris, Bibliothèque nationale de France, Fonds lat. 1771, dating from the first half of the ninth century, written in Northern Francia, cited in Pilsworth, 'Representations', p. 23, n. 5.

[50] Ramsey, *Ambrose*, p. 195.

> and came near Rome, the same spirit that had possessed him before began to trouble him [again].[51]

It could be argued that this was not, in fact, a healing miracle at all, since the relief was only temporary. Rather, it was a case of sanctity by proximity. By implication, however, it was also the combination of saint and place — Milan — that is potent here. In chapter forty-three another servant, this time of the powerful Roman-barbarian General Stilicho, is possessed, but completely cured and staying at the basilica under Ambrose's protection. It is discovered, however, that he has been forging documents:

> When [Ambrose] questioned him and discovered that he was responsible for such a great crime he said that he ought to be handed over to Satan for the destruction of his flesh [...] at the very moment when these word were still on the bishop's lips an unclean spirit seized him and began to tear him into pieces [...] In those days we saw many others purged of unclean spirits when he imposed his hands and commanded [them to depart].[52]

This stands in stark contrast to the healing miracles of other Northern Italian episcopal *vita* where the recipients go on to lead exemplary Christian lives: Ambrose heals and protects someone who is subsequently proved unworthy, although the sin is primarily against the State by forging letters of the tribuneship. As discussed above, whenever a writer is attempting to construct a *vita* of a recently dead individual, particularly in the case of someone as politically

[51] 'Per idem tempus, cum vir inlustris Probus puerum suum notarium, qui spiritu inmundo graviter vexabatur, direxisset ad episcopum, egressum urbem dimisit diabolus, timiens ad virum sanctum perduci. Atque ita puer quandiu Mediolannii apud episcopum fuit, nulla in illo diaboli dominatio apparuit; sed ubi egressus Mediolanio est et prope urbem pervenit, idem spiritus qui illum antea habuerat vexare coepit.' *Vita Ambrosii*, ch. 21, p. 80.

[52] 'Superioribus autem diebus, cum Stiliconis tunc comitis servus, qui daemonio laboraverat, in Ambrosiana basilica iam sanus maneret, commendatus a domino suo; ferebatur enim, quod libenter ab eodem haberetur, facere falsas epistulas tribunatus, in tantum ut tenerentur homines, qui ad ministrandum pergebant; sed ubi ad personam servi sui pervenit comes Stilico, ipse noluit in servo vindicare. Homines etiam qui decepti fuerant interventu sacerdotis dimisit, de ipso vero servo sacerdoti questus est. Quem vir sanctus, cum de basilica egrederetur, requiri fecit atque ad se perduci. Quem cum interrogasset et deprehendisset auctorem tanti flagitii, ait: "Oportet illum tradi Satanae in interitum carnis, ne talia in posterum audeat committere". Quem eodem momento, cum adhuc sermo esset in ore sacerdotis, spiritus inmundus arreptum discerpere coepit; quo viso, non minimo timore repleti sumus et admiratione. Multos etiam diebus illis, inponente illo manus et imperante, ab spiritibus inmundis vidimus esse purgatos.' *Vita Ambrosii*, ch. 43, p. 114.

well-connected and powerful of Ambrose, they often have to work with difficult or even unpromising material.[53]

Another unusual healing miracle in the *vita* is when Ambrose heals a lame man, named as Nicentius, by accidentally stepping on his foot at the altar.[54] As with the temporary exorcism of the secretary, Paulinus depicts Ambrose's sanctity as being innate, almost a physical presence — there are surely echoes here of the woman with the flow of blood being healed by touching Christ's cloak. This is very different to other, albeit legendary, Northern Italian bishops such as Apollinaris or Hermachora, whose hagiographers are always at pains to emphasize the centrality of faith and prayer (in both healer and supplicant) in harnessing divine power in order to achieve successful healing miracles.

After Ambrose's death his body is brought from the 'major church' (the cathedral) to Sant'Ambrogio, where:

> A crowd of demons made such a clamour that they were being tormented by him that their wailing could not be borne. Crowds of men and women also laid down their handkerchiefs and aprons so that they might come into some contact with the holy man's body.[55]

This is reminiscent of the crowds accompanying the procession of Syrus's body in Genoa, and may well echo contemporary practice. What is not clear in this passage, however, is if the crowds are jostling for contact relics in order to be healed, as pious souvenirs of a momentous occasion in the history of the city and/or to venerate in mini shrines in the home. Certainly such contact relics transfer sanctity into a domestic setting.[56] In chapter fifty-two a healing miracle does occur after touching relics, but, curiously, not Ambrose's.

[53] For Frankish examples of this see Fouracre and Gerberding, *Late Merovingian France*. On Ambrose's political context see N. McLynn, *Ambrose of Milan: Church and Court in a Christian Capital* (Berkeley, 1994).

[54] *Vita Ambrosii*, ch. 44.

[55] 'Sed lucescente die dominico, cum corpus ipsius, peractis sacramentis divinis, de ecclesia levaretur portandum ad basilicam Ambrosianam, in qua positus est, ita ibi daemonum turba clamabat se ab illo torqueri, ut eiulatus eorum ferri non possent. Quae gratia sacerdotis non solum in illo loco, verum etiam in plurimis provinciis usque in hodiernum manet. Iactabant etiam turbae virorum ac mulierum oraria vel semicinctia sua, ut corpus sancti aliquatenus ab ipsis contingeretur.' *Vita Ambrosii*, ch. 48, pp. 121–22.

[56] On the late Roman household and asceticism see K. Cooper, 'Approaching the Holy Household', *Journal of Early Christian Studies*, 15.2 (2007), 131–42; K. Cooper, *The Fall of the Roman Household: Religion, Gender, and the Household in the Sixth-Century* (Cambridge, 2007). On the representation of the household in hagiography see K. Sessa, 'Domestic Conversions:

> When we were receiving the remains of the martyrs Sisinnius, Martyrius, and Alexander (who attained the crown of martyrdom in our time — namely, after the death of the holy Ambrose — in the region of Anaunia, after having suffered under pagan men) with the deepest devotion at Milan, a certain blind man approached who touched the coffin in which the remains of the holy men were being carried, and on that same day he obtained his sight.[57]

The connection with Ambrose is somewhat tenuous: the blind man, from the Dalmatian coast, related how he saw Ambrose and companions, clothed in white, and was told by Ambrose himself to go to Milan to 'meet my brothers' and be healed. Significantly, however, in this vision, Ambrose, although not a martyr, is clearly classed alongside them, their equal, hence the reason for the inclusion of this vignette. Again it also showcases Milan as the holy city, full of relics with the ability to heal. As detailed above, it is surprisingly rare in early medieval Northern Italian hagiography to find such a specific claim made for the healing power of relics in a named city.

It is the curing of the lame Nicentius, however, which is the one healing miracle that makes it onto the sumptuous ninth-century gold reliquary altar commissioned by Archbishop Angilbertus of Milan (824–59). This altar survives in pride of place in the basilica of Sant'Ambrogio to this day, and is decorated on one side with scenes from the life of Christ, and on the other that of Ambrose.[58] The scenes from the life of Ambrose, however, face the celebrant at

Households and Bishops in the Late Antique "Papal Legends"', in *The Community, the Family, and the Saint: Patterns of Power in Early Medieval Europe*, ed. by J. Hill and M. Swan (Turnhout, 1998), pp. 79–114, and C. Leyser, '"A Church in the House of the Saints": Property and Power in the Passion of John and Paul', in *Religion, Dynasty and Patronage in Early Christian Rome 300–900*, ed. by K. Cooper and J. Hillner (Cambridge, 2007), pp. 140–62. On the early medieval household in general see the classic study by D. Herlihy, *Medieval Households* (London, 1985), ch. 3 and the selected proceedings on the household from the 2001 Leeds International Congress: C. Beattie, A. Maslakovic, and S. Rees Jones, eds, *The Medieval Household in Christian Europe, c. 850–c. 1550: Managing Power, Wealth, and the Body* (Turnhout, 2003).

[57] 'Sisinnii etiam, Martyrii et Alexandri martyrum, qui nostris temporibus, hoc est post obitum sancti Ambrosii, in Anauniae partibus persequentibus gentilibus viris martyrii coronam adepti sunt, cum reliquias Mediolanii summa cum devotione susciperemus, adveniente quodam caeco et referente cognovimus, qui eodem die tacto loculo, in quo sanctorum reliquiae portabantur, lumen recepit.' *Vita Ambrosii*, ch. 52, p. 124.

[58] See S. Bandera, *L'altare d'oro di Sant'Ambrogio* (Milano, 1995), the contributions in C. Capponi, ed., *L'altare d'oro di Sant' Ambrogio* (Milano, 1996), and C. Hahn, 'Narrative on the Golden Altar of Sant'Ambrogio in Milan: Presentation and Reception', *Dumbarton Oaks Papers*, 53 (1999), 167–87.

the altar, not the congregation.[59] Further, Hahn has convincingly argued that this scene was included in the altar primarily because of its eucharistic associations: Nicentius is approaching the altar when Ambrose steps on his foot.[60] Where Nicentius is cured, therefore, is as important in the overall narrative of the altar as the moment of healing itself. Even on the front of the altar only one scene depicts Jesus's healing ministry.[61]

This lack of emphasis on healing, despite the numerous and prestigious relics at Sant'Ambrogio, is reflected in a ninth-century reworking of the *Vita Ambrosii*, which may even have been composed by the anonymous author at the monastery attached to Sant'Ambrogio itself, although Archbishop Anspertus (868–81) and one of his predecessors, Angilbertus II (824–59) have been suggested as possible commissioners of this work.[62] As I have highlighted elsewhere, many of the chapters from Paulinus's original work omitted in the new version of the *Vita Ambrosii* are healing and exorcism miracles.[63] So Paulinus's account of Ambrose's healing of a paralysed woman in Rome, his exorcism of demons, even his cure of Nicentius's lameness, are all cut.[64] Only one exorcism and the healing miracles that demonstrate the sanctity of the relics of the martyrs Gervasius, Protasius, Nazarius, and Celsus are retained.[65] This is not to say that the second *Vita Ambrosii* is completely devoid of any reference to Ambrose's role as a healer. The anonymous author adds an episode where Ambrose heals the daughter of the Emperor Theodosius's general, Stilicho.[66]

Overall, the healing miracles omitted involve lower status individuals, whereas the new miracle involves the daughter of arguably the most powerful man in

[59] Hahn, 'Narrative', p. 170.

[60] Hahn, 'Narrative', pp. 176–77.

[61] Hahn, 'Narrative', p. 170, n. 13.

[62] On Anspertus as a possible commissioner see A. Paredi, *Vita e meriti di S. Ambrogio: testo inedito del secolo nono illustrato con le miniature del salterio di Arnolfo* (Milano, 1964), pp. 11–17. For a summary of the arguments, and a reaffirmation of the case for Angilbertus II see P. Tomea, 'Ambrogio e i suoi fratelli: Note di agiografia milanese altomedievale', *Filologia Mediolatina*, 5 (1998), 149–232 (pp. 177–87).

[63] Pilsworth, 'Medicine', pp. 260–61.

[64] *Vita Ambrosii*, chs 10, 16, 21, 28 and 44.

[65] *Vita Ambrosii*, chs 14 and 43.

[66] The second *Vita Ambrosii* has been edited twice, firstly by Angelo Paredi, with an Italian translation and introduction, and then in 1973 by Pierre Courcelle, with very useful notes on the sources used by the author of the text. Paredi, *Vita e meriti*; Courcelle, *Recherches sur saint Ambroise*, pp. 49–121.

the Roman Empire. The author of the second *Vita Ambrosii* is therefore keen to portray Ambrose as moving at the highest levels in both religion and politics.[67] In this context, the careful selection of healing miracles is a vital part of this 'rebranding' of Ambrose in the ninth century. If the commissioner of the work was indeed Archbishop Anspertus, he certainly would have much to gain from presenting Ambrose as a powerful political player with the power to both berate and heal those in the very highest positions. He had a protracted dispute with the papacy which eventually resulted in his excommunication.[68] The monastery of Sant'Ambrogio, founded at the basilica in the eighth century, may have been equally keen, however, to reflect the power of the monastery through this revised portrayal of Ambrose.[69]

One of the principal problems is that although the second *Vita Ambrosii* survives, very unusually, in a possibly near-contemporary manuscript copied in Milan: it is the only surviving *codex* of the text.[70] The manuscript itself is simple but handsome, carefully copied, with a portrait of Ambrose on the cover page.[71] We therefore do not know if it was ever intended for wider distribution or not, or whether the representation of Ambrose in the *vita* mirrors the way the cult of Ambrose was promoted at Sant'Ambrogio or not. We do know, however, that the first, fifth-century *Vita Ambrosii*, with its greater emphasis on Ambrose's healing powers, was popular, certainly in the ninth century, precisely when the second *vita* was being composed.[72] Whether that was a factor in its popularity, though, is impossible to say. There is also a relic bed of St Ambrose, designed to display his body, which may have been built somewhere between the fourth and the ninth century, although it is not attested in documents until

[67] Pilsworth, 'Medicine', p. 261.

[68] See Paredi, *Vita e meriti*, pp. 11–17 and Pilsworth, 'Representations', pp. 50–53.

[69] Pilsworth, 'Representations', p. 64. On the monastery see *Il monastero di Sant'Ambrogio*, and R. Balzaretti, *The Lands of Saint Ambrose: Monks and Society in Early Medieval Milan* (Turnhout, forthcoming).

[70] St Gallen, Stiftsbibliothek, 569. The attribution of the manuscript is cited from an unpublished letter of Bernard Bischoff by Paredi, *Vita e meriti*, p. 6. Paolo Tomea doubts, however, that the manuscript was necessarily close to the original given the number of errors. He suggests that the anonymous ninth-century corrector may have been collating this manuscript with another, more accurate exemplar. See Tomea, 'Ambrogio', p. 169.

[71] Pilsworth, 'Representations', p. 66. See also N. Ghiglione, 'Il libro nel territorio ambrosiano', in *Milano, una capitale da Ambrogio ai Carolingi*, ed. by C. Bertelli (Milano, 1987), pp. 149–54.

[72] See Paredi, 'Paulinus', p. 221; Ruggini, 'Sulla fortuna'; Ferrari, 'Manoscritti e cultura'.

1598, and was located in the chapel of St Vittore in Ciel d'Oro.[73] We are therefore in no doubt that Ambrose, along with the martyrs he discovered, were venerated in the early Middle Ages. It is the precise nature of that veneration which remains necessarily nebulous, given the possibly widely variant needs and expectations of those who visited the cult site.

An integral part of Sant'Ambrogio, and Ambrose's original reason for building the basilica, was the housing of the relics of Milan's martyrs discovered by himself. Indeed, Ambrose's sanctity arguably rests at least in part on his reputation as the finder of martyrs. Paulinus relates how Gervasius and Protasius were discovered:

> Around the same time the holy martyrs Protasius and Gervasius revealed themselves to the bishop. As a matter of fact they were located in the basilica where the bodies of the martyrs Nabor and Felix are today. The holy martyrs Nabor and Felix, however, were very popular, whereas neither the names nor the graves of the martyrs Protasius and Gervasius were known — so much so that everyone who wanted to go to the enclosure where the graves of the holy martyrs Nabor and Felix were protected from harm used to walk on top of the graves [of Protasius and Gervasius]. But when the bodies of the holy martyrs were exhumed and placed on biers, the illnesses of many were seen to have been cured there. There was even a blind man by the name of Severus, who up to this day serves devotedly in the same basilica, called the Ambrosian, where the bodies of the martyrs were brought: when he touched the martyrs' garments he at once received his sight. Likewise, bodies possessed by unclean spirits were healed and returned home with the deepest gratitude.[74]

[73] Hahn, 'Narrative', p. 179. See also E. Cattaneo, 'La devozione a Sant' Ambrogio', *Archivio ambrosiano*, 27 (1974), 85–110, and F. Reggiori, 'La lettera di Sant'Ambrogio', in *Antichi tessuti della Biblioteca Ambrosiana*, ed. by A. Capitani d'Arzago (Milano, 1941), pp. 107–16, cited in Hahn, 'Narrative', p. 179, n. 80.

[74] 'Per idem tempus sancti martyres Protasius et Gervasius se sacerdoti revelaverunt. Erant enim in basilica positi, in qua sunt hodie corpora Naboris et Felicis martyrum; sed sancti martyres Nabor et Felix celeberrime frequentabantur, Protasii vero et Gervasii martyrum ut nomina ita etiam et sepultura incognita erat, in tantum ut supra ipsorum sepulcra ambularent omnes qui vellent ad cancellos pervenire quibus sanctorum Naboris et Felicis martyrum ab iniuria sepulcra defendebantur. Sed ubi sanctorum martyrum corpora sunt levata et in lecticis posita, multorum ibi sanatae aegritudines perdocentur. Caecus etiam Severus nomine, qui nunc usque in eadem basilica quae dicitur Ambrosiana, in quam martyrum corpora sunt translata, religiose servit, ubi vestem martyrum attigit, statim lumen recepit. Obressa etiam corpora ab spiritibus inmundis curata summa cum gratia domum sepetebant.' Paul the Deacon, *Vita di S. Ambrogio: introduzione, testo critico e note a cura di Michele Pellegrino*, ed. by M. Pellegrino (Roma, 1961), ch. 14, pp. 70, 72.

This passage firstly makes clear that Nabor and Felix already had a successful cult in fourth-century Milan at the funerary sanctuary built by another early Milanese episcopal discoverer of relics, Bishop Maternus of Milan, known as the Naboriana.[75] The popularity implicitly implies that healing took place at this shrine, but it is not mentioned, since it is only incidental in Paulinus's narrative. (Neither of the two surviving versions of the *passio* of Nabor and Felix include healing miracles.)[76] Secondly, as with the body of Bishop Syrus of Genoa, healing miracles took place in the process of translation, outside of the basilica. Unlike the Libyan sailor in the *vita* of Syrus, however, who takes a contact relic which heals others, the blind man Severus is directly healed by touching Gervasius and Protasius's clothes. Paulinus's emphasis on the continuing presence of Severus in the basilica of Sant'Ambrogio demonstrates the importance of living testaments as proof of the healing powers of relics. While the healing of the possessed is a standard hagiographic *topos*, it is interesting that Paulinus describes them as returning home, extremely thankful. The meaning of this phrase, however, is opaque: did he envisage them having been cared for at home while possessed, or did their cure mark re-integration into their own families and households?

A hagiographic letter, claiming (entirely spuriously) to be written by Ambrose himself, fleshes out Gervasius's and Protasius's lives and deaths.[77] It is unlikely, however, to have been written in Milan: in this narrative Gervasius and Protasius, in contrast to their mosaic 'portraits' in Sant'Ambrogio, are depicted as brothers, with the Ravennese martyr Vitalis as their father.[78] Rather, this text creates a holy family from saints' relics venerated at Ravenna and depicted in the many mosaics in the city's churches.[79] There is no mention of healing in the text, but another Ravennese martyr, Ursicinus, is described as a doctor. He is brought before the pagan judge Paul, and wavers, but with Vitalis's encouragement, becomes a martyr.[80]

[75] G. Mackie, *Early Christian Chapels in the West: Decoration, Function and Patronage* (Toronto, 2003), p. 126.

[76] AASS, July III, 291–94.

[77] AASS, June III, 817–46. By the nineteenth century the spurious nature of this letter was well recognized: see F. Savio, 'Due lettere falsamente attribuite a Sant' Ambrogio', *Nuovo Bulletino di Archeologia Cristiana*, 3 (1897), 153–77. See also Zanetti, 'Les Passions'.

[78] Deichmann, *Ravenna*, III, figures 338 and 339 and F. Savio, *Gli antichi vescovi d'Italia dalle orgini al 1300 descritti per regioni. La Lombardia. I. Milano* (Firenze, 1913), p. 798.

[79] Pilsworth, 'Representations', pp. 82–83.

[80] Ursicinus's wavering is described as 'vellet male evadere', AASS, June III, 817–46, ch. 19.

Is this a hitherto unnoticed variation on the 'failed doctor' *topos* discussed above? It is certainly not considered noteworthy in itself that he is a doctor, and it is not clear if, as a doctor, he is considered as having more to lose by declaring himself a Christian. Gervasius and Protasius do not immediately become martyrs, however: they spend a decade reading and praying. This could point to a monastic context for the composition of this text, but the two 'brothers', together with Vitalis and Ursicinus, are all represented in the Ravennese archbishops' private chapel of Sant'Andrea, built in the early sixth century.[81] Clearly, whatever the aim of the text, healing is singularly unimportant to the sanctity of these saints in the eyes of the pseudo-Ambrosian author.

Gervasius and Protasius do, however, appear in another holy configuration in the Milanese *passiones* of fellow Ambrosian martyrs Nazarius and Celsus.[82] In the principal version of the *passio*, Gervasius, Protasius, Nazarius, and Celsus are all imprisoned by Emperor Nero, and eventually killed.[83] They jointly appear in a dream to a layman, Cereatius, questioning him as to why he has taken his bodies.[84] He replies that his only daughter, who was paralysed, has been healed. They persuade him to bury the bodies at 'Ad tres muros'.[85] This is obviously an *ad sanctos* healing, the sheer proximity of the relics, rather than a direct prayer or appeal to the saints, as they were apparently unaware of the effect their bodies are having! The author states that when Ambrose discovers their bodies, and takes them to the basilica, many cures are effected.[86]

The other principal basilica built by Ambrose in Milan was the *Basilica Apostolorum*, now called San Nazaro, built between around 382 and 386 in a prominent position outside the city walls on the road towards Rome.[87] The body of the martyr Celsus, found by Ambrose in the same garden as Nazarius,

[81] Pilsworth, 'Representations', p. 91.

[82] See *Analecta Bollandiana*, 2 (1883), 302–07, chs 1, 2, 5, 6, 7.

[83] BHL 6042, *AB* 2, chs 2 and 9.

[84] *AB* 2, ch. 9.

[85] *AB* 2, ch. 9.

[86] *AB* 2, ch. 10.

[87] B. Brenk, 'Der Kultort, seine Zugänglichkeit und seine Besuche', in *Akten des XII. Internationalen Kongresses für christliche Archäologie, Bonn 22–28 September 1991*, ed. by E. Dassmann and J. Engemann, 2 vols (Münster, 1995), i, 69–122 (p. 82); *Milano capitale dell'impero romano 286–402 D.C.* (Milano, 1990), pp. 119–24. See also S. Lewis, 'Function and Symbolic Form in the Basilica Apostolorum at Milan', *Journal of the Society of Architectural Historians*, 28.2 (1969), 83–98.

was also brought to the basilica.[88] It has been suggested that relics were probably situated in the floor of the apse, given the location of surrounding prominent burials.[89] Indeed, the basilica was adapted by Ambrose to accommodate his newly found martyr relics with a large apse, in the centre of which would have been Nazarius's tomb.[90] Beat Brenk argues that while San Nazaro was not an international pilgrim destination in the early Middle Ages, within the region it was likely to have been well visited as a martyr church and burial place of several Milanese bishops.[91] A silver reliquary in the shape of a cube, decorated with biblical scenes and said to have been used by Ambrose to house the relics of apostles, still survives in Milan's cathedral treasury.[92] Further, a short part of the Roman Itinerary (pilgrim guide), the *Notitia ecclesiarum urbis Romae*, actually relates to Milan and was possibly originally a separate text.[93] Picard argues for a seventh-century date for this itinerary, which mentions saint Nazarius, along with Ambrose, Gervasius and Protasius, Victor, Nabor and Felix, Celsus, Valeria, and selected early bishops and other martyrs.[94] The itinerary is laconic in the extreme: it simply lists where the tombs or relics of notable saints and bishops can be found: these guides do not say what pilgrims might have done when they got there!

Among those mentioned in the Itinerary, but not included in the hagiographic 'holy families', either in Milan or Ravenna, are Nabor and Felix, discussed above, and the martyr Victor, whose chapel predates Sant'Ambrogio, but is now part of it. Even here, though, Ambrose's martyrs are omnipresent. Fifth-century mosaics in this chapel depict, apart from Victor, Ambrose with the martyrs Gervasius and Protasius, and another early Milanese bishop,

[88] *Vita Ambrosii*, ch. 33.

[89] Brenk, 'Der Kultort', p. 85 and p. 122. See also M. Mirabella Roberti, 'Sepolture privilegiate nelle chiese paleocristiane di Milano', in *L'inhumation privilégiée du IVe au VIIIe siècle en Occident*, ed. by Y. Duval and J.-C. Picard (Paris, 1986), pp. 157–61. The 1990 *Milano capitale* exhibition book, however, sees two foci of veneration: the altar containing the apostolic relics, and Nazarius's remains at 'capite templi' (presumably the apse). See *Milano capitale*, p. 119.

[90] Picard, *Le souvenir*, pp. 52–53.

[91] Brenk, 'Der Kultort', p. 86. The bishops buried there were: Venerius, Marolus, Glycerius, and Lazarius, all dating from the fifth century. See Picard, *Le Souvenir*, p. 53.

[92] Milan, Tesoro del Duomo, Inv. 1427. See *Milano capitale*, p. 122.

[93] Picard, *Le Souvenir*, p. 20. See also C. Leyser, 'The Temptations of Cult: Roman Martyr Piety in the Age of Gregory the Great', *Early Medieval Europe*, 9.3 (2000), 289–307 (pp. 296–97).

[94] Picard, *Le Souvenir*, pp. 20 and 24.

Maternus, alongside Nabor and Felix, whose cult he probably developed.[95] This chapel was also, however, a memorial chapel, as it was where Ambrose's brother Satyrus was probably buried.[96] As Mackie has outlined, the focus of the decoration of the chapel is on death and resurrection, with Victor at the forefront.[97] Victor's relics were moved to the church of St Vittore al Corpo by 777, and Satyrus, although a layman, enjoyed a cult centred on St Vittore in Ciel d'Oro in the martyr's absence.[98] What we do not know, in common with virtually all the other sacred spaces discussed in this chapter is to what extent, if at all, they were associated specifically with healing.

Certainly the only surviving early medieval hagiographical text dedicated to Victor, the *Passio Victoris*, sheds little light on this question. It was probably composed in the eighth century: Picard has speculated that it was written when Victor's relics were moved to their new home.[99] If this was the case, however, the *passio* was written to celebrate Victor's status as a martyr rather than directly allude to the efficacy of his relics. This text is notable in having no miracles of any kind attributed to Victor at all. Rather, his suffering as a persecuted Christian soldier in the time of Emperor Maximinus is his principal claim to sanctity. The *passio* is also full of references to Milanese landmarks: the *Porta Vercellina*, *Porta Ticinensus*, and the *Porta Romana*. In keeping with the pagan setting of the narrative they are secular rather than ecclesiastical landmarks. In this case, the principal aims of this text were to celebrate Victor's feast day, inspire the faithful in their Christian life and everyday sacrifices, and proclaim Milan as the home of martyrs: healing does not come into it.

Therefore, while Milan was undoubtedly an important stop on pilgrimages to Rome from Francia, and probably also had a steady flow of more local 'relic tourists', it is not clear if many came with the express purpose of being healed. Further, under the Lombards it was Pavia, not Milan, which was the seat of secular power. Could the proximity of Lombard kings (once converted to Catholicism from Arianism) have helped the development of cultic healing sites there?

95 Picard, *Le souvenir*, pp. 38–40.

96 Mackie, *Early Christian Chapels*, pp. 127–28.

97 Mackie, *Early Christian Chapels*, p. 129.

98 Picard, *Le Souvenir*, p. 130; Mackie, *Early Christian Chapels*, pp. 128–29.

99 Picard, *Le Souvenir*, p. 130.

Pavia

Two generations before the Lombards invaded Italy, a late antique church dedicated to the doctor-saints Cosmas and Damian in Pavia was probably built partially under the episcopate of Ennodius, but completed by Crispin, his successor.[100] We do not know, though, to what extent it became a centre for healing, if at all.

However, turning to St Sebastian, Paul the Deacon relates how, under the Lombards, the population in the late seventh century were suffering with the pestilence. A man had a vision in which he was told that the epidemic would only end when an altar honouring St Sebastian was established in the church of St Peter of Chains. The man acquired the necessary relics from Rome, and created an altar dedicated to St Sebastian as instructed, upon which the epidemic dissipated.[101] Even if, at the distance of a century, with Paul writing about Lombard Italy through the prism of Carolingian rule, this vignette tells us less than we might think about disease and piety in Pavia in the 680s, it shows that by the second half of the eighth century at the very latest Sebastian was seen as a potential protector for plague sufferers.[102] Lester Little has suggested that Sebastian became associated with the plague in particular for two central reasons.[103] Firstly although Sebastian is often depicted in Christian art through the ages as being martyred with arrows, this attack did not in fact kill him, and according to his legend a Christian widow restored him to good health, only for Sebastian to helpfully again present himself to the Emperor and be beaten to death.[104] He therefore (initially at least) escaped almost certain death. Secondly, however, arrows have a long association with destruction and suffering: in Homer's *Iliad* Apollo wreaks vengeance on Agamemnon and his army

[100] Christie, *From Constantine*, p. 107.

[101] Paul the Deacon, *Historia Longobardorum*, 6.5, p. 166; *Le Liber pontificalis: texte, introduction et commentaire*, ed. by L. Duchesne, 2 vols (Paris, 1886–92), English translation as *The Book of Pontiffs (Liber pontificalis): The Ancient Biographies of the First Ninety Roman Bishops to AD 715*, trans. by R. Davis (Liverpool, 1989), pp. 193–94, cited in Little, 'Life and Afterlife', pp. 28–29.

[102] See, for example, R. McKitterick, 'Paul the Deacon and the Franks', *Early Medieval Europe*, 8.3 (1999), 319–39, and the conference proceedings, *Paolo Diacono e il Friuli altomedievale (secc. VI–X): atti del XIV Congresso internationale di studi sull'Alto Medioevo, Cividale del Friuli, Bottenico di Moimacco, 24–29 settembre 1999*, Atti dei congressi 14 (Spoleto, 2001).

[103] Little 'Life and Afterlife', pp. 28–29.

[104] Little 'Life and Afterlife', pp. 28–29.

for nine days with the arrow of death.[105] The story also, however, handily provides a watertight justification for why Roman relics of an important Roman saint found their way to Pavia.

What this vignette depicts, though, is the establishment, or more accurately perhaps, the legend for the establishment of a cult in Pavia, for a very specific purpose, healing and protection from plague. This, therefore, was an extraordinary event, rather than a site for the healing of more everyday, commonplace ailments. Have we perhaps been looking in the wrong place? Were rural cultic sites more focused on healing?

Rural Cultic Sites: The Case of Pedona and Bobbio

Another saint with, like Victor or Ambrose, both an ecclesiastical structure and an early medieval *vita* dedicated to them is the now somewhat obscure saint, Dalmatius of Pedona. The monastery of St Dalmazzo, a seventh-century Lombard foundation, occupied a key location on the road between Byzantine Liguria and the Lombard kingdoms.[106] There is debate concerning the date and different versions of the saint's life of Dalmatius. Nick Everett seeks to resolve this in his important 2000 study of Lombard hagiography: the earliest version of the text is BHL 2082, preserved in an early tenth-century manuscript, Milan, Biblioteca Ambrosiana, MS P113 Sup., fols 1–6, but Everett suggests an early eighth-century date for the original redaction of the text.[107] As with so many other Northern Italian hagiographical texts of this date, demonstrating apostolic links is one of the key concerns of the anonymous monk of St Dalmazzo who composed the text.[108] However, unusually for Northern Italian hagiographical texts, Dalmatius performs both pre- and post-mortem healing miracles. The first is the daughter of a *magister militum* (literally, master of soldiers), of the town of Albensium, who had been ill for a long time and was close to death.[109] As with Apollinaris's healing miracles, healing here is explicitly linked to spiritual health, that is conversion to Christianity.[110] In

[105] Little, 'Life and Afterlife', p. 30.

[106] Cantino Wataghin, Destefanis, and Uggé, 'Monasteri e territorio', pp. 311–16. See also A. M. Riberi, *S. Dalmazzo di Pedona e la sua abazia (Borgo San Dalmazzo) con documenti inediti* (Torino, 1929), pp. 367–80.

[107] Everett, 'Hagiography', pp. 74 and 79.

[108] Everett, 'Hagiography', p. 79. For the text, see Ribieri, *S. Dalmazzo*, pp. 367–80.

[109] Ribieri, *S. Dalmazzo*, ch. 8, pp. 373–74.

[110] Ribieri, *S. Dalmazzo*, ch. 8, p. 374.

Milan Dalmatius heals a boy with blood flowing from his nose, who is possessed: in a high voice the demon declares that if Dalmatius does not come, he will never leave the boy.[111] The most significant miracle, however, occurs after his death, at his tomb, and therefore is very unusual in early medieval Northern Italian hagiography.

> A certain most illustrious woman [...] called Deinopa, was gripped by a most serious illness, so that no pulse was living in her, and she died [...] one of the servants of Saint Dalmatius advised that she [...] be brought to the church of the aforementioned holy man [...] and coming into the church, they placed her on the floor, with the head of the woman (facing) towards the tomb of the holy man [...] from the third to the eighth hour of the day.[112]

Dalmatius then appears in a vision to one of those who served there. He declares that Dalmatius had said: '(She) who is above my altar (should) be washed with water, and drink, and arise.'[113] After the instructions are followed, Deinopa duly revives, and all praise God. This is a classic depiction of the ancient and medieval practice of incubation, sleeping at the tomb/temple in order to be healed.[114] An unusual aspect of this miracle, however, is the emphasis on the lack of a pulse to denote that Deinopa really has died. Assessing the pattern of a patient's pulse was a well-known and ancient diagnostic tool, even though it was obviously not associated with the circulation of blood, as that had to wait for the Englishman William Harvey in the seventeenth century.[115] It appears to have been included to demonstrate the Deinopa really was (in early medieval terms at least) dead, and not just unconscious. The fact that the woman is named is also designed to reassure an audience that this was an actual healing miracle that had taken place at Dalmatius's tomb.

[111] 'Sic diabolus cum magno fremitu alta voce clamare coepit: "Si Dalmatius huc non venisset, de isto puero numquam exieram."' Ribieri, *S. Dalmazzo*, ch. 11, p. 375.

[112] 'Nunc quaedam illustrissima femina [...] iam Deinopia nomine, dum gravissima teneretur aegritudine, sicque ut iam nullus in illa pulsus vivendi esset et mortua [...] Tunc veniens unus de serventibus sancti Dalmatii, dedit consilium ut ea [...] ad supradicti sancti viri ecclesiam deportaretur [...] Cumque intrantes in ecclesiam, posuerunt corpus in pavimentum, caput mulieris ad sepulcrum sancti viri, et ianuis clausis, omnes proiecti foras, ab hora diei tertia usque ad horam octavam.' Ribieri, *S. Dalmazzo*, ch. 15, pp. 377–78.

[113] 'Quod est super altario meo lavetur ex aqua et bibe et surge.' Ribieri, *S. Dalmazzo*, ch. 16, p. 378.

[114] Nutton, *Ancient Medicine*, pp. 103–04.

[115] On ancient discussion of the pulse, see Nutton, *Ancient Medicine*, pp. 126–27, 237–38. On William Harvey, see R. French, *William Harvey's Natural Philosophy* (Cambridge, 1994).

The healing of women also would appear to be the cornerstone of Saint Columbanus's credentials as a healer, alongside the curing of fevers. He founded the monastery of Bobbio in 616, situated in a valley on one of the main routes between Piacenza and Genoa in North West Italy.[116] Pilgrims and travellers came from as far afield as Ireland and the Middle East.[117] Columbanus's *vita*, written by Jonas, a monk of Bobbio, some twenty-five years after Columbanus's death.[118] The *vita* of Columbanus himself is largely dedicated to events outside of Italy, particularly his volatile relationship with the Merovingian dynasty.[119] Columbanus does find time, however, for the occasional healing miracle. The first occurs when Columbanus — having been invited by a Merovingian king who Jonas probably wrongly identifies as Sigibert — is living with some companions in the remote but beautiful Vosges region in what is now North East France.[120] A monk who is with him falls ill with a fever, and the other monks fast and pray for him.[121] On the third day a man unexpectedly appears, bringing much needed food supplies, and tells them about his wife, who has long been suffering from a fever.[122] Columbanus and the monks pray for her. On the man's return he discovers his wife, 'seated' at home, and learns that the fever left her at the very hour when the man of God had been praying for her.[123] Presumably

[116] E. Destefanis, *Il monastero di Bobbio in età altomedievale: Ricerche di archeologia altomedievale e medievale* (Firenze, 2002), p. 1.

[117] Destefanis, *Il monastero*, pp. 47 and 98.

[118] I. Wood, *The Missionary Life: Saints and the Evangelisation of Europe 400–1050* (Harlow, 2001), p. 35; edited by B. Krusch, MGH SRM, 4 (Hannover, 1905), pp. 65–108.

[119] See H. B. Clark, and M. Brennan, eds, *Columbanus and Merovingian Monasticism* (Oxford, 1981); Wood, *Missionary Life*, pp. 31–35.

[120] I. Wood, *The Merovingian Kingdoms, 450–751* (London, 1994), p. 195.

[121] 'Eo ergo in loco virum Dei cum suis commorantem, subito unum e fratibus [...] vis febrium coepit flagellare [...] coepit omnium animos adspirare, ut pro egri fratres sospitate ieiunio omnes et oratione vacarent.' *Vita Columbani*, I, ch. 7, p. 73.

[122] 'Tertia iam die peracto ieiunio, nihil habentibus, unde fessa corpora reficerentur, subito conspiciunt virum quendam, cum panum supplimento vel pulmentorum aequos honeratos, ante fores, adstare [...] Oblatis itaque viro Dei quae detulerat, coepit cum cordis humilitate deposcere, ut vir sanctus pro coniuge sua Dominum deprecaretur, quam per anni circulum tanta ignis febrium urebat, ut iam non crederetur superis reddi.' *Vita Columbani*, I, ch. 7, p. 73.

[123] 'Cumque ille cum suis orationem conplesset, statim ea quae periculum mortis in propatulo habebat sanitati est reddita. At vero cum vir eius, largita sibi a viro Dei benedictione, domum remeasset, invenit coniugem suam domi sedentem, sciscitatusque, qua hora eam febrium vis reliquisset, repperit ea hora sanatam fuisse, qua vir Dei pro ea Dominum deprecasset.' *Vita Columbani*, I, ch. 7, p. 73.

the significance of the fact that she is seated is that previously, being in danger of death (*periculum mortis*), she would have been in bed.

However, Jonas's work was more ambitious than simply writing Columbanus's *vita*. Jonas envisaged Columbanus at the head of a holy chain of Abbots and nuns following his example at the various monastic foundations he had been involved with in Francia and Northern Italy.[124] The type of healing miracles they perform also mirror Columbanus's, in that they focus on the curing of fevers. Athalo, Abbot of Bobbio, is approached by the anxious parents of a small boy 'in extremis' with a fever, who is healed after the Abbot prayed for him at several churches and visited him secretly at home.[125] Eustasius of Luxeuil also cured a brother called Agilus of a fever through prayer.[126] Even Abbot Bertulf of Bobbio was himself struck with a fever on his return from Rome to Bobbio but was healed by St Peter.[127] Nuns at one of Columbanus's Frankish foundations

[124] See Wood, *Merovingian Kingdoms*, pp. 184–89.

[125] 'Hisdem etenim vir cum quodam in tempore ad Mediolanum urbem venisset, ibi quidam puerolus in extremis febrium anxietatibus positus, vitae tantum expectabat exitum; cuius parentes, audito beati Athale adventum, festino ad eum properant cursu eumque precantur, ut illis subveniat. Quod cum vir Dei dissimulare voluisset, fletibus ac terribilibus sacramentis eum conpellantur, ut prius p. 117 eat quam noxia ardor suppremas eum privet ab auras. Anxius ergo et popularis favores rumores fugiens: 'Ite', inquid, 'ego, ut potuero, vos prosequar.' Veniens ergo basilicas et sanctorum loca circuit, pro infirmo precatur, ut protinus sospitate reddatur. Deinde, ut promisse fidei impleret effectum, ad infirmum festinus venit; ne quis largitori muneris praeco existeret, domum latenter ingressus, infirmum adtigit, moxque virtus divina sanctis precibus favens sospitati pristinae egrum reddit. Grates simul parentes conditori referunt, qui sic suorum ad petitiones famulorum pietatis suae accommodat aures.' *Vita Columbani*, ch. 4, pp. 116–17.

[126] 'Cumque progressus inde coeptum iter perageret, quendam fratrem Agilum nomine, qui modo Resbacensis coenubii praesul existit, vehemens febrium ignis p. 123 coxit. Quem Eusthasius adtigit interventuque orationum sanavit ac pristinae statim sospitati reddidit. Deinde pervenit ad supradictum coenubium; ibi tam plebem interius quam vicinos populos ad christianum vigorem excitare studet multosque eorum ad paenitentiae medicamenta pertraxit.' *Vitae Columbani*, II, ch. 8, pp. 122–23.

[127] 'Appennina attigimus rura et propter castrum cui Bismantum nomen est venissemus, tanta vis febrium Bertulfum oppressit, ut omnino morte praeveniri crederetur. Aeger enim ab Urbe progressus fuerat. Oppresserat omnes maestitia tam longevi itineris quam labor aegri patris, nec prorsus eius de sospitate spem habentes, tenso tentorio, aspera in loca, undique vallati maestitia nec omnino de sospitate paterna fidentes, metati sumus. Erat enim vigilia passionis beatorum Petri et Pauli apostolorum. Cumque iam atra nox inruerit, ille inter ignes febrium me arcessivit ac curis mens dedita de nocturna vigilia sciscitavit [...] Cumque ergo cuncta silentia operissent, beatus apostolorum princeps Petrus advenit ac super stratum aegri patris adstetit: "Surge", inquid, "et sospes tuos ad sodales perge."' *Vita Columbani*, pp. 145–46.

North of the Alps were also depicted by Jonas as suffering from fevers.[128] Living in close proximity to each other, infectious diseases are likely to have been common in early medieval monasteries, and a fever is often one of the most common (and visible) signs of illness. However, similar phrases are used repeatedly by Jonas, raising the possibility that he is using the term 'fever' to denote illness in general — he never, unlike contemporary medical texts, denotes the type of fever e.g. quartan, tertian, that they might be suffering from.

Jonas's aim, therefore, is to demonstrate, through the motif of the curing of fevers, that all the monasteries founded by Columbanus — and the monks and nuns who lived in them — were holy, and patterning themselves on their founder's example. Jonas's writings therefore do not provide direct evidence of a cult of healing specifically at Bobbio — pilgrims may have been principally attracted to the monastery as a shrine to a great monastic founder.

Conclusion

Depictions of sickness and holy healing in Northern Italian texts, therefore, were invariably bound up with the very earthly concerns of ownership and rights. There is no doubt that shrines were visited in the hope of a cure, churches built and donations made in gratitude. However, we must also take seriously, in the light of the Northern Italian evidence, Peregrine Horden's suggestion that healing at a shrine was an option only taken up by a minority.[129] Repeated references in the hagiographic texts to the care of the sick in the home are, I argue, too numerous and varied simply to be discussed as biblical homage. They are undoubtedly influenced by biblical *topoi*, but also surely point to the true centre of gravity for the *locus* of the home in which most people experienced illness, and, if they were lucky, healing, by whatever means.[130] It is a truism, though, that things are found most often when they are not sought: did healing take place in hostels (*xenodochia*) even if it was not the primary aim of either these institutions or their guests? This, together with those healers who were not sanctioned by the ecclesiastical authorities, is the subject of chapter five.

[128] Gibitrudis and Ercantrudis: *Vita Columbani*, pp. 131–33.

[129] Horden, 'Sickness and Healing', p. 2.

[130] On the importance of 'self-help' or 'home healing' see Horden, 'Sickness and Healing', p. 2.

Chapter 5

The Age of Anxiety? Homes, Hostels, and Unsanctioned Healers

While saints' shrines may have not been the first port of call for the majority of the sick in early medieval Northern Italy, they did at least — from an ecclesiastical point of view — have the advantage of being in full sight of the clergy, and little mention is made of the unregulated shrines that could be a problem elsewhere in Europe.[1] Early medieval households, however, while by no means private spaces in the sense we would understand it, nevertheless could potentially be a more difficult arena for the clergy to successfully intervene in.[2] The home was a space or concept about which early medieval Italian writers and compilers felt highly ambivalent. It was where both miraculous saintly cures and proscribed rituals with chants and bundles of herbs could take place.[3] It was also simultaneously the potential 'consulting room' for soothsayers and witches and the *locus* of family care for the sick and disabled. The home therefore remains the true Cinderella location for healing,

[1] On failed and unregulated shrines in medieval Europe, see B. Ward, *Miracles and the Medieval Mind: Theory, Record and Event 1000–1215* (London, 1982).

[2] For an overview of the very large body of work on this subject, see Beattie and others, *The Medieval Household*.

[3] The recitation of charms while picking or using herbs has a long, pre-Christian history in Italy, and is by no means restricted just to the home or lay/lower status users — see L. T. Olsan, 'Charms and Prayers in Medieval Medical Theory and Practice', *Social History of Medicine*, 16.3 (2003), 343–66 (p. 359).

rarely discussed by early medieval historians of medicine, despite the fact that it was almost certainly where the vast majority of treatment and healing took place throughout the Middle Ages and beyond.[4] Indeed, much of the discussion in Part I on lawcodes and medical recipes, which include magico-medical material, and occupational injuries, could as easily have been included in this chapter.

Concern about unregulated, 'dodgy' healers might be an expected response from both secular and ecclesiastical legislators, but there was also considerable anxiety about hostels, *xenodochia*, themselves often converted houses founded by laymen. They were founded and endowed invariably for the sake of the fate of the souls of either deceased relatives or the founders themselves. However, their foundations were at risk of being plundered, misused, or simply neglected by their nearest and dearest. They were also, if the evidence of the Carolingian capitularies is to be believed, often failing in their duty to provide practical assistance to pilgrims and the poor, let alone physical or spiritual improvement.

What healing in the home and hostel care also have in common, apart from their domestic origins, is that we are reliant predominantly on legal sources — secular and ecclesiastic — for almost all our information. One type of text in particular, the penitential, detailing potential sins of the faithful and appropriate punishment, was itself a concern for the ecclesiastical authorities if not an approved work: sexual misdemeanours and 'dark' practices required careful handling.[5] Approved or not, these sources shaped how unsanctioned healing and healers were defined and perceived.

Penitentials as a Source for Early Medieval Medicine

Although rarely considered alongside the secular legal codes, which I discussed in chapter one, Christian bishops in the early medieval period also sought dominion over the populace's moral infractions through the distribution and use — by bishops, monks, and priests alike — of penitentials.[6] It is also surely sig-

[4] See Horden, 'Sickness and Healing', pp. 416–32 (p. 416). For a recent example of how such activities can be analysed, see M. Cabré, 'Women or Healers? Household Practices and the Categories of Health Care in Late Medieval Iberia', *Bulletin of the History of Medicine*, 82.1 (2008), 18–51. I am grateful to Monica Green for this reference.

[5] On concerns about penitentials see R. Pierce (later R. McKitterick), 'The "Frankish" Penitentials', in *The Materials, Sources and Methods of Ecclesiastical History: Papers Read at the Twelfth Summer Meeting and the Thirteenth Winter Meeting of the Ecclesiastical History Society*, ed. by D. Baker (Oxford, 1975), pp. 31–39 (pp. 32–33).

[6] For the debate on precisely how, and by whom, early medieval penitentials were used, see R. Meens, 'The Frequency and Nature of Early Medieval Penance', in *Handling Sin: Confession*

nificant that secular law codes and penitential literature were sometimes transmitted together.[7] These handbooks detailed sins ranging from assault to abortion and listed the commensurate periods and types of penance to atone them.

There has been much debate about who exactly used these guides. Some contemporaries felt that they should be abolished altogether as uncanonical, but they continued to be written, copied, and revised regardless of any church Council decrees.[8] Originally it was assumed that were used by priests but that not all the provisions necessarily reflected common contemporary practice.[9] Kerff then argued that they were principally used by bishops at synodal inquisitions.[10] However, both Rob Meens and Sarah Hamilton have demonstrated that penitentials were used in many contexts, from the monastic or ascetic setting to practical pastoral use by priests and bishops. The key to determining this, for Hamilton and Meens, is to consult as large a number of surviving penitential manuscripts as possible, and to then analyse manuscript content, layout, any annotations or adaptations and so on to provide clues as to their uses and intended audiences.[11] Several different versions of penitentials copied in Northern Italy in the early Middle Ages survive, indicating both a lively inter-

in the Middle Ages, ed. by P. Biller and A. J. Minnis (York, 1998), pp. 35–61; R. Meens, 'Penitentials and the Practice of Penance in the Tenth and Eleventh Centuries', *Early Medieval Europe*, 14.1 (2006), 7–21, and S. Hamilton, *The Practice of Penance, 900–1050* (Woodbridge, 2001), especially p. 22. See also R. Kottje, 'Busspraxis und Bussritus', in *Segni e riti nella chiesa altomedievale occidentale*, Settimane di studio del Centro Italiano di Studi sull'Alto Medioevo, 33 (Spoleto, 1987), pp. 369–403. For selected translations of the penitentials see J. T. McNeill, and H. M. Gamer, eds, *Medieval Handbooks of Penance: A Translation of the Principal Libri Poenitentiales and Selections from Related Documents* (New York, 1938).

[7] See, for example, München, Bayerische Staatsbibliothek, Codices Latini Monacenses 3853, second half of the tenth century — provenance unclear — which includes part of the *Lex vaicariorum*, *Lex alamannorum*, and Halitgar, Bede-egbert double penitential, Hrabanus Penitential; cited in R. Kottje, *Die Bussbücher Halitgars von Cambrai und des Hrabanus Maurus: ihre Überlieferung und ihre Quellen* (Berlin, 1980), p. 38. Halitgar, *De Ordine Peonitentium*, in *Patrologiae cursus completus: series latina*, ed. by J.-P. Migne, CV (1851), cols 649–710.

[8] P. Payer, *Sex and the Penitentials: The Development of a Sexual Code 500–1150* (Toronto, 1984), p. 9.

[9] Payer, *Sex and the Penitentials*, p. 119.

[10] F. Kerff, 'Mittelalterliche Quellen und mittelalterliche Wirklichkeit: zu den Konsequenzen einer jüngst erschienenen Edition für unser Bild kirchlicher Reformbemühungen', *Rheinische Vierteljarhsblätter*, 51 (1987), 275–86.

[11] Meens, 'The Frequency', pp. 35–61, especially at pp. 41–46; Hamilton, *Practice*, especially pp. 45–52.

est in, and adaptation of, these texts and other works of canon law.[12] The main penitential texts themselves, however, which have survived in Northern Italian manuscripts originate from Francia or Anglo-Saxon England or Ireland. Those copied in Northern Italy include the Merseburg penitential and, from the ninth and tenth centuries respectively, Halitgar's and the Vallicelliana.[13] Since early medieval episcopal councils rail against anonymous, 'unauthorized' penitentials, the surviving manuscript record almost certainly gives us a somewhat curtailed, perhaps even sanitized version of early medieval penitential literature, and some of these anonymous penitentials may have been Northern Italian in origin. Many of these, I suspect, though, may have themselves been compilations and adaptations based on existing models. The fact that the principal penitentials in use in northern Italy in this period were not written there, however, does not completely negate their usefulness as a source. Parchment was too expensive for copying on a mere whim or for all but the wealthiest of institutions to commission a manuscript simply to look pretty or be stored in a chest.

Further, the surviving manuscripts include many different combinations of texts, which suggest that they were carefully tailored to the needs of the communities or individuals for which they were designed. Their content is therefore relevant for early medieval Northern Italy, whatever the ultimate origin of some of the texts themselves. It was the many 'unnatural' practices the penitentials described which could make them potentially dangerous literature to have

[12] See Meens, 'The Frequency', pp. 41–61; Kottje, *Die Bussbücher*, pp. 16–76; Kottje, *Paenitentialia minora*, xxv–xxxiii; G. Hägele, *Das Paenitentiale Vallicellianum, I: Ein oberitalienischer Zweig der frühmittelalterlichen kontinentalen Bussbücher: Überlieferung, Verbreitung und Quellen* (Sigmaringen, 1984), especially at p. 93; L. Körntgen, 'Ein italienisches Bussbuch und seine fränkischen Quellen: das anonyme Paenitentiale der Handschrift Vatikan Archiv. S. Pietro H. 58', in *Aus Archiven und Bibliotheken: Festschrift für Raymund Kottje zum 65. Geburtstag*, ed. by H. Mordek (Frankfurt, 1992), pp. 189–205. Northern Italian manuscripts of Halitgar's penitential include: Berlin, Deutsche Staatsbibliothek, Hamilton 290, second half of the tenth century; Novara, Biblioteca Capitolare, 18 (LXXI), mid–third quarter of the ninth century; Oxford, Bodleian Library, 516 (2570), third quarter of the ninth century; Città del Vaticano, Biblioteca Apostolica Vaticana, MS Vaticani latini 5751, end of the ninth century; Vercelli, Biblioteca Capitolare, CXLIII (159), second half tenth century; Verona, Biblioteca Capitolare, LXIII (61), mid-tenth century; Paris, Bibliothèque nationale de France, Fonds nouvelle acquisition latin 281 (folios 92–94, 99–101, 110, 119) tenth/eleventh century; Barcelona, Biblioteca de la Universidad, 228, second half of the tenth century; Merseburge, Dombibliothek, 103, first half of the eleventh century; Milano, Biblioteca Ambrosiana, L 28 sup, last third of the ninth century. These are listed in Meens, 'The Frequency'.

[13] See above, n. 6.

in naive hands: too much detail could 'put ideas in people's heads', yet too little would not allow the 'crime' to be suitably atoned.

Interestingly, similar concerns did not seem to be raised for the secular law codes, even though they dealt with many of the same phenomena, albeit in sometimes different language: witches, abortion, and magic. It could be argued that penitentials and secular lawcodes were aimed at very different audiences, yet the fact that they were sometimes copied together contradicts this hypothesis. One explanation could be that the underlying anxiety for bishops and higher clergy is not with the penitentials themselves but less well-educated members of the clergy, perhaps in isolated areas, who might struggle with the boundaries between orthodoxy, heresy, and magic. As I shall show, the secular law codes show that local attitudes to so-called 'witches' might not have been as hard line as law makers would have wished.

Magical Practices, Unsanctioned Healers, and the Home

Many historians have sought to define the term magic.[14] For the purposes of this discussion, I shall use Henry Maguire's definition: 'unsanctioned dealings with supernatural forces that stood outside of the official practices of church and state'.[15]

This definition has the advantage of being both wide ranging and value neutral: as we will see, though, even within one genre or one king's law codes, writers and compilers themselves could have multiple and often inconsistent views and definitions. Further, by its very nature, the 'unsanctioned' supernatural was intimately bound up with views on, and definitions of, what constituted 'orthodox' Christian belief and practice. This too could easily shift, albeit perhaps subtly, between regions and time periods. The figure of the witch or sorcerer, in particular, has been rich in rhetorical significance in textual and figurative sources throughout history. This means that their frequent appearance in early medieval sources may tell us more about what rulers and/or communities feared rather than giving us any realistic idea of the role(s) and methods of healers outside of the church or the medical elite. However, if something is

[14] See, for example, the discussion in K. Jolly, *Popular Religion in Late Saxon England: Elf Charms in Context* (London, 1996), pp. 96–102; R. Kieckhefer, *Magic in the Middle Ages* (Cambridge, 2000), pp. 8–16. Valerie Flint, in her book *Rise of Magic*, defines magic as 'the exercise of a preternatural control over nature by human beings', p. 3.

[15] H. Maguire, 'Magic and Money in the Early Middle Ages', *Speculum*, 74.4 (1997), 1037–54 (p. 1037).

purely a literary construct, it arguably has a unity, smoothness, or 'sameness' that is often lacking when writers are struggling to mould or mesh the messiness of reality to an ideal or established *topos*. The best we can therefore hope for is to sometimes glimpse possible practices in the 'gaps' between inconsistent representations.

What is clear is that from an early date, Christian leaders and writers identified the home as a *locus* for the performance of these 'unsanctioned dealings': in the fourth century John Chrystomum was particularly exercised by mothers and nurses marking children's foreheads with mud or attaching bells to their arms to protect them from harm or death.[16] John's concern, though, was as much with women as with the potentially unregulated space of the household, and women were frequently identified with magical practices in both literary and legal sources in the early Middle Ages.[17] This may not simply be a literary trope. Female graves in Northern Europe have been found which contain possibly 'magical' items such as rings, herbs, or cloth scraps, enclosed in small boxes.[18] However, in an Italian context, what might more neutrally be termed 'ritual' objects such as bird talons or dog and toad skeletons have been found associated with child burials at a fifth-century site at Teverina, Central Italy.[19] Soren and Soren argue that the burials may be a result of malaria and that the finds suggest the use of 'black magic and witchcraft' to protect the living.[20] Pliny's *Natural History* mentions the use of toads to ward off various diseases, including fevers.[21] Certainly the objects may have been one means for the community — who were not necessarily pagan — to attempt to protect themselves from disease.[22] Of course we have no way of knowing the circumstances in which these animal parts were buried: was it the parents, and/or a local wisewoman (or man), or even other community members, who insisted on including these items for burial? Protective symbols in the fabric of a late antique villa have also been found in the course of excavations in what is now Albania, facing

[16] Cited in Maguire, 'Magic and Money', p. 1038.

[17] Riché, *Daily Life*, p. 184; McNeill and Gamer, *Medieval Handbooks of Penance*, p. 42.

[18] A. Meaney, 'Women, Witchcraft and Magic in Anglo-Saxon England', *in Superstition and Popular Medicine in Anglo-Saxon England*, ed. by D. Scragg (Manchester, 1989) pp. 9–40 (pp. 9–12, 29–30). See also, L. M. C. Weston, 'Women's Medicine, Women's Magic: The Old English Metrical Childbirth Charms', *Modern Philology*, 92.3 (1995), 279–93.

[19] Soren and Soren, *A Roman Villa*, p. 463.

[20] Soren and Soren, *A Roman Villa*, p. 517.

[21] Pliny, *Historia Naturalis* XXII, 49, cited in Soren and Soren, *A Roman Villa*, p. 517.

[22] See Christie, *From Constantine*, pp. 112–13.

the Italian peninsula.[23] As many commentators have pointed out, it would be a mistake, though, to separate such practices from learned medicine or elite practitioners: examples abound throughout the Middle Ages of medical authors, from Alexander of Tralles to Gilbertus Anglicus, including charms and other supernatural remedies, in their work. How though, did female practitioners in particular become associated with unregulated and magical practices?

In the Roman Empire, there was a bewildering array of what might be termed health practitioners — male and female — in the broadest sense. Apart from the elite, the *medici* (including some female *medicae* although their precise role is disputed), there were also *chirurgi* (surgeons), specialists such as *auricularii* (ear doctors), *pharmacopiae* (potion sellers), *maiai* and *obstetrices* (midwives), *atraliptae* (medical attendants), *rhizotmoi* and *herbarii* (root cutters, herbalists), *gymnastai*, *magi* (magic-workers), *mathematici* (astrologers), and *aniles* (wise women).[24]

The biggest change between the Classical and early medieval period, however, is that, throughout the West, the diverse Classical associated health practitioners such as the root gatherers or even midwives become shadowy bit-part players in much of the written record, leaving only the term *medicus* and scattered references to witches, storm-raisers, wisewomen, and herb-gatherers in law codes, penitentials, and literary sources, the precise interpretation and significance of which, as I shall show, is complex.[25] Have such practitioners simply

[23] J. Mitchell, 'Keeping the Demons out of the House: The Archaeology of Apotropaic Strategy and Practice in Late Antique Butrint and Antigoneia', in *Objects in Context, Objects in Use: Material Spatiality in Late Antiquity*, ed. by L. Lavan, E. Swift, and T. Putzeys (Leiden, 2007), pp. 273–310. I am grateful to Peregrine Horden for this reference.

[24] R. Flemming, *Medicine and the Making of Roman Women: Gender, Nature and Authority from Celsus to Galen* (Oxford, 2000), pp. 33, 38, 44, and for the debate concerning the status and role of the female *medica* see p. 36. On Roman medicine in general see Nutton, *Ancient Medicine*; Cruse, *Roman Medicine*. See also V. Nutton, 'Archiatri and the Medical Profession in Antiquity', *Papers of the British School at Rome*, 45 (1977), 191–226 (repr. in V. Nutton, *From Democedes to Harvey: Studies in the Social History of Medicine* (London, 1988)).

[25] See, for example, Gregory of Tours' use of the term '(h)arioli' in *The Miracles of St Martin*, I, 26, '[...] ut mos rusticorum habet, a sortilegis et ariolis ligamenta ei et potiones deferebant', cited in MacKinney, *Early Medieval Medicine*, p. 71, or the use of the term 'masca' (witch) in the Lombard law codes. Gregory the Great writes to Archbishop Ianuarius of Caralis, Sardinia, Ep. IX, 204, in 599 that 'We vehemently exhort your fraternity to maintain your pastoral vigilance against idol-worshippers and soothsayers and magicians; to preach publicly among the people against the men who do such things.' Cited in Christie, *From Constantine*, p. 73. See also *Paenitentialia minora*, ed. by Kottje, Merseburgense A, p. 132, lines 13–19, 28: 'Si quis ariolus fuerit vel aliquas divinationes fecerit, V annos peniteat, III in pane et aqua.' Kottje, *Die*

become symbolic echoes of either the lost Roman Empire in the West or, in the case of diviners and storm-raisers, superstitious and semi-pagan practices? Or rather do they represent an ongoing reality in early medieval Europe? We know from the evidence of herbal recipes and monastic writings and plans that herbs continued to play a central role in early medieval medical practice, and some births would have continued to need experienced intervention, so the need for such services did not disappear with the fall of the Roman Empire. We can therefore safely discount a mass retirement of associated medical practitioners when Augustus Romulus was himself 'retired' as emperor in 476.

Even so, it can be argued that the shrinking of the Classical plethora of medical practitioners in the contemporary sources does point to a weakening of the occupational identities of these groups in the early medieval ages with a more 'part-time' approach to these roles.[26] This has already been identified as a key problem in particular for female medical practitioners in the early modern period (*c.* 1500–1800) in Western Europe, but its roots, I suggest, lay many centuries earlier, and also apply to lower status males involved in medical care.[27] In practice, this 'weakening of occupational identity' means, for example, that a local woman experienced in assisting at births in her community might also play a role in her family's business, for example, and therefore not term herself, or indeed be termed by others, as a *obstetrix* even though she effectively functioned as such. However, again the surviving evidence must surely play a role, as women, while participating in legal transactions, are much less numerous than men in early medieval Italian charters, for example.

The choice of location for healing could also affect the visibility of practitioners. As I shall discuss in chapter six, even elite doctors rarely appear in the surviving evidence in the direct context of their medical practice. Therefore, where exactly *medici* were undertaking patient consultations is never stated. However, the assumption in the Lombard laws is that the *medicus* is brought to the patient, wherever they might be, rather than *vice versa*.[28] We might therefore surmise that 'home visits' were the norm for early medieval *medici*. Similarly,

Bussbücher, p. 267; Ex concilio Bracarense (fol. 82r); McNeill and Gamer, *Medieval Handbooks of Penance*, p. 41. On the use of penitentials, see Meens, 'The Frequency'; Hamilton, *Practice*; Hägele, *Das Paenitentiale Vallicellianum I.*; Cosentino, 'La figura del medicus'.

[26] Horden, 'Sickness and Healing', especially at pp. 422–23.

[27] See, for example, S. Mendelson and P. Crawford, *Women in Early Modern England 1550–1720* (Oxford, 1998), pp. 301–27.

[28] See chapter six.

an ancient provision was included in Justinian's *Digest* whereby midwives were summoned to the house to ascertain whether or not a woman was pregnant.[29] Particularly in the case of labour we have no reason to suppose women, whether in the Classical or early medieval period, regularly gave birth outside of their own home.[30]

However, in the case of other types of practitioners such as wisewomen, storm-raisers, and those involved in predicting the future, it would appear that customers sought them out in their homes/places of work, rather than the other way round. In Liutprand's laws issued in the fifteenth year of his reign (727 AD) it was decreed that:

> He who, unmindful of the wrath of God, goes to sorcerers or witches for the purpose of receiving divinations or answers of any kind whatsoever from them, shall pay to the royal fisc as composition half of the price at which he would have been valued if someone had killed him, and in addition, shall do penance according to the established canon [...] Moreover, he who sends his man or woman slave to such sorcerers or witches for the purpose of seeking responses from them, and it is proved, shall pay composition as abovementioned. If indeed the man or woman slave goes to the soothsayer or witch without the consent of his or her lord and so without his authority, likewise for the purpose of seeking responses, then his or her lord ought to sell him or her outside the province. And if his or her lord neglects to do this, he [the lord] shall be subjected to the punishment noted above.[31]

[29] The Examination of pregnant women and the observation of delivery, Justinian, *Digest*, Book 25, 4, 1: In the time of the deified brothers, a husband said his wife was pregnant, but the wife denied it (already divorced). The deified brothers replied 'it will be best for the house of an extremely respectable woman to be chosen into which Domitia will go, and that three skilled trustworthy midwives selected by you examine her.

[30] M. Green, 'Bodies, Gender, Health, Disease: Recent Work on Medieval Women's Medicine', *Studies in Medieval and Renaissance History*, 3.2 (2005), 1–46. See also Cabrè, 'Women or Healers?'.

[31] 'Si quis timoris Dei immemor ad ariolus aut ad ariolas pro aruspiciis aut qualibuscumque responsis ab ipsis accipiendis ambolaverit conponat in sagro palatio medietatem pretii sui, sicut adpretiatus fuerit, tamquam si eum aliquis occisissit et insuper agat penitentiam secundum canonum instituta. Simili modo et qui ad arbore quam rustici sanctivum vocant atque ad fontanas adoraverit aut sagrilegium vel incantationis fecerit similiter mediaetatem pretii sui conponat in sagro palatio Et si quicumque sciens ariolum aut ariolam, non eos manefestaverit, aut illos celaverit, qui ad ipsos vadent et non manefestaverit, supra scriptae poene subiaceat. Qui autem servum suum aut ancillam ad ipsos ariolus aut ariolas transmiserit ad aliqua responsa ab eis recipienda, et provatum fuerit, suprascripta poenam conponat. Si vero servus aut ancilla sine volontate dominorum suorum, et tantum ex sua auctoritatem ad ariolum aut ariola ambolaverit, similiter ad aliqua responsa accipienda, tunc dominus eorum venundare eos deveat foris

Other related practices, however, such as the recitation of charms and incantations before gathering a herb or taking a remedy, could take place in an individual's own home and garden.[32] Did it really matter though, who said charms, and where? The kind of practices that so disturbed John Chrystomum, or the placing of objects in a grave, did not necessarily have to be carried out by what might be termed a specialist of the supernatural. Nevertheless, the legal and literary sources both name numerous types of practitioners. For example, while no one is likely to sign themselves as a witch or even wisewoman in a charter, they appear repeatedly in the legal codes, an indication that they were symbolically important whatever the reality on the ground might have been.[33] Patricia Skinner argues that the references to witches (*mascae/strigae*) in both Rothari's mid-seventh-century Lombard law code and the supplementary code in the eighth century by Liutprand demonstrate a tenacious belief in witches by the general population — but not necessarily the rulers themselves — despite Christianization.[34] Rothari even tries to dissuade attacks on servile female *mascae*, brushing aside the belief that 'a woman (can) [...] eat a living man from within'.[35] This may seem to have little to do with healing.

However, what was a 'witch' in the terms of the legal code? Obviously from this particular law it was believed they could harm or kill enemies. However, in the same law code is an intriguing clause concerning duels and 'witch's herbs':

> When a man participates in a duel, he may not have upon himself witch's herbs or like things. [...] If it is suspected that a man carries such prohibited things secretly, they shall be searched for by the judge and if they are found on him, they shall be torn out and cast aside.[36]

provincia. Et si neglexerit dominus eorum hoc facere, suprascriptae poenae subiaceat.' *Leges Luitprandi*, Bluhme, 84. I, pp. 141–42.

[32] On charms see L. T. Olsan, 'Charms and Prayers in Medieval Medical Theory and Practice', *Social History of Medicine*, 16.3 (2003), 343–66.

[33] On witchcraft and the Lombard legal code see Skinner, *Women*, p. 42.

[34] Skinner, *Women*, p. 42.

[35] 'Nullus presumat haldiam alienam aut ancillam quasi strigam, quem dicunt mascam, occidere; quod christianis mentibus nullatenus credendum est, nec possibilem ut mulier hominem vivum intrinsecus possit comedere.' *Edictus Rothari*, Bluhme and Boretius, ch. 376, p. 87; trans. by Drew, *Lombard Laws*, p. 127. On cannibalistic witches in other law codes see V. Flint, *The Rise of Magic in Early Medieval Europe* (Princeton, 1991), p. 291, cited in Skinner, *Women*, p. 42, n. 17.

[36] 'Nullus camphio praesumat, quando ad pugnando contra alium vadit, herbas quod ad maleficias pertenit, super se habere, nec alias tales similes res, nisi tantum arma sua, quae

What the 'like things' might have been we can only guess: perhaps animal parts or scraps of cloth similar to items found in the graves discussed above? Whatever they might be, they are not dismissed as mere superstition, but something that could give an opponent a significant and unfair advantage. Clearly in this case herbs are intended to act as a protective charm and/or harm the duellist's opponent.[37] From this, however, it is arguably only a short step for *mascae* to provide remedies for physical ailments, since knowledge of herbs — which can protect, which can heal — is implied in this clause. In Alamannic law this connection is perhaps a little more explicit, since the term 'herbaria' is used alongside 'stri(g)a'.[38] This role, however, would not be without its risks, since knowledge of herbs includes those that can kill as well as heal, and if a remedy fails to work, or something unexplained happens in the community, the 'wisewoman' could rapidly metamorphosize in the community's eyes into the vampiric 'masca' of Rothari's law code. It would also appear that accusations of witchcraft could be made for monetary gain or personal animosity: Rothari's edict also deals with guardianship issues where a free girl or woman has been unjustly accused of being a witch (*striga*) by her own guardian.[39]

However, a law issued by Liutprand in 727 suggests that local officials may often have been less than assiduous in seeking out sorcerers or witches, raising the possibility that they were an accepted part of the community as long as they were not perceived as doing harm. The motivation for protecting witches, though (however they were defined), would appear to be complex:

> And if it becomes clear that the judge or the schultheis or the forester or the deganus of the place where those sorcerers or witches are found has not condemned them or has taken a bribe or has absolved them as if for piety or any other reason, then he shall pay his entire wergeld as composition to the sacred palace.[40]

convenit. Et si suspicio fuerit, quod eas occulte habeat, inquiratur ad iudicem, et si inventa super eum fuerit, evellantur et iactentur.' *Edictus Rothari*, Bluhme and Boretius, ch. 368, p. 85; Drew, *Lombard Laws*, p. 125.

[37] On protective charms see Kieckhefer, *Magic*, pp. 75–80.

[38] 'Si femina aliam stria aut erbaria clamaverit sine rixam, sine absente hoc dixit, solvate solidos 12.' *Leges Alamannorum*, ed. by K. Lehmann, MGH Leges Nationum Germanicarum, 5.1 (Hannover, 1888), Fragmentum II, 31, p. 23. See also the definition of 'herbaria' in A. Souter, *A Glossary*, p. 172.

[39] *Edictus Rothari*, Bluhme and Boretius, ch. 127, p. 30; Drew, *Lombard Laws*, p. 90. See also Riché, *Daily Life*, p. 184 for politically motivated accusations of witchcraft.

[40] 'Et si manefestatum fuerit, quod sciat iudex aut sculdahis vel saltarius aut deganus, ubi ipsi arioli aut ariolas sunt, et eos non condemnaverit aut premium tolerit, aut quasi causa

There was obviously money to be made out of those considered witches or sorcerers for avaricious local officials. More puzzling is the phase 'has absolved them as if for piety'. Does this mean they forgave them as a Christian duty, or, rather, considered them as if not a quasi-saint, then at least as an important (and valuable) member of the local community? If they used Christian incantations, for example, when picking or administering herbs, the lines between 'healer' and 'witch', not to mention 'pagan superstition' and 'Christian practice' were perhaps more blurred than the Lombard lawcode compilers would have had us believe.

There is also, significantly, a mismatch between the terms in the Lombard laws (*masca* and *striga* for witch/enchantress) and those used in the penitentials and other literary texts. In penitential texts themselves the most frequently used terms are for *aruspices* and *(h)arioli*, soothsayers or fortune tellers, although Souter translates *hariolus* as mountebank (quack).[41] Although a fortune teller is not a healer per se, we can assume that at least some of the questions people had were about health and the progress of an illness or condition, whether their own or a friend or relative's. They therefore should be included in any discussion of supernatural forms of healing. Unlike *masca* or *striga*, in the penitentials the masculine forms of *haruspex* and *hariolus* tend to be used. These terms were in use at least from the Classical period as they were recorded in the works of Pliny and Cicero: they therefore have ancient (and pagan) overtones as well.[42] Having said that, Charlemagne's 789 *Admonitio Generalis* highlights the biblical injunctions against fortune telling.[43] The terms *haruspex* and *hariolus* were widely used in the early Middle Ages: as well as penitential texts they can also, as mentioned above, be found in the work of Gregory of Tours.

Yet, despite the divergent terminology between the Lombard/Alamannic lawcodes and the penitentials/Church councils, there are hints that these different genres of texts may not be discussing completely culturally or linguis-

piaetatis vel pro qualicumque genio eos absolserit: tunc integro wirgild suo in sagro palatio conponat.' *Leges Liutprandi*, Bluhme, 727, 85. II, p. 142; Drew, *Lombard Laws*, p. 181.

[41] Souter, *A Glossary*, p. 169.

[42] Lewis and Short, *A Latin Dictionary*: haruspex = 'a soothsayer, diviner, inspector of the entrails of victims'; hariolus = 'a soothsayer, prophet'.

[43] 'Item habemus in lego Domini mandatum: "non auguriamini"; et in deuteronomio: "nemo sit qui ariolos sciscitetur vel observet vel ad auguria intendat"; item: "ut sit maleficus non incantatore nec ithones consolatur". Ideo praecipimus, ut cauculatores nec incantotores nec tempestarii vel obligatores non fiunt; et ubicumque sunt, emendentur vel damnentur.' *Capitularia regum Francorum*, I, 65, pp. 58–59.

tically specific phenomena. In the penitentials, more often than naming the occupation of an individual, they usefully tend to describe proscribed behaviour. For example, in the Merseburg Penitential, one section discusses those 'who make amulets (literally bundles, *ligatura*) from herbs': their rituals also included Christian chants.[44] Who is saying the charm, though: a relative or a wisewoman?

The bundle of herbs, however, also recalls the would-be duellists in Lombard law, discussed above, who were allegedly hiding herb amulets in their clothes before combat. Further, reference to love (and possibly by implication fertility) potions are made in both penitentials copied in Northern Italy and Carolingian penitentials.[45] In the case of the love potions, it is specified that 'women' make them themselves: it is unclear for the herb amulets whether a *masca*/*striga* is implied as the original maker or not. Clearly, the penitential compilers, like John Chrystomum, disapproved and perhaps also feared what they would term the superstitious practices of mothers as much as wisewomen or soothsayers. The early medieval penitentials repeatedly include an injunction from Theodore's Anglo-Saxon penitential against mothers placing their children on top of a roof or oven to heal them. Even if it was a practice in Northern Italy too, was it essentially a naturalistic cure in an attempt to 'sweat out' a fever or restore humoral balance, or was it a ritual to appeal for supernatural aid (from whatever source)?[46] We are on safer ground with the bundles of amuletic herbs, since they appear in different textual contexts. What we do not know is if 'witches',

[44] 'Si quis ligaturas fecerit per herbas vel qualicunque ingenio incantauerit et super christianum ligauverit, sciat se fidem Christi amisisse, III annos peniteat, I ex his in pane et aqua.' Kottje, *Paenitentialia Minora*, ch. 41, lines 472–81; ch. 36, lines 472–81, p. 136.

[45] 'Quia pestiferas adhuc stirpes et reliquias artis magicae in tantum vigere ad nos perlatum est, ut quaedam maleficae inlicitum amorem aliorum mentibus, aliis vero odium inmittere dicantur, quaedam etiam ita venerariae sunt, ut quosdam peremisse multo populi rumore deferantur, huiusmodi diavoli ministras diligenti examinatione proditas sub acerrima penitentia redigendas statuimus, et in ipso tantum exitu, si tamen prius dina poenitentiae opera fecerint, reconciliandas esse permittimus.' *Capitularia regum Francorum*, II, ch. 23, p. 122; 'Si qua mulier semen viri sui in cibum miscens aut inlicitas causas fecerit, ut inde plus eius amore suscipiat, III annos peneteat.' Kottje, *Paenitentialia minora*, lines 1236–42, ch. 103; ch. 92, lines 1236–42, p. 156.

[46] 'Si qua mulier infantem suum super tectum aut in furnace ponit et vult sanare eum, V annos peneteat.' Kottje, *Paenitentialia minora*, p.155 99. ME1 line 1212. In Biblioteca Apostolica Vaticana, MS Vat. lat. 5751, the clause reads: 'Si mulier infantem suum super pectum suum posuerit aut in funem super puteum propter sanitatem, V annos peniteat.' Kottje, *Paenitentialia minora*, p. 155 V23 88, lines 1212–18. 88. See R. Meens, 'Children and Confession', in *The Church and Childhood*, ed. by D. Wood (Oxford, 1994), pp. 53–65 (p. 60), cited in Hamilton, *Practice*, p. 204.

'wisewomen', and 'soothsayers' concentrated on protective charms, love potions (and possibly poisons), and foretelling the future rather than the direct healing of ailments. Even if activities were restricted to these 'spheres of influence', the unsanctioned (or liminal) supernatural would appear to have been part of peoples' everyday experience in order to prevent, if not cure, injury and illness.

Potions, Poisons, and the Control of Fertility

The making, selling, and using of poisons and potions was of great concern to both Roman and 'Barbarian' legislators alike.[47] Justinian's legal compendium discusses the selling of potentially lethal concoctions.

> Someone is punished who sells baneful potions to the public or possesses them for the purpose of homicide [...] 2. The addition of the phrase 'baneful drugs' indicates that there are certain drugs which are not baneful. The term is therefore neutral, covering as much a drug prepared for the purpose of healing as one for the purpose of killing, as also that which is called an aphrodisiac [...] It is however, regulated by *senatus consultum* that a woman who, not admittedly maliciously but inadvisably, has administered a fertility drug from which the recipient dies shall be relegated. 3. It is laid down by another *senatus consultum* that dealers in cosmetics are liable to the penalty of this law if they recklessly hand over to anyone hemlock, salamander, monkshood, pinegrubs, or a venomous beetle, mandragora, or, except for the purpose of purification, Spanish fly.[48]

This clause carefully elucidates the principle that the seller of a drug (and apart from cosmetic dealers these are not specified) is responsible for its effects, even if it was intended to heal rather than harm. However, the punishment appears to be far more severe for those who sell known poisonous substances such as

[47] M. Elsakkers, 'Reading Between the Lines: Old Germanic and Early Christian Views on Abortion' (unpublished doctoral thesis, Amsterdam University, 2010), pp. 357–65. I am grateful to Marianne for supplying me with a copy of her thesis so that I could take account of her work as I was completing final revisions on this book.

[48] 'Quinto, qui uenenum necandi hominis causa fecerit uel uendiderit uel habuerit, plectitur [...] Adiectio autem ista 'ueneni mali' ostendit esse quaedam et non mala uenena. Ergo nomen medium est et tam id, quod ad sanandum, quam id, quod ad occidendum paratum est, continent, sed et id quod amatorium appellatur [...] Sed ex senatus consulto relegari iussa est ea, quae non quidem malo animo, sed malo exemplo medicamentum ad conceptionem dedit, ex quo ea quae acceperat decesserit. Alio senatus consulto effectum est, ut pigmentarii, si cui temere cicutam salamandram aconitum pituocampus aut bubrostim mandragorum et id, quod lustramenti causa dederit cantharidas, poena teneantur huius legis.' Justinian, *Digest*, Book 48,8,3.1.

hemlock or monkshood to the public without being sure of the use to which it will be put.

The Roman law makers are therefore obviously familiar with the principal poisons, whether derived from plants or animals, in use in their day. They agree that there is a difference between poisons and drugs intended to heal, but recognize that the effects of these drugs can be similar, and that the seller bears some responsibility for deaths caused by drugs they sold. They also are dealing with a multiplicity of sellers, including those promising to improve people's sex lives or provide a much needed heir as well as those designed to kill or heal. The fact that these extracts were included in Justinian's legislation indicate that control of the drug trade was in all probability still a concern, even if the sellers and drugs were less multivalent in early medieval Italy and Byzantium than the Roman Empire at the height of its powers.

This may be reflected in the Lombard law codes, where the emphasis is on those who administer poisons rather than those who sell them. In Rothari's seventh-century edict it is decreed that:

> Whoever gives another poison in his drink and that one dies shall pay as composition a sum equal to the full wergild of the dead man in accordance with his rank [...] If a freeman or free woman gives another poison in his drink but that one does not die, he who gave the poison shall pay as composition a sum equal to half the wergild at which that one would have been valued had he been killed.[49]

This may indicate that many lay people had sufficient knowledge of poisonous plants to concoct their own recipes, and the edict suggests that poisonings were not always completely successful, as sometimes the intended victim recovered. However, in a further clause on poisoning in Rothari's *Edict* the shadow of a poison-seller can perhaps just be discerned:

> If a man or woman slave gives someone poison and that one does not die, then the slave's lord shall pay as composition a sum equal to half of the wergild at which he who got the poison is valued.[50]

[49] 'Si liber aut libera venenum alii dederit ad bivendum, et qui acceperit, ex ipso veneno mortuus non fuerit, conponat qui venenum dedit, medietatem praetii ipsius, quod adpraetiatus fuerit, si eum occidissit [...] Si quis venenum ad bivendum dederit, et qui acceperit, mortuos fuerit, praetium mortui secundum qualitatem personae in integrum conponat.' *Edictus Rothari*, Bluhme and Boretius, chs 140 and 141, p. 32; Drew, *Lombard Laws*, p. 74.

[50] 'Si servus aut ancilla venenum alicui dederit, et ille qui accepit mortuos non fuerit, conponat dominus servi vel ancillae medietatem praetii, quod ipse valuerit, qui accepit.' *Edictus Rothari*, Bluhme and Boretius, ch. 142, p. 32; Drew, *Lombard Laws*, p. 74.

No mention is made, though, of where, or from whom precisely the slave might have got the poison, and there does not seem to be a specific penalty for selling poison. Like Justinian's compilers and their Roman sources, however, Rothari and his advisors appear to have been very concerned about death by poison, perhaps because of its ease of application. This would explain why the punishment for slaves who were deemed to have administered poison are particularly harsh in the *Edict*, since many household slaves at least would presumably have had access to a master's or guest's food stores or prepared food and drink at one time or another.

What is missing from the discussion of poisoning in both Justinian's *Digest* and Rothari's *Edict*, however, is how to distinguish between poisoning and a death from natural causes. The eighth-century Lombard king Liutprand addresses this issue directly in his section 'on using poison to kill a freeman':

> In the past we and our judges decreed that he who kills a freeman shall lose all his property (Liutprand 20, 62). As a result there have been some men who sought to prove by combat — as provided by the earlier law — that one of their relatives who had suffered some illness and died in his bed was actually deliberately killed. However, it seems to us to be a very serious thing that a man should lose his entire substance as the result of a duel fought by one man. Therefore we now decree that if in the future such a case arise, he who wishes to prove by means of a duel that the death of one of his relatives was caused deliberately, then, those things having been observed which were prescribed in the earlier edict [Liutprand 71], he should take oath on the gospels that he does not press his suit with evil intent, but as the result of a definite suspicion. Then he shall have the right to prove his charge by duel, as has been provided before. If the blow falls upon that man who was charged with the crime or upon the champion whom he secured, he shall not lose all of his property but shall pay composition to [his accuser] according to the quality of the person [who had died] just as the earlier law of compositions provided. For we are uncertain concerning the judgment of God [in this matter] and we have heard that many men have unjustly lost their cause through combat; however, on account of the customs of the Lombard people we are unable to abolish this law.[51]

[51] 'Recolimus enim, quod statuimus cum nostris iudicibus, ut qui hominem liberum occiserit, omnem substantiam suam amittat. Modo vero dum repetirent singuli homenis, cui forte aliquam duritiam detenebant, quod parentis eius, qui in lectulum suum mortuos fuerat, per veninum occisissit, et dum per pugnam ipsam causam, sicut antiqua fuerat consuitudo, querere disponebat: gravis causa esse nobis conparuit, ut sub uno scuto per pugnam omnem substantiam suam homo amitterit. Ideoque statuere previdemus, ut si amodo talis causa emerserent, quis ille mortem parentis sui querere per pugnam voluerit, quod eum per veninum occisissit, observata ea, quae in anteriorem edicto scripsemus, ut per euangelia firmit, quod non asto animo causam ipsam querat, nisi quod certa ei sit suspectio: potestatem habeat querere per pugnam, sicut antea

Liutprand's concern here is not so much to determine whether someone did die of natural causes or not: he does not represent himself as having much faith in the ordeal by duel system, although this distancing of himself from this tradition may be designed to placate angry, destitute duel-losers. Certainly his adjustment to his own law seems to suggest this: limiting the compensation does not, as the clause itself states, prove guilt: it is a classic case of social compromise to identify a blame figure while allowing that figure to maintain their status and former life. No discussion of the possible signs of poisoning is included, implying that the physical symptoms are considered unknowable.

One type of 'recipe' not mentioned in the legal sources explicitly but which appears in the penitential literature is love potions or aphrodisiacs. In the anonymous Merseburg penitential, probably originally Frankish in origin and preserved in three manuscripts, two of which are from Northern Italy, it is stated that: 'if a woman mixes the semen of her man (husband) into food for illicit reasons, in order to receive more love from him, (she should do) penance for three years.'[52] This obviously does not require the services of a rootcutter or other practitioner, and would have been carried out by the woman herself.

However, another magico-medical practice which does include herbs is also included in the Merseburg penitential. The author declares that: 'whoever makes a bundle of herbs [...] and then says a charm above a Christian should do three years of penance, one on bread and water.'[53] There is no mention here

fuit consuitudo. Et si ei ferita venerit, cui crimen ipsum inmettitur aut ad camphionem ipsius, quem conductum habuit, non amittat omnem substantiam suam, sed conponat eum secundum qualitatem personae, sicut antea fuit lex conponendum. Quia incerti sumus de iudicio Dei, et multos audivimus per pugnam sine iustitia causam suam perdere; sed propter consuitutinem gentis nostrae Langobardorum legem ipsam vetare non possumus.' *Leges Liutprandi*, Bluhme, 118. II, Drew, *Lombard Laws*, pp. 195–96.

[52] 'Si qua mulier semen viri sui in cibum miscens aut inlicitas causas fecerit, ut inde plus eius amore suscipiat, III annos peneteat.' Kottje, *Paenitentialia minora*, p. 156 ME1 lines 1236–42, 103. The two Northern Italian copies of this anonymous penitential, possibly written in Francia, are: Città del Vaticano, Biblioteca Apostolica Vaticana, MS Vat. lat. 5751, possibly copied in Verona at the end of the ninth century and Merseburg, Archiv des Domkapitels, MS 103, dating from the ninth century and also of Northern Italian origin. See Kottje, *Paenitentialia minora*, pp. xxiv–xxxiv. On this clause about aphrodisiacs, see Payer, *Sex and the Penitentials*, p. 32.

[53] Città del Vaticano, Biblioteca Apostolica Vaticana, MS Vaticani latini 5751: 'si quis ligaturas fecerit per herbas vel qualicunque ingenio incantauerit et super christianum ligauverit, sciat se fidem Christi amisisse, III annos peniteat, I ex his in pane et aqua.' Merseburg, MS 103: 'si quis legatura fecerit in erbas vel qualibet ingenio malo incantaberit et super christianum ligaberit, scias eum fidem dei amisisse, III annos peneteat, I ex his in pane et aqua.' Kottje, *Paenitentialia minora*, p. 136, nos 36 and 41 respectively, lines 472–81.

of whether the person concerned collected the herbs. Nor is it made clear if the individual saying the charm is envisaged as being a relative or a local wisewoman.[54] It would be a mistake, however, to view this as a 'popular' practice in the sense of being used principally by those of lower status. Rather, it was popular in the sense that it formed part of medical practice for all types of medical practitioners, including the elite.[55]

The type of herbal recipe in penitential texts and elsewhere which has received the most attention from scholars, however, is those designed as contraceptives or abortifacients.[56] The Merseburg penitential simply states that 'if a woman has voluntarily produced an abortion, she should do penance for three years with bread and water'.[57] With this type of penance a diet of bread and water is only eaten on specific days rather than every day.[58] Presumably the word 'voluntarily' is added to distinguish from miscarriages due to natural causes.[59] However, no mention is made of by what means the abortion might be carried out, or whether anyone else is expected to have aided the woman. Perhaps to remedy this and to prevent any loopholes being found by would-be-penitents, in the version of this penitential as preserved in Città del Vaticano, Biblioteca Apostolica Vaticana, MS Vat. lat. 5751, the compiler spells out in precise terms what is meant by this: 'if a woman aborts voluntarily, that is, by whatever cause at her own hand or others, so that she does not conceive or kills the conceived (embryo), she should do penance for three years on bread and water.'[60]

In this particular manuscript the term 'aborsum' includes contraceptive measures as well as abortion of an embryo, no matter how early on in the preg-

[54] Olsan, 'Charms', pp. 343–66; Kieckhefer, *Magic*; Flint, *The Rise of Magic*.

[55] See for example Horden, 'Medicine and Healing', p. 6 on Alexander of Tralles and amulets.

[56] See in particular Riddle, *Contraception and Abortion* and its critique by Elsakkers, 'Reading Between the Lines', pp. 461–62.

[57] 'Si qua mulier aborsum fecerit voluntariae, III annos peneteat cum pane et aqua.' Kottje, *Paenitentialia minora*, p. 135, ME1, lines 445–53, no. 33. On dating, p. xxvii.

[58] Payer, *Sex and the Penitentials*.

[59] Marianne Elsakkers points out that in recipes the word 'aborsum' can be ambiguous, indicating miscarriage as well as abortion. See M. Elsakkers, 'Abortion, Poisoning, Magic and Contraception in Eckhardt's *Pactus Legis Salicae*', *Amsterdamer Beiträge zur Älteren Germanistik*, 57 (2003), 233–67; Elsakkers, 'Reading Between the Lines', pp. 461–62.

[60] 'Si quis mulier voluntarie aborsum, id est qualecunque causa sibi aut alii fecerit, ut non concipiat aut conceptos occidat, III annos in pane et aqua peniteat. Et si fornicauerit et occiderit, quod nascitur, X annos peniteat', Kottje, *Paenitentialia minora*, V23, p. 135, lines 445–56, no. 38.

nancy. However, in Classical medical literature and some secular legal codes, such as *Lex Alamannorum*, in force for Alamans in early medieval Northern Italy, an embryo is considered unformed and therefore not a human life for forty days after conception for males and ninety days for females.[61] Alamannian law also makes the distinction in terms of whether it is possible to discern the sex of the foetus or not.[62] Marianne Elsakkers suggests in relation to this passage in Alamannian law that the language used has similarities with Macrobius and possibly also Augustine's discussion of formed foetuses.[63] In Pliny the boundary is also forty days, but in Hippocratic works and Galen it is placed at three months for males, four months for females.[64] An addition to the Merseburg penitential, perhaps surprisingly, acknowledges and uses this basic concept of a boundary: 'A woman, if she kills a son in the uterus before 50 days, (should do) penance for a year, (but) if it is (more than) fifty days from conception, she (should do) penance for three years as for homicide.'[65] No explicit mention is made here of the distinction between an unformed embryo and a foetus, nor — unlike the influential late seventh-century Anglo-Saxon penitential ascribed to Theodore, for example — is the thorny issue of ensoulment discussed.[66] At the very least, however, the compiler of this addition to the Merseburg penitential is placing greater value on a foetus after fifty days than before. Perhaps this is a

[61] Niederhellmann, *Arzt*, p. 134. See also M. Elsakkers, 'The Early Medieval Latin and Vernacular Vocabulary of Abortion and Embryology', in *Science Translated: Proceedings of the Leuven Congress 2004*, ed. by M. Goyens, P. De Leuvens, and A. Smet (Turnhout, 2008), pp. 367–403. On Visigothic law and the distinction between formed and unformed foetuses and abortion see M. Elsakkers, 'Gothic Bible, Vetus Latina and Visigothic Law: Evidence for a Septuagint-based Gothic Version of Exodus', *Sacris Erudiri*, 44 (2005), 37–76 (pp. 38–41).

[62] 'Si quis aliquis mulierem prignantem (*sic*) aborsum fecerit, ita ut iam cognoscere possis, utrum vir an femina fuisset: si vir debuit esse, cum 12 solidis conponat; si autem femina, cum 24.' *Leges Alamannorum*, Merkel, p. 150, cod A LXXXVIIII 1. 'De eo, qui mulieri pregnanti abortivum fecerit. 1. Si quis mulieri pregnanti abortivum fecerit, ita ut iam cognoscere posit, utrum vir an femina fuit: si vir debuit esse, cum 12 solidis conponat; si autem femina, cum 24.' Merkel, p. 150 cod B XCL. See also Niederhellmann, *Arzt*, pp. 121–22.

[63] Elsakkers, 'Latin and Vernacular Vocabulary', p. 12.

[64] Niederhellmann, *Arzt*, p. 134. See also Elsakkers, 'Latin and Vernacular Vocabulary', pp. 3–10.

[65] 'Mulier, si occiderit filium in utero ante XL dies, annum I peneteat, si post XL dies conceptionis, ut humicida III annos peneteat.' Kottje, *Paenitentialia Minora*, p. 166, Appendix ME 1 lines 65–67, no. 164.

[66] On this point in Theodore's penitential see Elsakkers, 'Latin and Vernacular Vocabulary', p. 14.

dose of *realpolitik* on behalf of the compiler, admitting that the ecclesiastical hierarchy was fighting a losing battle to persuade everyone that all human life was the same from the moment of conception. Following late antique Church Councils most early medieval penitential literature generally makes no such distinction and some penitentials even equate herbal abortions with witchcraft.[67] However, the compiler of the Merseburg penitential, in contrast, connects abortion more prosaically with sex outside marriage. It is stated that if a woman who has fornicated aborts the infant or kills it after birth, she should do penance for ten years.[68]

The barbarian law codes make no connection between abortion and either witchcraft or fornication. Rather, they do not see abortion as a legal matter.[69] Rothari's mid-seventh-century Lombard *Edict* does use the term 'avortum' (*sic*), but in the sense of a miscarriage as a result of a blow: fines are given for causing this in cows, horses, and servants alike: 'He who strikes a woman slave large with child and causes a miscarriage shall pay three solidi as composition. If, moreover, she dies from the blow he should pay composition for her and likewise for the child who died in her womb.'[70] No distinction is made between a blow aimed specifically to end a pregnancy (in other words a means of forcing a woman to abort, or perhaps even at her instruction) and that as punishment or an attack for other reasons. Given the fact that the clauses concerning miscarriage in cows, horses, and slave women are grouped together, the central concern here is loss of potentially valuable property rather than the value or sanctity of life as such. A further section of Rothari's *Edict*, section 75, also deals with the death of a foetus in the womb. The language, however, is markedly different to those clauses dealing with slavewomen and livestock:

> If a child is accidentally killed while still in the mother's womb, and if the woman is free and lives, then her value shall be measured in accordance with her rank, and

[67] Niederhellmann, *Arzt*, p. 132, p. 135 and p. 139.

[68] 'Si qua de mulieribus, que fornicantur, occiderit, quod nascitur, aut avortiuum (*sic*) facere festinare, X annos peneteat.' Kottje, *Paenitentialia Minora*, pp. 140–41, lines 658–60.

[69] Niederhellmann, *Arzt*, p. 130.

[70] 'De ancilla praegnante. Si quis percusserit ancilla gravida et avortum fecirit. Conponat solidos tres. Si autem ex ipsa percussura mortua fuerit, conponat eam, simul et quod in utero eius mortuum est.' *Edictus Rothari*, Bluhme and Boretius, no. 334; Drew, *Lombard Laws*, p. 117. On pregnant cows and horses see nos 332–33. On similar provisions in Visigothic law see M. Elsakkers, 'Inflicting Serious Bodily Harm: The Visigothic Antiquae on Violence and Abortion', *Tijdschrift voor Rechtsgeschiedenis: The Legal History Review*, 71 (2003), 55–63.

> composition for the child shall be paid at half the sum at which the mother is valued. But if the mother dies, the composition must be paid for her according to her rank in addition to the payment of composition for the child killed in her womb. But thereafter the feud shall cease since the deed was done unintentionally.[71]

The difference in language: the phrase 'accidentally killed' ('nolende [...] occisus fuerit') is used rather than the word 'avortum' may be related to the fact that this clause relates to free rather than slave women and therefore is more delicately phrased. It is also clear that the aim of this clause, in contrast to those on miscarriage in horses, cows, and slavewomen, is to attempt to prevent, or at least limit, blood feuds (*faida*). This could explain the emphasis on the supposedly accidental nature of any miscarriage caused by a blow. In itself, however, this perhaps indicates that the woman or woman's family at least did not always consider this to be the case. Again no discussion is entered into about possible circumstances that would result in a pregnant woman being hit in the stomach, or other means of deliberate abortion.

Alamannian law also uses the term 'abortivum' in its clause on miscarriage resulting from a blow: 'If some man strikes a pregnant beast, and causes a miscarriage, so that the foal lies dead, [he should pay] one solidus in compensation.'[72] For a woman the penalty is much stiffer: 'If a woman is pregnant, and by the act of another the infant is born dead, or if he/she is born alive but does not survive nine nights [...] compensate with 40 solidi or the oaths of twelve men.'[73]

In Justinian's *Digest* Ulpian is cited on abortion. Ulpian was, like the compilers of the various versions of the Merseburg penitential, concerned to distinguish between miscarriages and deliberate abortion, but is unspecific about the

[71] 'Si infans in utero matris suae nolende ab aliquem occisus fuerit: si ipsa mulier libera est et evaserit, adpretietur ut libera secundum nobilitatem suam, et medietatem quod ipsa valuerit, infans ipse conponatur. Nam si mortuus fuerit, ponat eam secundum generositatem suam, excepto quod in utero eius mortuum fuerit, ut supra, cessante faida, eo qoud nolende fecit.' *Edictus Rothari*, Bluhme and Boretius, no. 75; Drew, *Lombard Laws*, p. 65.

[72] 'De eo, qui pregnum iumentum ferierit, et abortivum fecerit. Si autem aliquis homo ictu ferierit pregnum iumentum, et abortivum fecerit, ita ut iactet ipsum poledrum mortuum, unum solidum conponat.' *Leges Alamannorum*, Merkel, cod B LXXIII. p. 134.

[73] 'Si qua mulier gravida fuerit, et per factum alterum infans natus mortuus fuerit, aut si vivus natus fuerit et novem noces non vivit [...] 40 solidos solvate aut cum 12 medicos electos iuret, *Lex Alamannorum*, Merkel, Cod. A, LXX; Si qua mulier gravida fuerit, et per factum alterius infans natus mortuus fuerit, aut si vivus natus fuerit et octo dies non vivet, cui inputatum fuerit, 40 solidos solvate aut cum duodecim mediis electis iuret.' Cod. B, LXXVII. p. 137. Niederhellmann, *Arzt*, p. 124.

means: 'if it is proved that a woman has done violence to her womb to bring about an abortion, the provincial governor shall send her into exile.'[74]

Possibly one of the ways to discern if it was a miscarriage or abortion was to try and find the seller of the abortifacient, if indeed that was how it was carried out. This would certainly fit with the preoccupation in the Justinian *Digest* with the sellers of poisons. The number of herbal recipes for contraceptive or abortive purposes in contemporary copies of Herbals and recipe collections — including St Gallen, Stiftsbibliothek, MS 217, pages 253 and 256 — together with the attention paid to the practice in the penitentials and legal material does seem to support Riddle's argument that they were a regular part of medical practice.[75]

Having said this, it is unclear how many mothers in early medieval Northern Italy, if any at all, 'placed their infant either on top of a roof or oven to look to heal him' as detailed in the Merseburg penitential, which itself took this clause (perhaps via other penitentials) from the Anglo-Saxon penitential of Theodore.[76] It is also not made explicit if this is included in penitentials because it was considered by the ecclesiastical hierarchy as a magical, pagan practice, or because it could result in the death of the infant. It is likely to be the former as other clauses in the penitential literature specifically deal with the accidental killing of infants. The Merseburg penitential, in the version preserved in MS Vat. lat. 5751 states that 'if a woman suffocates an infant through negligence without baptism, (she should) do penance for three years, one of those on bread and water, two without meat and wine'.[77] The Merseburg version of this penitential simplifies this to baldly state that if a woman suffocates her infant

[74] 'Si mulierem uisceribus suis uim intulisse quo partum abigeret, constiterit, eam in exilium praeses prouinciae exiget.' Justinian, *Digest*, Book 48, 8, 8.

[75] Riddle, *Contraception*, pp. vii-viii and pp. 104–05. See also Sigerist, *Studien*, p. 25, p. 43 and p. 140, cited in Riddle, *Contraception*. Beccaria, *I codici*, p. 370, no. 2a.

[76] 'Si qua mulier infantem suum super tectum aut in fornace ponit et uult sanare eum, V annos peneteat.' Kottje, *Paenitentialia minora*, ME1, p. 155 line 1212, no. 99. In Città del Vaticano, Biblioteca Apostolica Vaticana, MS Vaticani latini 5751 the clause reads: 'Si mulier infantem suum super pectum suum posuerit aut in funem super puteum propter sanitatem, V annos peniteat.' Kottje, *Paenitentialia Minora*, V23, p. 155, lines 1212–18, no. 88. See R. Meens, 'Children and Confession', p. 60, cited in Hamilton, *Practice*, p. 204.

[77] 'Si qua mulier infantem oppressent per neglegentiam sine babtismo (*sic*), III annos peniteat, I ex his in pane et aqua, II sine carne et vino.' Kottje, *Paenitentialia Minora*, V23, p. 131, lines 262–69, no. 21.

she should do three years penance, one of those on bread and water.[78] No distinction is made here between deliberate and accidental killing.

However, in another penitential copied in Northern Italy at the same time as the Merseburg penitential, Oxoniense (Oxford) II, hereafter the Oxford penitential, the compiler is at pains to stress the accidental nature of infant deaths.[79] 'Of a woman, who faithfully did not wish to suffocate her infant. If a woman undoubtedly did not wish to suffocate (her infant) she (should) fast for fourteen weeks.'[80] What is notable is that the penance is significantly lighter — measured in weeks rather than years — than those listed for similar circumstances in the Merseburg penitential. Further, the compiler of the Oxford penitential carefully distinguishes between different causes of infant death: 'Of a woman, who discovers her infant dead next to her. If she does not hold it on her conscience that she caused the death of the infant she should fast for four weeks to purify her soul.'[81] The inclusion of the phrase 'next to her' suggests that this clause refers to cases where the baby dies after sharing a bed with his or her mother. Death therefore could be caused by accidental suffocation, although the circumstances are not specified. (In today's terms, one possible cause is Sudden Infant Death Syndrome (SIDS) as sleeping with an infant is today known as one factor that can increase the risk of SIDS if precise instructions for safe co-sleeping are not followed.)[82] In the Oxford penitential if an infant is suffocated while the mother is drunk, the punishment is more severe than the previous set of circumstances: twenty weeks of fasting.[83]

[78] 'Si quis uxorem suam infantem opresserit, III annos peneteat, I ex his in pane et aqua.' ME1 p. 131, lines 262–68, no. 18.

[79] One of the manuscripts into which this penitential was copied originates from Northern Italy at the turn of the eighth and ninth centuries. It now survives only as a fragment in Darmstadt, Hessiche Landes-u. Hochschulbibliothek, MS 895. See Kottje, *Paenitentialia minora*, p. xxxvi and pp. 181–205.

[80] 'De muliere, si fidele infantem suffugauit nolendo. Si autem certe mulier, qui suffocauit nolendo, illa ieiunet ebdomada XIV.' Kottje, *Paenitentialia minora*, p. 195, lines 443–44, no. 26.

[81] 'De mulieris, si inuenerit iuxta se infantem mortuum. Si non tenet eam conscientiam eius, ut per eam mortuum fuisset infans, sed tamen ad purificandum animam suam ieiunet ebdomada IV', p. 195 lines 439–42, no. 25.

[82] J. J. McKenna and S. Mosko, 'Mother-Infant Cosleeping: Toward a New Scientific Beginning', in *Sudden Infant Death Syndrome: Problems, Progress, and Possibilities*, ed. by R. Byard and H. Krous (London, 2001), pp. 258–74.

[83] 'De eam, qui aebriam suffogauit infantem. Si autem mulier ebria suffogauit infantem fideles per neglegentiam suam, illa ieiunet ebdomada XX.' Kottje, *Paenitentialia minora*, p. 196, lines 453–56, no. 29.

More obscure is the clause concerning the unintentional suffocation of a foreign (*gentilem*) child, where the tariff is greater than for that while inebriated.[84] It could be that the sense here is 'foreign' in the sense of a child that is not a woman's own rather than being from a distant land. If this is the case this clause may be intended to deal with the deaths of babies which occurred while they were being looked after by a woman who was not their mother — a wet nurse even? The Oxford penitential also discusses circumstances when a child is dropped and left during times of conflict or invasion: in these cases it concludes that the woman is not to blame, but can still fast for three weeks. In the context of late eighth or early ninth-century Northern Italy, apart from localized conflicts between landowners, for example, this clause was unlikely to be needed. However, the Carolingians had only invaded a few decades previously, and in the South of Italy Arab incursions were an ongoing reality.[85] Finally, the compiler also considers intentions as well as actions: 'of her, who wishes to suffocate another's child, she should fast for forty weeks with tears and groans.'[86]

The compiler of the Oxford penitential obviously had a particular concern for the correct response of a confessor to the various causes of infant death. This may of course simply spring from a desire to be systematic and comprehensive, but the compiler may also be responding to requests for guidance on these matters by those for whom the penitential was intended. It is unfortunately unclear where this penitential originates from: it could be either Northern Italy or the North East of the Frankish Empire in the circle of the Anglo-Saxon missionary Willibrord.[87]

While individual lawcodes and penitentials therefore all had their own individual preoccupations in relation to the making of potions and the causes and punishments for abortion, miscarriages, and stillbirths, they also share more common ground in approach and attitude than one might expect. Both secular lawcodes and the penitentials recognize a difference in the severity of the offence dependent on how developed the foetus was, and that a distinction needs to be made between accidental and deliberate acts that result in the death

[84] 'De ea, qui gentilem infantem suffogauit (*sic*) ille ieiunet ebdomada XXVIIII.' Kottje, *Paenitentialia minora*, p. 195, lines 445–46, no. 27.

[85] Brown, 'Byzantine Italy, c. 680-c. 876', pp. 320–48, and Brown, 'Lombard and Carolingian Italy'. See also La Rocca, *Italy*, especially chapter 1, W. Pohl 'Invasions and Ethnic Identity', at pp. 27–33 and chapter 3, S. Gasparri, 'The Aristocracy', at pp. 59–84.

[86] 'De eam, qui gentilem suffugauerit infantem volendo, illa ieiunet ebdomada XL cum lacrimis et gemitum.' Kottje, *Paenitentialia Minora*, p. 196, line 457, no. 30.

[87] Kottje, *Paenitentialia minora*, p. xxx.

of a foetus or infant. It is not the penitential handbooks, however, which focus on hostels, *xenodochia*, despite being pious foundations. As I shall show, it is secular legislators for whom these often wayward institutions caused the most headaches.

From Home to Hostel: Health and the Xenodochium

Xenodochia have received an increasing amount of attention over recent decades, usually in the context of the history of the hospital.[88] As mentioned above, *xenodochia* were often themselves converted homes, and were usually founded for the health of the donor's soul in the afterlife, to be run either by monks or clergy. Even in histories of the hospital it has been recognized that the aim of *xenodochia* was not primarily to provide medical care. Instead, the term, derived from Greek, literally means 'house of strangers', and although their function varied, generally *xenodochia* provided bed and board for pilgrims and the poor.[89] As we shall see in chapter six, there are cases where *medici*, such as Gaidoald and Leo at Pistoia, are associated with a particular *xenodochium*. We do not know if part of their involvement included *pro bono* medical work or whether they were purely donors or associates of the *xenodochium*. However, as Peregrine Horden has pointed out, we should look at the overall structure of the institution, not just the personnel.[90] As detailed in previous chapters, contemporaries envisioned healing by many 'non-medical' means, not least diet, and the provision of food for pilgrims and poor was one of the *xenodochium*'s principal functions in the early medieval West.[91]

As seen in the previous chapter on saints' shrines, although a basilica or chapel could be designed or adapted to receive the faithful to view and even touch the relics of a revered saint, we are reliant on texts or inscriptions to shed

[88] See, for example, A. Crislip, *From Monastery to Hospital: Christian Monasticism and the Transformation of Health Care in Late Antiquity* (Ann Arbor, 2005); P. Horden, *Hospitals and Healing from Antiquity to the Later Middle Ages* (Aldershot, 2008); B. Bowers, ed., *The Medieval Hospital and Medical Practice* (Aldershot, 2007); J. Henderson, P. Horden, and A. Pastore, eds, *The Impact of Hospitals, 300–2000* (Oxford, 2007).

[89] P. Horden, 'The Earliest Hospitals in Byzantium, Western Europe, and Islam', *Journal of Interdisciplinary History*, 35.3 (2005), 361–89, especially at p. 366.

[90] Horden, 'The Earliest Hospitals', p. 377.

[91] P. Horden, 'A Non-Natural Environment: Medicine without Doctors and the Medieval European Hospital', in *The Medieval Hospital and Medical Practice*, ed. by B. Bowers (Aldershot, 2007), pp. 133–45.

more light on how a particular shrine may have been used or viewed in practice. Only for certain shrines, however, such those in Milan, do we have copious documentary evidence. Even this, as I have shown, is not necessarily conclusive in determining the importance of healing as opposed to just veneration at these basilicas and chapels. Cantino Wataghin and Pani Ermini face similar frustrations in tracing early pilgrims: apart from accounts and itineraries, principally for Rome or the Holy Land, we know very little about pilgrims visiting shrines outside the Holy Cities.[92] Albert has also shown in his recent study of pilgrimage that 'pilgrims' and 'the poor' could often be synonymous terms.[93]

All this is relevant for *xenodochia*, since they hosted pilgrims and the poor, and are often only attested briefly in foundation or endowment charters. About their actual role and activities, in particular whether they followed the wishes of the original founder or not, we often know very little. Indeed, it could be argued that *xenodochia* have little to do with healing, since they were essentially hostels. One foundation charter from Piacenza does mention the 'debilem' — variously defined in Lewis and Short's dictionary as the 'lame, disabled, crippled, infirm, debilitated, feeble, frail and weak', but there is no indication whether they received any different care to pilgrims or the poor.[94]

However, research on modern populations has established a strong link between poverty and ill-health (and indeed disability and poverty).[95] The connections are obviously complex and at least partially culturally dependant, not to mention potentially nebulous in the light of divergent definitions of 'poverty' or even 'health'. Nevertheless, however defined there is no reason to suppose that some interconnection did not exist in earlier periods, since poor or no accommodation, and a limited or erratic diet all would have contributed to making an individual particularly vulnerable to disease and developing chronic conditions. In these circumstances, even a roof over one's head and a meal could

[92] G. Cantino Wataghin and L. Pani Ermini, *Santuari martiriali e centri di pellegrinaggio in Italia fra Tarda antichita e Alto medioevo, Akten des XII Internationalen Kongresses für christliche Archäologie* (Münster, 1995), i, 136.

[93] B.-S. Albert, *Le Pélerinage à l'époque Carolingianne* (Louvain, 1999), p. 21.

[94] 'Similiter etiam xenodochium debilium et adventantium peregrinorum pro remedio et mercede anime', 874, Piacenza, cited in T. Szabo, 'Xenodochia, Hospitäler und Herbergen — kirchliche und kommerzielle Gastung im mittelalterlichen Italien (7. bis 14. Jahrhundert)', in *Gastfreundschaft, Taverne und Gasthaus im Mittelalter*, ed. by P. Peyer (München, 1983), pp. 61–92 (p. 65).

[95] The classic study is E. A. Winslow, *The Cost of Sickness and the Price of Health* (Geneva, 1951), and modern studies proliferate on the link between diseases and conditions as diverse as AIDS, mental illness and blindness.

have a positive impact on an individual's health. Further, as discussed in Part I, diet was considered one of the key tools for maintaining or restoring health in premodern Western medicine.

What has generally been agreed by historians, however, is that medical treatment, in the sense of consultations by *medici*, were not routinely offered in *xenodochia*, exceptions notwithstanding.[96] However, as I shall discuss in chapter six, groups or successive generations of *medici* could be associated with specific monasteries or *xenodochia*. What is unclear is whether this simply reflects contemporary fashions in donations and patronage, an early medieval version of 'keeping up with the Jones's', or alternatively, if *medici* are consciously defining themselves as a group by forging connections with the same institution. Whatever the motivation, it is not beyond the bounds of possibility that *medici* might have offered (or been persuaded) to occasionally provide their services *pro bono* at the *xenodochia* they were connected with, whether for the monastic or clerical personnel of the hostel or its guests.

Xenodochia were not just a possible *locus* for physical healing though, whether it was achieved with bread and vegetables, or a bed for the night. Firstly, the very act of founding these institutions was invariably to safeguard the donor's spiritual health, and their popularity in Italy (as elsewhere in Europe and the East) in the first millennium surely has much to do with the fact that it was a safe, 'arms-length' and — for those with the means — apparently straightforward way to imitate Christ by caring for the sick, the poor, and the dispossessed.[97] They could be run by monks, clerics, or a *praepositus* (head/overseer): spiritual healing was therefore, in theory at least, an integral part of the *xenodochium*'s *raison d'être*.[98]

The origin of the *xenodochium*, like the word itself, derived from the Greek, and it was in the East where they first emerged around the middle of the fourth century.[99] In the West, Jerome mentions the foundation of a *xenodochium* by Pammachius and Fabiola on the coast outside Rome in two of his letters, dated

[96] See Horden, 'Sickness and Healing' for examples where *medici* were associated with *xenodochia*, pp. 426–47.

[97] Brown has argued that bishops used pious foundations for the poor as a means to promote their authority and leadership — see P. Brown, *Poverty and Leadership in the Later Roman Empire* (London, 2002), especially pp. 45–73 and also the comments of P. Horden, 'The Earliest Hospitals in Byzantium, Western Europe, and Islam', *Journal of Interdisciplinary History*, 35.3 (2005), 361–89 (pp. 362–64).

[98] See Horden, 'Sickness and Healing', p. 426.

[99] Horden, 'The Earliest Hospitals', p. 366.

397 and 399.[100] As has been recognized, however, the term *xenodochium* is a general one, and their precise function varied depended on their location and, with luck, the wishes of the founder. The spelling of the term 'xenodochium' in legal documents also varies considerably, and the terms *diaconia* and *hospitale/hospitales* (*pauperum*) are also used, often interchangeably.[101] Those institutions can also be termed 'oraculum' or 'ecclesia' in the same document.[102] Albert in his recent book on pilgrimage has argued that *xenodochia* on major pilgrimage routes to Rome were probably primarily intended for pilgrims (with the poor often accepted too), but outside of these routes, for *xenodochia* in early medieval Italy the converse was true, with the poor the principal recipients.[103]

While probably true overall, this division obscures the many different systems of organization and prioritization envisaged by the founders of early medieval *xenodochia*. For example, the archpriest Dateus founded a *xenodochium* in Milan that was designed to cater primarily for abandoned children but in the event that not enough parents were deserting their offspring, the doors would then be opened to the poor and pilgrims.[104] In other cases, though, several different categories of potential 'customers' are listed, with no apparent prioritization unless the order in which they are given is significant: the *xenodochium* of St Silvestro at Lucca, founded in 720 AD, was to receive pilgrims and to console 'the poor, widows and orphans' as well.[105]

[100] Horden, 'The Earliest Hospitals', p. 367. On Roman xenodochia see also H. W. Dey, 'Diaconiae, Xenodochia, Hospitalia and Monasteries: "Social Security" and the Meaning of Monasticism in Early Medieval Rome', *Early Medieval Europe*, 16.4 (2008), 398–422.

[101] See Albert, *Le Pélerinage*, pp. 324–26 for his discussion of how the term '(h)ospitale' is context dependant, and can denote either a general *xenodochium* or an institution specifically for pilgrims. He also argues that the difference between the terms *xenodochium* and *hospitales pauperum* relate more to the category of founder than of function. In a charter dated 730 AD, a 'diaconia' is instituted by three brothers outside the walls of Lucca, specifically for the reception of pilgrims: in the last few lines, however, it is referred to as a 'senodochium' (*sic*), suggesting that the terms, in this context at least, were interchangeable. See Albert, as above, and *ChLA 2nd ser.*, 58, no. 907, pp. 74–75.

[102] Szabo, 'Xenodochia', especially at p. 67.

[103] Albert, *Le Pélerinage*, pp. 347–48.

[104] Szabo, 'Xenodochia', p. 165.

[105] 'Donamus [...] hecclesie Beati Sancti Silvestri fundamento ipso cum casa quem sinedoco constituemus [...] et ita [...] ut [...] esset peregrinus recipiendum, pauperis, viduuis et orfanis consolandum', 720, Lucca, cited in Szabo, 'Xenodochia', p. 65, n. 27. See also E. Coturri, 'Gli ospedali lucchesi del periodo longobardo', in *Atti del primo Congresso Italiano di storia ospitaliera* (Reggio Emilia, 1957), pp. 148–62.

Even in the original founding charters, however, the remit of these *xenodochia*, at times perhaps no more than a converted house of modest size, could be quite limited. We should not necessarily envisage an 'open door policy' for all comers. The founders — lay as well as clerical — could specify the number of individuals to be helped, and for how many times a week. For example, in March 777 a certain Toto, 'for the sake of his soul and that of his parents', made arrangements for his house to become a *xenodochium* after his death, under the care of the Milanese basilica of Sant'Ambrogio and Archbishop Thomas and his successors.[106] Toto's servants/slaves were to have the status of *aldii* (semi-free) and give produce annually for the benefit of the *xenodochium*, which was legally responsible for them.[107] The *praepositus* of the institution was to provide meals to twelve poor people on Wednesdays and Fridays in Lent, and to the poor on saints' feast days.[108] Also in Milan, some thirty years early, another *xenodochium* was founded, this time with the specific aim of distributing aid to paupers.[109] The wording in these particular charters would seem to suggest that these *xenodochia*, at least, were perhaps more soup kitchen than residential hostel. Indeed, in a document from Monza, dated 769, the *xenodochium* or *oraculum* of St Felice was called a 'mensa pauperum' (literally, 'table of the paupers').[110]

Another *xenodochium*, however, the subject of a royal document dated 825, and now preserved in the state archives at Turin, was explicitly designed to

[106] 'Ego iamdicto Toto [...] instituo atque decerno ut, a presenti diae ovitus meis, esse debeat domum habidationis meae in suprascripto loco Campelionis, Christo propitio, exenedochium, confirmante me inibi omnibusque rebus meis [...] ita ut post meum dicessum cuncta, ut dectum est, deveniatur potestati et domniationis eiusdem aecclesiae Beati Ambrosii atque iam fati domni Thomae archiepiscopi ordinandi et defensandi.' Milan, 8 March 777, *ChLA 2nd ser.*, 56, no. 22, p. 61, lines 5–8; it is also edited by A. Natale, *Il museo diplomatico dell'Archivio di Stato di Milano* (Milano, 1971), I, no. 25.

[107] 'Et confirmo ut omnes servos et ancellas meas [sint] aldiones et perteneat mundium eorum ad ipso exenedochium [...] Et ita volo ut illi homines meis, qui consueti sunt cum suas anonas operas mihi faciendi, ut cum anona eidem exenedochii operas ipsas perficiant.' *ChLA 2nd ser.*, 56, no. 22.

[108] 'Et pro anima mea atque parentorum meorum remedium, per ipsius ponteficis ordinationis vel per quem ab eo inibi ordinatus fuerit prepositus, pascantur inibi omni tempore pauperes, omnibus diebus veneris, quod est per singolas eodemata die uno, nomina duodicem insimul et, quatraginsime tempus, similiter die veneris et die mercoris ipsi pauperes inibi reficiantur, unde nobis meaneat gautium sepiternum.' *ChLA 2nd ser.*, 56, no. 22, p. 61, lines 8–10.

[109] Natale, *Il museo diplomatico*, I, no. 13.

[110] Cited in Szäbo, 'Xenodochia', p. 65, *Codice Diplomatico Longobardo*, ed. by L. Schiaparelli, 2 vols (Roma, 1929–33), II (1933), no. 194.

receive pilgrims/foreigners (*peregrini*) and the poor daily and was well placed in a high valley outside Turin, Monte Cisino.[111] Further, the cluster of *xenodochia* in and around Lucca suggest that they were designed primarily to provide overnight accommodation for pilgrims, as Lucca was a principal stop en route to Rome.[112] For example, in 730 Liutprand confirmed a *xenodochium* founded for pilgrims by three noble Lombard officials outside Lucca's walls.[113] Such pilgrims presumably arrived with their fair share of infections and medical conditions. Nobles, bishops and princes as well as laymen and the clergy all founded *xenodochia*, and at the other end of the spectrum from the converted dwelling, San Satyro in Milan was supposed to feed a hundred people a month.[114] Important monasteries in the region, such as Bobbio, could own a substantial number of *xenodochia*: we often know little about these institutions, however, beyond their name, location, and, where relevant charters survive, the name and wishes of the original founder.

How did this vast range of institutions work in practice, though? In the case of small, converted-house *xenodochia* like Toto's, what happened on the days when food was not being distributed? Was it effectively like a small estate, or, in the case of monastic *xenodochia*, a type of daughter monastery? We do not know, in the case of those primarily catering to pilgrims, whether visitors stayed a mere handful of nights, or longer: a longer stay arguably could have had a greater impact on an individual's health. Further, court judgements demonstrate that complications could arise after the founder's death, with relatives of the deceased apparently frequently being keener to pocket the revenues from the land and properties of the *xenodochia* than provide bed and board to those on the fringes of society.[115]

The wearily persistent legislation of successive Carolingian rulers, bemoaning the ruined state or poor management of *xenodochia* suggests that many were

[111] 'Igitur comperiat cuntorum fidelium sanctae dei Ecclesiae seu nostrorum strenuitas quia dum ad domni et genitoris nostri Hludouuici serenissimi atque religiosissimi augusti sanctosanctum votum in monte Ciniso quoddam hospitale in honore domini Dei ac salvatoris nostri Iesu Christi seu et beatissime semper virginis Marie ad peregrinorum receptionem eo iubente fieret constructum, voluit tanta illud rerum propriarum substanti locupletare per quam sufficeret diurnus papuerum Christi concusus tolerari.' *ChLA 2nd ser.*, 57, no. 13, p. 70, lines 3–5.

[112] Albert, *Le Pélerinage*, p. 361. See also above, n. 152.

[113] *ChLA 2nd ser.*, 30, no. 109, pp. 73–75, cited in Albert, *Le Pélerinage*, pp. 324–25. See also above, n. 152.

[114] Albert, *Le Pélerinage*, p. 351.

[115] See Albert, *Le Pélerinage*, pp. 327–33, particularly at pp. 329 and 331.

not run as originally intended by their founders.[116] For example, in the 780s and 90s Pippin of Italy's capitularies repeatedly mention *xenodochia*: he states that he wishes 'to conduct those things that have been destroyed, depending on quality of the conditions, to their original place, so that the poor of the Lord might be refreshed'.[117] Some eighty years later, Carolingian officials, *missi*, were being instructed 'and thus the *xenodochia*, where they have been neglected, are to be revived to their original state; indeed hostels of the poor, as much in the mountains as wherever they are known to have been, should be restored fully and with diligent care'.[118] Obviously concern for the welfare of the poor and pilgrims was expected of a Christian king, but the frequency with which this topic is revisited in the legal material suggests both that it was a genuine concern and that attempts to improve the situation from the centre were often ineffective. The mention of 'mountains' in the capitulary to the *missi* probably refers to hostels for pilgrims in the Alpine passes.[119]

However, it may also point to a division between suburban or urban *xenodochia* and their rural counterpoints: hostels in busy pilgrim route towns such as Lucca or even on well-trodden routes over the Alps were arguably far less likely to fall into disrepair (and were more visible if they began to be misused) than a small rural converted-house *xenodochium*, for example. Where houses were converted, like Toto's house, they may not have been located where they were most needed, and therefore became most useful primarily as sources of revenues from any estates endowed with them. Likewise, their effectiveness in improving the lives (and health) of the poor and pilgrims would have varied greatly, dependant both on location and the quality of administration and oversight in place. It is equally difficult to judge if those that continued to operate as they were intended were able to meet demand. For the majority, family networks and 'home remedies' must surely have remained the primary, and preferred, 'safety net' during periods of poverty and/or ill-health. It is also interesting that if there was a spiritual dimension to care in *xenodochia*, it is not

[116] See *Capitularia regum Francorum*, I and II, nos 91, 92, 95, 170, 180, 217. See also the comments of Albert, *Le Pélerinage*, pp. 281–86.

[117] 'Que vero destructa sunt secundum qualitatem temporum ad priore cultum perducere cupimus, ut ibi pauperes Domini reficiantur.' *Capitularia regum Francorum*, I, no. 92, 3, p. 195.

[118] 'Senodochia autem sic, ubi sunt neglecta, ad pristinum statum revocent; hospitales vero pauperum tam in montanis, quam et ubicumque fuisse noscuntur, pleniter et diligenti cura restaurentur.' *Capitularia regum Francorum*, II, no. 217, p. 94.

[119] Albert, *Le Pélerinage*, pp. 349–51.

mentioned in the legal sources. For supernatural aid, not just saints, but also wisewomen, witches and soothsayers, had to be sought out.

Conclusion

A very real question mark remains, however, as to what extent the majority of Northern Italy's early medieval inhabitants regularly used hostels, witches, or soothsayers alike. The key issue is whether the anxieties of secular lawmakers and penitential compilers about magic, unregulated healers and dysfunctional hostels are principally 'strawdogs', or whether they were responding to wider community problems and concerns. I would certainly argue that the concerns of the lawmakers and compilers in the surviving early medieval Northern Italian manuscripts do go beyond the expected rhetorical disapproval and worry for unregulated practices and institutions. What is likely, however, is that many of the 'witches' and 'sorcerers' of the legal sources would be termed as healers and wisewomen by their local communities, at least until something went wrong and a scapegoat was needed. Similarly, the vast majority of the population, unlike legislators, may have seen no contradiction as Christians in concocting remedies at home using the copious recipes discussed in chapter three, and simultaneously boosting its efficacy with a muttered charm. The legislative evidence would also suggest that remedies could also be 'bought in', whether to mend a broken leg or a broken heart. The frequency with which rulers legislated on *xenodochia* suggests that while they were not, unlike secular householders, associated with unregulated practices or healers, they often struggled to move much beyond their domestic origins to provide effective care for the poor, sick or pilgrims. For early medieval Northern Italians, if they had sufficient means, the first port of call, once 'self-help' at home had failed, was not the shrine, soothsayer or *xenodochium*, but the doctor. This, I shall argue in the following chapter, is testament to the strong Roman traditions in Italy even centuries after the last Roman Western emperor had been deposed. The higher status of doctors also ensures their greater visibility in a wider range of sources, particularly legal transactions, allowing us to move beyond the laws and penitentials which are now are our only witness to the many shadowy — often female — low status healers and potion makers of early medieval Italy.

Chapter 6

Doctors: In Search of the Early Medieval 'Medicus'

Some doctors charge the most excessive prices for the most worthless medicines and drugs, and others in the craft attempt to deal with and treat diseases they obviously do not understand. Gargilius Martialis, *Materia Medica*.[1]

So writes the third-century North African horticultural writer and Roman soldier Gargilius, whose writing on gardening, at least, was certainly known in early medieval Italy.[2] The key question for this chapter is whether the population of early medieval Northern Italy shared Gargilius's low opinion of doctors or not. Since we have no direct evidence of the medical practice of doctors in early medieval Italy, we are reliant on legal codes and transactions, although I shall argue that these sources are the key to determining doctors' social status in the region. The roots of medical practice in Italy, however, and the way doctors were perceived, lie in its Imperial Roman past.

Part of the traditionally low and usually derogatory view of doctors in the Classical world may well be snobbery — many doctors in the early Roman Empire were slaves. In Korpela's 1987 study of medical practitioners in ancient

[1] 'Quibusdam vilissima remedia ingentibus pretiis vendentibus, aliis ea quae curare nesciebant cupiditatis causa suscipientibus.' Preface, 7, in *Gargilii Martialis medicinae*, ed. by V. Rose (Leipzig, 1875), p. 7. See J. Riddle, 'Gargilius Martialis as a Medical Writer', *Journal of the History of Medicine and Allied Sciences*, 39.4 (1984), 408–29, and R. Tapper, 'The *materia medica* of Gargilius Martialis' (unpublished doctoral thesis, University of Wisconsin, Wyoming, 1980).

[2] J. Riddle, 'Gargilius Martialis', p. 409.

and late antique Rome, in the second century BC, using both inscriptions and literary sources, 4% of doctors were listed as freeborn, 41% freedmen, 13% slaves, 4% foreigners, 26% with three names, and 11% uncertain.[3] In the Roman Empire as a whole, Nutton's 1970 dissertation asserted that 80% of attested doctors were either slaves, freed, or foreigners but by the third century AD the percentage of freed/slave doctors had decreased to 25%.[4] This trend is also reflected in the Roman data analysed by Korpela.[5] Korpela convincingly argues, however, that legal status cannot be equated exactly with social and economic status, as even among slaves, for example, status could vary widely depending on the type of slave/household, and little difference in wealth, as demonstrated through gravestone evidence, could be discerned between the different legal groups.[6] Further, among doctors there were privileged or specialist groups such as chief physicians, the *archiatri*, or army doctors, which again could cut across legal status.[7]

Whatever century you are looking at, therefore, the term *medicus* encompassed practitioners of varying status and origin, which cannot easily be distilled into a single vignette or epigram.[8] A late antique funerary inscription from Concordia records a Greek doctor called Flavius Aristo, while an Egyptian doctor is buried in Milan and another from Asia Minor is recorded in an epitaph at Verona.[9] In terms of status the doctor Aelius Gentilis, buried in Bolsena in Central Italy is described as a *vir laudabilis* and being of *honesta fama*, a similar status to merchants and skilled craftsmen.[10] Inscriptions therefore indicate that

[3] J. Korpela, *Das Medizinalpersonal im Antiken Rom: ein sozialgeschichte Untersuchung* (Helsinki, 1987), p. 39.

[4] V. Nutton, 'The Medical Profession in the Roman Empire from Augustus to Justinian' (unpublished doctoral thesis, University of Cambridge, 1970), cited in R. Flemming, *Medicine and the Making of Roman Women: Gender, Nature and Authority from Celsus to Galen* (Oxford, 2000), p. 51. See also Nutton, *Ancient Medicine*, pp. 164–65.

[5] Korpela, *Das Medizinpersonal,* p. 111.

[6] By the second century AD, 8% of attested doctors were freeborn, 12% freed, 12% slaves, 14% foreigners, 31% three-named, 22% uncertain: Korpela, *Das Medizinpersonal*, pp. 34–35.

[7] Korpela, *Das Medizinpersonal*, pp. 140–41.

[8] V. Nutton, 'From Galen to Alexander, Aspects of Medicine and Medical Practice in Late Antiquity', in *Symposium on Byzantine Medicine*, ed. by J. Scarborough (Washington, DC, 1985), 1–14 (p. 11), n. 91, cited in Cosentino, 'La figura del medicus', p. 368.

[9] Cited in Nutton, 'From Galen to Alexander', p. 12.

[10] *Inscriptiones Christianae Italiae septimo saeculo antiquiores* (Bari, 1986–), I: *Regio VII, Volsinii*, ed. by C. Carletti, 6–7, cited in Cosentino, 'La figura del medicus', p. 373 n. 70.

at least some *medici* in the Roman Empire — bearing in mind that more attestations survive from the Eastern half of the Empire than in the West — were both reasonably wealthy and prominent members of their local communities.[11] Was this the case in post-Roman Italy too, and did the term 'medicus' shift in meaning at all? To attempt to answer these questions this chapter first surveys evidence from the literary and legal codes — both Roman and 'Barbarian'. I shall then focus on the underused resource of charters — records of legal transactions — to assess the status, educational level and social (and possibly professional too) circle of early medieval Northern Italian doctors.

The Figure of the 'Medicus' in Early Medieval Roman and 'Barbarian' Legal Codes and Letters

Starting with the reign of the Ostrogoth Theodoric (493–526) we have several independent references to Theodoric's own physician, the deacon Helpidius. Far from just being a lowly functionary, he appears to have had influence with Theodoric and his court: he helped Bishop Ennodius of Pavia obtain a house in Milan.[12] He also sent a letter to Bishop Avitus of Vienne, is mentioned in Cassiodorus's *Variae*, and is characterized as a close confidant of Theodoric's in Procopius's account of the Gothic Wars.[13] He even receives a small role in the *vita* of Caesarius of Arles, where his house is said to have been exorcised by the saint sprinkling holy water.[14] He is named as doctor and deacon, and

[11] Nutton, 'From Galen to Alexander', pp. 12–13. See also the epitaph of Caelius Benedictus from Spoleto, *Inscriptiones Christianae Italiae septimo saeculo antiquiores* (Bari, 1986–), VI: *Regio VI, Umbria*, ed. by G. Binazzi, 101, cited in Cosentino, 'La figura del medicus', p. 373 n. 70.

[12] Ennodius, *Opera*, ed. by F. Vogel, *Magni Felicis Ennodi Opera*, MGH AA, 7 (Berlin, 1885), ed. by W. Hartel, CSEL 6, letter 9.21. See also letter 7.7 and cf. Moorhead, *Theoderic*, p. 168.

[13] Avitus of Vienne, *Opera*, ed. by R. Peiper, *Alcimi Ecdicii Aviti Viennensis episcopi Opera*, MGH AA, 6 (Berlin, 1883), Letter 38; Procopius, *Bellum Gothicum*, 1.1.38, ed. and trans. by H. B. Dewing (London, 1914–40); Cassiodorus, *Variae* 4.24, in *Cassiodori Senatoris Variae*, ed. by T. Mommsen, MGH AA, 12 (Berlin, 1894), translated as Cassiodorus, *The 'Variae' of Magnus Aurelius Cassiodorus Senator, the Right Honourable and Illustrious Exquaestor of the Palace, Ex-ordinary Consul, Ex-master of the Offices, Praetorian Prefect and Patrician: Being Documents of the Kingdom of the Ostrogoths in Italy Chosen to Illustrate the Life of the Author and the History of his Family*, trans. by S. Barnish (Liverpool, 1992). Cited in Moorhead, *Theoderic*, p. 167.

[14] *Vita Caesarii*, 1.41 in *Passiones vitaeque sanctorum aevi Merovingici et antiquiorum aliquot*, ed. by B. Krusch, MGH SRM, 3 (Hannover, 1896), p. 473.

is therefore a prestigious 'catch' for exorcism as a royal doctor.[15] As with the *medici* named in the later charter material, however, Helpidius appears in these sources as a fully formed elite physician: nothing is said of his origins or training. Further, in the sources he is included because he plays a key political role in the Ostrogothic court, not because he is a medical practitioner. Of course, almost certainly he built his position at court through close access to Theodoric as his physician, but his social origins or diplomatic skills may have been just as important in his rise. Moorhead argues that Helpidius's name would suggest that he was a Catholic and a Roman, rather than an Arian Christian like his Ostrogothic master, but as Moorhead himself points out, 'Hilpidius' is a Gothic name in origin (and early medieval spelling can be extremely flexible).[16] In any case, names alone are no reliable guide to ethnicity.[17] In terms of Helpidius's training, the fact that he is a deacon would suggest that at least some of his education was obtained in an ecclesiastical school of one kind or another, but this does not preclude an apprenticeship-style training with a *medicus* or even attending a medical *schola* at Ravenna, for example.

He obviously has disposable income as a letter preserved in Cassiodorus's *Variae* demonstrates. Cassiodorus, who was Praetorian Prefect and *quaestor* to Theodoric and his successors, collected together in 537/8 letters, edicts and formulae drafted by himself to form the *Variae*.[18] The letter in question, sent to the deacon Helpidius by Theodoric in 507/11, informs Helpidius that Theodoric is happy to grant him permission to restore the baths there.[19]

[15] *Vita Caesarii*, 1.41, Krusch, p. 473.

[16] Moorhead, *Theoderic*, p. 167.

[17] Moorhead, *Theoderic*, p. 86. On Ostrogoths and ethnic identity see P. Amory, *People and Identity in Ostrogothic Italy 489–554* (Cambridge, 1997) and W. Pohl and H. Reimitz, eds, *Strategies of Distinction: The Construction of Ethnic Communities, 300–800* (Leiden, 1998); W. Pohl, *Le origini etniche dell'Europa* (Roma, 2000).

[18] Fridh, *Variarum*.

[19] 'Petitionis tuae proinde tenore comperimus loca in Spoletina ciuitate, quae iam longo situ squalor uetustatis obnuberat, splendorem reparationis expetere, ut rebus antiquitate confusis nouitatis facies adulta reddatur et beneficio tuo rediuiua consurgant, quae annositate inclinata corruerant. [...] Atque ideo petitioni tuae robur praesenti humanitate largimur, ut porticum cum areola post Turasi thermas, si tamen publico usui non deseruit, absoluta liberalitate potiaris: quia in licentiam reparationis accipiuntur potius praemia quam donantur. Hac igitur auctoritate suffultus in supra dictis locis aedificandi sume fiduciam nec aliquam in posterum metuas quaestionem, cum te et ciuitatis tuetur utilitas et reuerenda principis voluntas.' Fridh, *Variarum* IV, XXIV, p. 158. See also on baths and bathing in early medieval Italy, P. Squatriti, *Water and Society in Early Medieval Italy, AD 400–1000* (Cambridge, 1998), pp. 44–65.

Two other letters in Cassiodorus's collection relate to *archiatri*. The first is addressed to the *archiatrus* Iohannes, chief physician, and concerns a legal case involving the Vicar of Rome, Vivianus.[20] The second is a formula, a model letter, for the *comes archiatri*, count of the *archiatri*.[21] In it the attributes of the elite doctor are elucidated, and medicine is described as that most useful of arts.[22] An *archiatrus* examines a patient's urine and takes their pulse.[23] Talking and listening to the patient, however, is another important element.[24]

Under Theodoric, Roman law still prevailed: he was careful to issue only edicts rather than laws. The *Theodosian Code*, which was originally issued in 438, contains several provisions concerning the privileges of physicians. Book VI of the Theodosian code details the status and honours, including ennoblement, accorded to chief physicians of the Imperial palace, both active and retired.[25] Book thirteen focuses on the exemptions accorded to physicians:

[20] 'Propositum regale est pressis labe fortunae pietatis remedio subuenire et acerbos casus iniuriae meliore sorte mutare. Data siquidem supplicatione conquereris uirum spectabilem Viuianum legume artificio, quo callet, elatum, personam tuam obiectis criminiationibus insecutum et eo usque peruentum, ut indefensus contra iuris ordinem uicarii urbis Romae sententia damnareris: nunc autem religiosae mentis affectu odia mundane damnasse auctorique suo tuum displicuisse periculum. Et ideo, si nullis impugnationibus eneruantur asserta, laesionem non patimur miseris inhaerere, quam suis constiterit machinatoribus displicere. Quapropter in abolitum missa sententia, quae a uicario urbis Romae super hac parte cognoscitur promulgata, patriae te rebusque omnibus nostra reddit auctoritas, nec ullo tempore calumniam super hac parte formides. Sed ne cuiusquam forsitan plectenda temeritas in te impetus reparare possit audaciae, patricii Albini saluis legibus tuitio te deputata communiet, quia nihil fieri uolumus inciuile, cuius cottidianus labor est pro generali quiete tractare.' Cassiodorus, Fridh, *Variarum*, IV, XLI, pp. 169–70.

[21] Cassiodorus, Fridh, *Variarum*, VI, XIX, pp. 248–50.

[22] 'Utillimas artes [...] Obscura nimis est hominum salus, temperies ex contrariis umoribus constans: ubi quicquid horum excreuerit, ad infirmitatem protinus corpus adducit. Hinc est quod sicut aptis cibis ualitudo fessa recreatur, sic uenenum est, quod incompetenter accipitur. Habeant itaque medici pro incolumitate omnium et post scholas magistrum, uacent libris, delectentur antiquis: nullus iustius assidue legit quam qui de humana salute tractauerit.' Cassiodorus, Fridh, *Variarum*, VI, XIX, pp. 248–49.

[23] 'Perito quidem archiatro uenarum pulsus enuntiat, quod intus natura patiatur: offeruntur etiam oculis urinae, ut facilius sit vocem clamantis non aduertere, quam huius modi minime signa sentire.' Cassiodorus, Fridh, *Variarum*, VI, XIX, p. 250.

[24] 'Requirant rudes, quos uisitant aegrotantes, si dolor cessauit, si somnus affuerit: de suo vero languore te aegrotus interroget audiatque a te uerius quod ipse patitur.' Cassiodorus, Fridh, *Variarum*, VI, XIX, p. 250.

[25] *Codex Theodosianus*, ed. by T. Mommsen and P. Meyer, 3 vols (Berlin, 1905), translated

> We command that physicians, grammarians, and other professors of literature, together with the property which they possess in their own municipalities, shall be exempt from public obligations and that they shall perform the duties of honourable offices. We forbid also that they be summoned into court or suggest any indignity, and if any person should molest them, he shall pay to our treasury one hundred thousand coins.[26]

Another section also accords exemptions to chief physicians, who worked in the imperial bureaucracy:

> All chief physicians and ex-chief physicians [...] shall remain free and exempt from all public tax payments, and they shall not be called to any payment of gold, silver, or horses, obligations which on occasion are assessed upon the aforesaid municipal senates and dignitaries. Moreover, we decree that the indulgence of this sanction shall devolve also upon their children.[27]

This does not mean, however, that such a system remained in Italy under Theodoric. However, we do know from Cassiodorus's *Variae* that Theodoric at least continued to pay the salaries of teachers, including those teaching medicine.[28] The Theodosian Code also contains references to abuses of a physician's skills that may have continued to have had resonance in Ostrogothic Italy as well as in the Byzantine Empire: it exhorts physicians to treat the poor as well as the wealthy.[29]

Justinian's *Institutes* included, as in the Theodosian code, reference to physicians and other teachers in Rome.[30] In the *Institutes*, however, the focus is on the status and exemptions of foreign professionals: 'grammarians, rhetori-

as *The Theodosian Code and Novels and the Simondian Constitutions*, trans. by C. Pharr (Princeton, 1952), Book VI, 16.

[26] 'Medicos, grammaticos et professores alios litterarum inmunes esse cum rebus, quas in civitatibus suis possident, praecipimus et honoribus fungi; in ius etiam vocari eos vel pati iniuriam prohibemus, ita ut, si quis eos vexaverit, centum milia nummorum aerario inferat.' *Codex Theodosianus*, Mommsen and Meyer, Book XIII, 3, p. 740.

[27] 'Archiatri omnes et ex archiatris [...] a praestationibus quoque publicis liberi immunesque permaneant nec ad ullam auri et argenti et equorum praestationem vocentur, quae forte praedictis ordinibus aut dignitatibus adscribuntur. Huius autem indulgentiam sanctionis ad filios quoque eorum statuimus pervenire.' *Codex Theodosianus*, Mommsen and Meyer, Book XIII, 3. 2.

[28] Moorhead, *Theoderic*, p. 140.

[29] *Codex Theodosianus*, Mommsen and Meyer, Book XIII, 3. 2.

[30] Justinian, *Institutes*, XXIV, 15.

cians, and physicians at Rome, and those who exercise such professions in their own country, and are within the number authorized, are exempted from being tutors or curators.'[31] This gives us some idea of the cosmopolitan nature of late antique Rome, and the restrictions in place. It is not clear from this, however, whether the physicians mentioned are simply practicing and are not involved in any teaching at all. Justinian's *Digest* includes a similar provision.[32] In Roman law, a 'tutor' or 'curator' is a legal obligation of guardianship rather than a tutor in the modern sense.[33] How common this was in Byzantine Italy, however, is doubtful.

Of course, some elements of Roman law are perhaps more likely to remain the same over the centuries than others: in the section on legacies Cassius writes that eye lotions, plasters, and other things of that kind are included in the *instrumentum* of a doctor.[34] The problem is that, with the exception of the 572 Ravenna papyrus charter, the principal evidence we have for the existence of *medici* in Byzantine Italy comes from Southern Italy: *medici* are recorded in Sicily and Rome between 594 and 608.[35] This also tells us nothing about the nature of their practice or the bureaucratic framework, if any, in which they worked. The Byzantine legal material is so vast, whether in terms of chronological, geographical or topical range that the actual applicability of specific laws relating to doctors is very difficult to assess with any certainty.

In this respect, as discussed in chapter one, the Lombard law codes are far more specific both in terms of the geographical area and individuals which they are intended to cover, and when they are issued: subsequent Lombard kings supplement and alter the original code.[36] For the treatment of injuries the Lombard legal codes only ever refer to *medici* being called, not any other kind

[31] 'Item Romae grammatici, rhetores et medici et qui in patria sua id exercent et intra numerum sunt, a tutela uel cura habent uacationem.' Justinian, *Institutes*, XXIV, 15.

[32] Justinian, *Digest*, Book 27, 6.1.

[33] A tutor is appointed for a pre-pubescent child, a curator for an adolescent/young adult up to the age of twenty-five. See *Institutes* XXII and XXIII on this, and on other aspects of tutor-/curator-ship see XIII, XV, XVI, XVII, XX, XXI.

[34] Justinian, *Digest*, Book 33, 18, 10.

[35] Gregory the Great's *Register* includes references to an 'Anastasius (7) medicus' (V, 4) in Palermo in 594, an 'Archaelaus medicus' (IX, 32) the following year in Syracuse. Gregory's *Dialogues* include a 'Coposius medicus' (IV, 5) in Rome in 593 while the *Liber pontificalis* refers to the *medicus* Iohannes in Valeria (I, 317, Pope Boniface IV). Cited in T. S. Brown, *Gentlemen and Officers*, pp. 251, 253, 256, 265.

[36] Drew, *Law and Society* and Drew, *Lombard Laws*.

of medical practitioner. This is included in various clauses because the principal was that the attacker paid for the medical costs of the victim, depending on the type of injury and the victim's social status. Indeed, the whole bedrock of the Lombard legal code was the paying of compensation adjusted according to the victim's social position (to which a value, a *wergild*, was attached). Ideally, from the king's point of view at least, justice was to be administered by his own officials rather than directly by the dukes.[37]

The circumstances in which a *medicus* is called, however, appear to be somewhat arbitrary. To begin with, the focus is on slaves and the half-free (*aldii*), rather than free-born victims.[38] Is this because it is assumed that the free born or freed will have access to their own doctor and can afford their own fees, if required, from the compensation that will be paid to them by the attacker according to their status? Perhaps attention centres on slaves because this was the arena in which extra financial burdens for the attacker were most contested, and that the compensation would normally be paid to the owner or *dominus* rather than to the servile victim themselves.[39] It also confirms what could have already been guessed, that Rothari's 643 law code primarily reflects the concerns of the land and slave owning elite who wanted to be compensated fully for the impairment or loss of what was in their eyes an economic asset, namely their slaves.

As can be seen from Table 1, a doctor should be called for both household/semi-free and field slaves for the cutting off of a nose or ear, head and chest injuries, broken hips, pierced or broken arms, and pierced legs.[40] For the gouging out of eyes, or cutting off hands or feet, however, a doctor is not mentioned in relation to any type of slave. Why is this? It could be because it is thought that these injuries often resulted in death anyway. For example, Bernard of Italy died after a politically sanctioned blinding in 818.[41] Additionally, even if the slave survived the blood loss and risk of infection, the loss of eyes, hands, or feet would almost certainly prevent them from continuing in their former role anyway. Arguably the types of injuries, such as broken bones, for which a doc-

[37] Drew, *Lombard Laws*, pp. 25–26.

[38] On the different kinds of slaves/semi-free see Drew, *Lombard Laws*, pp. 29–31.

[39] Drew, *Lombard Laws*, p. 30.

[40] See also now L. Oliver, *The Body Legal in Barbarian Law* (Toronto, 2011), which arrived just as I was making final revisions to this book.

[41] R. McKitterick, *The Frankish Kingdoms under the Carolingians 751–987* (London, 1983), p. 135.

Table 1. Doctor's fees mentioned in Lombard laws.

Injury	**Rothari's Edict (643) Chapter Number**	**Aldius (half-free) or household slave**	**Field Slave**
Beating	78/125	Yes	No
Hitting head	79	Yes	Yes
Cutting off nose	80/106	Yes	Yes
On cutting off ears	83/107	Yes	Yes
On cutting off lips	84	Yes	No
Concerning broken arms	87/112	Yes	Yes
On broken hips	94/112	Yes	Yes
Concerning injuries to the chest	101/111	Yes	Yes
On piercing arms and legs	102/110	Yes	Yes
On gouging out eyes	81	No	No
Concerning molar teeth	86	No	n/a
Concerning teeth	85	No	No
On cutting off hands	88	No	No
Concerning first fingers (thumbs) of the hand	—	Yes	No
Concerning second fingers	90	No	No
Concerning third fingers	91	No	No
Concerning fourth fingers	92	No	No
Concerning fifth fingers	93/118	No	Yes
On cutting off feet	119	No	No
Concerning first (big) toes	120	Yes	No
Concerning second toes	121	No	No
Concerning third toes	122	No	No
Concerning fourth toes	123	No	No
Concerning fifth toes	124	No	No

tor is called are those in which there is a realistic chance that the slave could be 'patched up' and returned to duty within a reasonable length of time.

It is also clear from the table that household/half-free slaves had a higher economic and social value than a field slave. For example, a doctor should be summoned when a household or half-free slave is beaten, has his or her lips cut off, or loses a thumb or big toe, but this does not apply to field slaves. Obviously the loss of a thumb or big toe has a greater impact on dexterity and balance, and hence economic value, than other digits, but surely this would also apply to the value of a field slave? Even here though, there is an anomaly. A doctor is mentioned in relation to the cutting off a field slave's little finger, but not for a household or semi-free slave. The rationale for this, if any, is obscure. It even raises the possibility that at times the calling of a doctor is implicit even when it is not actually stated.

What is clear however, is that the Lombard legal codes take as a given that *medici* existed and were numerous enough to be summoned as required. It is also assumed that a doctor would travel to the patient rather than vice versa. Was this schema ever actually implemented, however? Certainly chapter 128 of Rothari's edict (643) would suggest that there was a serious intention, at least, to make this system work on the ground:

> He who struck the blow should seek the doctor; if he has neglected to do this, the man struck or his lord should find the doctor. And he who broke the head or struck the abovementioned blows shall pay for the work lost and an amount for the doctor's fee as adjudged by learned men.[42]

Rothari's edict and later supplements also use Lombard vernacular terms for wounds and body parts rather than Latin terms (despite the edict being issued in Latin).[43] Lawmakers were therefore obviously keen that their provisions for the calling of doctors and the paying of compensation for specific injuries should be clearly understood. To move beyond the generic term 'medici' in law-codes, however, to put 'faces to names', we need to look to the charter evidence.

[42] 'Qui plagas fecerit, ipse querat medicus, et si neclexerit, tunc ille qui plagatus est aut dominus eius inveniat medicum. Et ille qui caput rumpit aut suprascriptus plagas fecit, et operas reddat et mercedes medici persolvat, quantum per doctos homines arbitratum fuerit.' Rothari's edict, *Edictus Rothari*, Bluhme and Boretius, ch. 128; Drew, *Lombard Laws*, p. 72.

[43] For example, *murioth*, *trero*, and *lagi*. Cited in Niederhellmann, *Arzt*, p. 9.

The Charter Evidence for Doctors in Late Antique and Early Medieval Italy[44]

Charters, 'carta' or 'chartula', literally meaning a sheet of parchment, were essentially records of transactions between individuals or institutions.[45] Most commonly these transactions involved the buying, selling or division of land, wills or the making of pious donations to churches and monasteries. Records of the settlement of legal disputes were called *placita*, while royal edicts were called capitularies, and royal charters (as opposed to private charters) granted privileges and made donations.[46] The earliest surviving private charters are from Ravenna, and date from the sixth century.[47] For the rest of Northern Italy, the earliest surviving charters date from the early eighth century, the vast majority in the original, which allows us to judge the basic literacy of *medici* and other witnesses.[48] Although most were preserved by ecclesiastical institutions, many relate to lay transactions involving land that only later came into Church hands.[49] The numbers of surviving charters rise steeply between the eighth and eleventh centuries: over a hundred for eighth-century Northern Italian charters, but over three thousand for the same region by the eleventh century.[50] Coverage across Northern and Central Italy is uneven however, with a large proportion of the

[44] A version of part of this section has appeared as C. Pilsworth, 'Could You Just Sign This for Me John? Doctors, Charters and Occupational Identity in Early Medieval Northern and Central Italy', *Early Medieval Europe*, 17.4 (2009), 363–88.

[45] A. Bartoli Langeli, 'Private Charters', in *Italy in the Early Middle Ages, 476–1000*, ed. by C. La Rocca (Oxford, 2002), pp. 205–19 (p. 212). All pre-ninth-century Italian charters are edited in the monumental series *Chartae Latinae antiquiores* (*ChLA*), and in the same series editions of ninth-century Italian charters are in progress (*ChLA 2nd ser.*).

[46] Azzara and Moro, eds, *I capitolari*; Bougard, *La justice*; Everett, *Literacy*, p. 186.

[47] Bartoli Langeli, 'Private Charters', p. 206. For Ravenna's charters see *ChLA 2nd ser.*, 54, and J.-O. Tjäder, *Die nichtliterarischen Lateinischen papyri Italiens aus der Zeit 445–700*, 3 vols (Lund, 1954–82).

[48] On literacy in early medieval Italy, for a starting point see Everett, *Literacy*; A. Petrucci and C. Romeo, *'Scriptores in urbibus': Alfabetismo e cultura scritta nell'Italia altomedievale* (Bologna, 1992); A. Petrucci, *Writers and Readers in Medieval Italy: Studies in the History of Written Culture*, ed. and trans. by C. Radding (London, 1995).

[49] On lay archives see W. Brown, 'When Documents are Destroyed or Lost: Lay People and Archives in the Early Middle Ages', *Early Medieval Europe*, 11.4 (2002), 337–66; A. Ghignoli, 'Su due famosi documenti pisani dell'VIII secolo', *Bulletino dell'Istituto Storico Italiano per il medio evo*, 106.2 (2004), 1–69. I am grateful to Thomas Granier for this reference.

[50] Bartoli Langeli, 'Private Charters', p. 206.

eighth-century surviving charters conserved in Lucca, for example.[51] Charters, particularly before the ninth century, were often drawn up by scribes who did not class themselves professional notaries: they might be the local presbyter, for example.[52] The charter had to be witnessed, and these witnesses would either sign their names, or simply mark a cross and have their names written in for them if they were not literate.[53] From eighth-century witness evidence Petrucci concludes that at least basic literacy was widespread among the clergy and urban (male) middle and upper classes.[54]

Perhaps partly due to their evocation of the minutiae of daily life such as the selling of an apple orchard or the allocation of a quantity of grain to the poor, the temptation has been to see charters as a more 'true' or at least more accurate picture of early medieval life than the edicts of lawcodes, for example, despite the fact that both are in fact highly codified.[55] Charters are structured using *formulae*, set phrases into which individual details of a transaction or agreement are woven. Further, it must be remembered that charters or *placita* (legal judgements) represent the 'official' version of a transaction or judgement, simplifying what may in some cases be a far more complex series of negotiations and agreements than are now visible to us.

Crucially, regionally based scribal practices can also affect how charters are phrased, and what details were included or omitted, particularly concerning a witness's profession. For example, Piacenza charters from the first half of the ninth century included several professions or titles, from merchant to judge.[56] In contrast, ninth-century charters from Ravenna still tended to use Classicizing

[51] P. Cammarosano, *Storia dell'Italia medievale: dal VI all'XI secolo* (Roma, 2001), p. 150 and pp. 160–61; Bartoli Langeli, 'Private Charters', p. 206. See also A. Petrucci, *Medioevo da leggere: guida allo studio delle testimonianze scritte del medioevo italiano* (Torino, 1992) and C. Scalon, ed., *Libri e documenti d'Italia: dai Longobardi alla rinascita delle città* (Udine, 1996).

[52] Everett, *Literacy*, p. 142; Bartoli Langeli, 'Private Charters', p. 208.

[53] Bartoli Langeli, 'Private Charters', p. 215 and see also P. Supino Martini, 'Alfabetismo e sottoscrizione testimoniali al documento privato nell'Italia centrale (sec. VIII)', in *Escribir y leer en Occidente*, ed. by A. Petrucci and F. M. Gimeno Blay (Valencia, 1995), pp. 47–61.

[54] A. Petrucci, 'Book, Handwriting and School', in A. Petrucci, *Writers and Readers in Medieval Italy: Studies in the History of Written Culture*, ed. and trans. by C. Radding (London, 1995), pp. 59–76 (originally published as 'Libro, scrittura e scuola', in *La scuola nell'occidente latino dell alto medioevo* (Spoleto, 1972), pp. 313–38).

[55] On this issue see Skinner, *Women*, particularly at pp. 12–13 and see also Skinner, 'A Cure', p. 300.

[56] *ChLA 2nd ser.*, 64, nos 2, 22, 25, 31, 33, 39.

titles such as 'vir clarissimus' rather than list professions as often.[57] This is of course partly a reflection of the mosaic of post-Roman states — Ostrogothic (489–552), then Byzantine (552–751), Lombard (568–773) and finally Carolingian (773/774 onwards) — that made up early medieval Northern and Central Italy. Stitched into this complex and shifting political framework, however, were even more localized regional scribal (and legal) traditions, with the result, as I shall show, that the charter evidence is almost certainly therefore 'hiding' some *medici* who acted as witnesses but whose profession is not listed.

Beginnings: The Learned Doctor in Late Antique Ravenna

By far the earliest Northern Italian charter which includes the term *medicus* dates to 572 when Eugenius, son of Leontius 'medici ab schola greca' was a witness in a papyrus charter now preserved in the British Library.[58] This charter recorded the sale by the farmer Domninus of a portion of two properties near Rimini (on the North Eastern coast of Italy, in Byzantine territory) to the court official Deusdedit. Eugenius was essentially a work colleague of the buyer Deusdedit, since they were both listed as being a *palatinus sacrarum largitionum*, that is a treasury official. It is the precise meaning of the term 'ab schola greca' that has received so much attention from scholars as it is ambiguous — Leo was a *medicus* from the Greek school rather than from a medical school *per se*. It is logical, but not automatic, to assume that the two are linked as he may have trained elsewhere before becoming a teacher.

If, however, we do consider the 'schola greca' to at least in part have included medical training as well as Greek language — the *lingua franca* of the Byzantine Empire — and literature, what precisely is meant by the term 'schola'?[59] Teaching may be held, for example, in more than building or location in the city, or could 'schola' even simply refer to a grouping of teachers? Evidence from Rome, though, suggests that 'schola' in this period could indeed refer to a physical building, although not necessarily with an educational focus: 'schola' was used in early medieval Rome to denote a hostel for visitors of a particular nationality, for example Saxon or Greek.[60] It can however, also specifically refer to a

[57] *ChLA 2nd ser.*, 54.

[58] London, British Library, MS Additional 5412, edited in Tjäder, *Die Nichtliterarischen lateinischen Papyri*, I (1954), 104–12.

[59] Brown describes Leontius as Greek, but Eugenius as being brought up in Ravenna. See Brown, *Gentlemen*, p. 77.

[60] Christie, *From Constantine*, pp. 105, 159, 180, 243, 508.

training institution such as the Roman *schola cantorum* (papal choir school).[61] In the Ravenna papyri it has been argued that the term is used in the sense of an order or corporation.[62]

It should not be assumed, however, that even within the papyri the term is being used in precisely the same sense in separate documents. 'Schola' or 'scola' can also be defined a 'learned conversation or debate, or a place for learned conversation or instruction, a school'.[63] If, in a sixth-century Ravennate context 'schola' does indeed relate to one building or complex devoted to education then it has never been identified in the archaeological record. Since the charter relates to Leo's son, it is also difficult to know if the *schola*, however constituted, was still in existence by 572. Certainly if anywhere in Northern Italy was to have a (Greek) medical school then Ravenna would be the most likely venue as centre of the Eastern Roman (Byzantine) Empire's campaign to reconquer and then hold territory in Italy and where many Classical Greek medical texts were translated.

Yet, discussion of the phrase 'scola greca', whether it refers to a Ravennate medical school or not, is almost always divorced from the context in which the phrase originally appears. However, this charter also has something to tell us about the status of the *medicus* Leontius's family. Firstly, the profession of *medicus* would not appear to have been followed by Leontius's son Eugenius, although Leontius may have had other children who followed in his footsteps. Instead, Leontius's son Eugenius worked for a key department in the Byzantine administration in Italy. Between the 530s and 550s the Eastern Emperor Justinian I waged his campaign of reconquest of lost provinces in Italy and North Africa, finally toppling the Italian Ostrogothic regime whose capital was in Ravenna, the city in which the Byzantine exarchate also then based itself.[64] From 568 onwards, however, the extent of the territory was once more drastically reduced, this time by the Lombards, particularly in the North where only Ravenna and its hinterland along the Adriatic coast remained.[65] 572, the year in which the charter was produced, was therefore part of a period of retrenchment for the Byzantine administration.

[61] Brown, *Gentlemen*, p. 185.

[62] Mazzini and Palmieri, 'L'ecole medicale', pp. 285–310: They translate the word as 'school' on the basis also of an inscription, CIL VI 29805.

[63] Lewis and Short, *A Latin Dictionary*, p. 1641. J. Niermeyer, *Mediae latinitatis lexicon minus* (Leiden, 1976), pp. 1232–33.

[64] See Brown, *Gentlemen*, pp. 1–10.

[65] Brown, *Gentlemen*, p. 5.

What we do not know from the charter itself is to what extent Eugenius owed his position in the Byzantine administration to his father's status and connections. The fact that not only his father's profession but also where presumably his father taught is mentioned, however, suggests that it was a source of pride rather than simply an identifier. It is possible, however, that it was linguistic ability in Greek, thanks to his father, that might have recommended Eugenius rather than his family's social status, although the majority of officials appear to have been drawn from local families rather than from those originating in the Eastern Roman Empire.[66]

Whatever the precise status of Leontius and his family, they arguably represent the end rather than the beginning of a prominent medical tradition in Ravenna, since there are no further references to *medici* in the charter material from Ravenna before 1000 AD, despite a relatively rich archive.[67] It should be remembered, however, as mentioned above, that Ravennate charters are not always very informative about the professions of donors or witnesses, often preferring Romanizing titles such as *vir clarissimus*.[68] In the Byzantine Empire on the Italian peninsula as a whole, however, there are several references to *medici* in their Southern Italian and Sicilian territories. The Byzantine writer Procopius mentioned an *iatros* (the Greek term for doctor) called Theoctistus who was attached to the garrison of Rome in 537 during Justininan's reconquest of Italy, but otherwise there is scant evidence on doctors in a military context in Italy.[69] Rather, several references to presumably civilian *medici* occur in the epistolary register of Pope Gregory the Great.[70] An Anastasius *medicus* of Palermo, Sicily, was recorded in Gregory's *Register* of letters in 594.[71] In 598 AD, an Archelaus *medicus* in Syracuse was mentioned in the same collection.[72] Also in the 590s, a certain Copiosus *medicus*, brother of the monk Iustus, appeared in Gregory's *Dialogues*.[73] Iohannes *medicus* from Valeria in the early seventh century was

[66] Brown, *Gentlemen*, p. 77.

[67] See Brown, *Gentlemen*, pp. 223–26.

[68] See Tjäder, *Die nichtliterarischen lateinischen Papyri* and *ChLA 2nd ser.*, 54, and 55.

[69] Cited in Cosentino, 'La figura del medicus', p. 373.

[70] Gregory the Great's *Register* is edited by p. Ewald and L. Hartmann, *Registrum epistolarum*, MGH Epistolae, 1–2 (Berlin, 1887–99), and, more recently, as Gregory the Great, *S. Gregorii Magni Registrum Epistularum*, ed. by D. Norberg (Turnhout, 1982).

[71] Gregory the Great, *Register*, V.4, cited in Brown, *Gentlemen*, p. 214 n. 19.

[72] Gregory the Great, *Register* IX. 32, cited in Brown, *Gentlemen*, p. 214 n. 19.

[73] Gregory the Great, *Dialogues* IV. 57, cited in Brown, *Gentlemen*, p. 256. Latin edition: *Dialogues*, de Vogüe.

mentioned in the papal *Liber pontificalis* as the father of Pope Boniface IV.[74] As far as we know they appear simply to have been regional doctors, and not have any direct connection to the Byzantine regime. This is in contrast to the first mention of a doctor in Lombard territory, to which I now turn.

By Royal Appointment: Pistoia and the Royal 'Medicus' Gaidoald

There is then a gap of over a hundred and fifty years before a *medicus* is mentioned again in a Northern or Central Italian charter. This reflects the turbulent political events which overtook early medieval Italy rather than a mass retirement of *medici*. In this period, as we have seen in relation to Eugenius and his father, the Byzantines gradually lost most of Northern and Central Italy to the invading Lombards in 568. Perhaps more surprisingly, the only *medicus* in surviving pre-tenth-century charters who actually initiates or is actively involved in donations and foundations, rather than just being a witness or leaser, is Gaidoald, doctor to the Lombard kings for over four decades.

In 726 in Pistoia, some miles north east of Lucca in Central Italy, the cleric Filipert, son of a blacksmith, sold to Gaidoald, *medicus* to the king, a stone-built Hall (described as a *sala* rather than the more prosaic *casa*), a courtyard, meadows and a kitchen garden outside Pistoia's walls for 100 *solidi*.[75] It is not clear why Gaidoald was involved in a transaction relatively far from the Lombard court at Pavia near Milan in Northern Italy: perhaps he had familial connections in Pistoia. The endowments he made, however, were spread more widely and, Stoffella argues, reflect his links with the royal family.[76] The only family we know about is a son called Gaiprand, mentioned in a much later charter.[77] Over forty years later, in 767, still in Pistoia, almost certainly the same Gaidoald (since he is described in this charter as the 'medicus regum'), by now at least in

[74] *Le Liber pontificalis*, Duchesne, I, Bonifatius IIII, ch. 69, p. 317, cited in Brown, *Gentlemen*, p. 215 n. 19. The province of Valeria is between what is now Lazio and Abruzzi and Molise — see J. Graesse, F. Benedict, and H. Plechl, eds, *Orbis Latinus: Lexikon lateinischer geographischer Namen des Mittelalters und der Neuzeit*, 3 vols (Braunschweig, 1972), III, 559.

[75] *ChLA*, 25, pp. 70–73. See also *Storia di Pistoia*, I: *Dall'alto medioevo all'età precomunale 406–1105* (Firenze, 1988), p. 116.

[76] M. Stoffella, 'Crisi e trasformazioni delle élites nella Toscana nord-occidentale nel secolo VIII: esempi a confronto', *Reti Medievali*, 8 (2007). This article is also available as a free download at http://www.retimedievali.it.

[77] 5 February 767, Schiaparelli, *Codice*, II, no. 203, p. 208, lines 14–16, cited in Rauty, *Storia di Pistoia*, I, 167.

Table 2. Charters and judgements involving medici in Northern/Central Italy 550–900 AD.

Date	Place	Name	Attribution
572	Ravenna	Eugenius	[...].filius Leonti medici ab schola greca
726	Pistoia	Gaidoaldus	Viro magnifico medico regie
748	Pistoia	[...] lfredus	Medicus
767	Pistoia	Gaidoaldus	Medicus
774	Chiusi	Iohannes (1)	Medicus
777	Lucca	Adelpert	Medicus
786	Lucca	Autpertus	Clericus et medicus
788	Lucca	Wito	Clericus
792	Asti	Rotcaus	Medicus
796	Pistoia	Leo	Medicus
796	Pistoia	Gaidoaldus	Bone memorie Gaidualdu medico
797	Pescia	Autchis	Filio Witi Clerici medici
811	Lucca	Autpertus	Clericus et medicus
812	Pistoia	Gaidoaldus	Medicus
816	Lucca	Iohannes (2)	Clericus
817	Lucca	Iohannes (2)	Clericus et medico (sic)
819	Lucca	Iohannes (2)	Clericus
821	Lucca	Iohannes (2)	Clericus et medico
822	Lucca	Iohannes (2)	Clericus et medico
823	Lucca	Iohannes (2)	Clericus et medico
824	Lucca	Iohannes (2)	Clericus et medico
824	Lucca	Iohannes (2)	Clericus et medico
824	Lucca	Iohannes (2)	Clericus et medico
824	Lucca	Gunpertus	Medicus
827	Lucca	Iohannes (2)	Clericus et medico
827	Pacilianu (Siena)	Radso	Clericus et medicu (sic)
831	Lucca	Bonifridus	Clericus et medicus
832	Lucca	Iohannes (2)	Clericus et medico
835	Lucca	Iohannes (2)	Clericus et medico
835	Lucca	Auripertus	Medicus
836	Lucca	Iohannes (2)	Clericus et medico

Date	Place	Name	Attribution
838	Lucca	Auripertus	Medicus
839–40	Lucca	Iohannes (2)	Clericus et medico
841	Lucca	Bonifridus	Clericus et medicus
843	Lucca	Bonifridus	Clericus et medicus
844 (Jan and April)	Lucca	Auripertus	Medicus
847	Lucca	Auripertus	Medicus
849	Lucca	Auripertus	Medicus
854	Verona	Ragibertus	Medicus
860	Caorso (Piacenza)	Iohannes (3)	Medico (sic)
862	Verona	Ragibertus	Medicus
864	Piacenza	Adellardus	Clericus et medicus
898	Piacenza	Leoprandus	Presbiter et medicus

his sixties and therefore elderly in early medieval terms, made arrangements for the monasteries and *xenodochia* (hostels/hospices) which he has founded in the area in the course of his life, the principal one being the monastery of San Bartolomeo.[78] He gave six estates and a church to San Bartolomeo, which Chris Wickham speculates may have consisted of half of his total property, concluding that Gaidoald was not particularly wealthy.[79] This may well be true in comparison with royal court circles or large landowners, but in local terms it was not insubstantial and included property scattered through Tuscany, including the area around Lucca, and Maremma.[80] Further, between 726 and 767 at least some of Gaidoald's money may have been spent on the monasteries and other institutions he had founded during the course of his life. Unfortunately, the 767 charter only survives as a twelfth-century copy, now preserved in Florence, but from the witness list it would appear that Gaidoald only made a sign of

[78] *Codice*, ed. Schiaparelli, II, 205–11. On life expectancies in the early middle ages see for example Riché, *Daily Life*, p. 47. On *xenodochia* in the West see Horden, 'The Earliest Hospitals'.

[79] C. Wickham, 'Rural Society and Economy', in *Italy in the Early Middle Ages, 476–1000*, ed. by C. La Rocca (Oxford, 2002), pp. 118–43 (p. 123). Cammarosano, *Storia dell'Italia medievale*, p. 119, describes Gaidoald as an eminent layman.

[80] Rauty, *Storia di Pistoia*, I, 167. See also S. Gasparri, 'The Aristocracy', in *Italy in the Early Middle Ages, 476–1000*, ed. by C. La Rocca (Oxford, 2002), pp. 59–84 (p. 71).

the cross rather than signing his own name.[81] This suggests that Gaidoald was either illiterate — which would be surprising given that without exception the other *medici* in the charter evidence always sign their own names — or was unable to sign due to illness, disability, or absence. The 726 charter, drawn up at Pistoia, does not provide any further information on this point: it is a damaged original and Gaidoald — very unusually — was not listed among the witnesses.[82] He was apparently present at the transaction as it is stated that the vendor 'accepisse et in presentia testium accepit ad Gaiduald [...] auri solidos [...]'. However, the charter itself may well have been drawn up after the fact, in Gaidoald's absence.[83]

Three decades later, in 796, Gaidoald's name appears once more, this time as the revered founder of St Bartolomeo.[84] Gaidoald at this point has been dead for presumably at least some decades, and was described as being of 'good memory', but was still identified by his profession, presumably quoted from the earlier charters. What is most striking about this particular charter, however, is that one of the witnesses was a certain 'Leo medicus'.[85] Was this a descendent of Gaidoald's, or, even more intriguingly, had St Bartolomeo developed into an institution particularly associated with local *medici*? Leo was literate, and wrote in new Italian cursive minuscule, indicating that he almost certainly was not just schooled at home in basic letter forms, but received training at some point in an ecclesiastical school and/or with a secular notary, as no clerical status is listed. St Bartolomeo, up to probably the mid-twelfth-century, appears to have consisted of three separate building complexes: the church, the monastery, and the *xenodochium*, built right next to the road.[86] As discussed in chapter five, *xenodochia* are usually characterized as hostels for foreigners and the poor, with food and a roof over their heads being the principal 'treatments'. However, the association of Leo with Gaidoald's foundation at least raises the possibility of

[81] Schiaparelli, *Codice*, p. 205.

[82] Schiaparelli, *Codice*, pp. 131–33.

[83] *ChLA*, 25, no. 794, p. 70. On the Spanish peninsula a number of charters were witnessed by a 'Reinoard' but he only signs with his own name in a few of them: see F. Udina Martorell, ed., *El Archivo Condal de Barcelona en los Siglos IX–X, studio critico de sus fondos* (Barcelona, 1951). See G. Feliu, and J. M. Salrach, eds, *Els Pergamins de l'Arxiu Comtal de Barcelona de Ramon Borrell a Ramon Berenguer I* (Barcelona, 1999), no. 46, with commentary, I, 319–20. Thanks to Jon Jarrett for discussion on this point and Martin Ryan for these references.

[84] *ChLA*, 25, no. 796, pp. 84–87.

[85] *ChLA*, 25, p. 86.

[86] Rauty, *Storia di Pistoia*, I, 117.

medici undertaking charitable medical work from time to time for a particular institution or institutions. Whether a more formal arrangement between *xenodochia* and *medici* ever existed is impossible to tell. Another Pistoian *medicus*, of which we now only have part of his name, [...]lfredus, witnessed the foundation of the monastery/*xenodochium* of Peter, Paul, and Anastasius in 748, which subsequently became subject to St Bartolomeo. Once more, though, we have no further details of whether this *medicus*'s involvement extended beyond witnessing duties.[87]

The final legal document in which Gaidoald's name is mentioned — like the 796 charter as the founder of the monastery — was a judgement from 812 about St Bartolomeo's abbot's military and other obligations.[88] By the time of these two final charters the Lombard dynasty who Gaidoald served had been ousted from power in Northern/Central Italy by the Carolingian dynasty from North of the Alps in 773–74, although there was not an immediate influx of Franks, and many Lombards, at least initially, retained their lands and offices.[89] All other references to *medici* in Northern and Central Italy in the charter material date from the 790s onwards and therefore must be viewed in this context. Gaidoald, from his name and role, was almost certainly a Lombard. Name evidence is notoriously slippery, however, and for the other *medici*, such as Leo, it is impossible to determine origin and family background from name alone. This is particularly true given that families could have mixed — Roman, Lombard, Alamannic, and, after 774, Frankish — backgrounds. There is even a certain Iohannes *medicus* with possible Visigothic connections witnessing a charter in Chiusi in 774 as the Lombard regime was collapsing around him.[90]

Doctors in the Provinces

Few *medici* would have achieved the status of Gaidoald as the doctor of kings, and as the founder of a *xenodochium* Gaidoald was unusual, perhaps even unique, among early medieval Northern Italian *medici*. Most appear to have lived their lives quietly in provincial towns, and the only way we know about them at all is through their witnessing of charters.

[87] Schiaparelli, *Codice*, no. 96, p. 280.

[88] C. Manaresi, *I placiti del 'regnum Italiae'* (Roma, 1955), no. 25, pp. 77–80. On *placita* see also Azzara and Moro, *I capitolari*.

[89] Christie, *From Constantine*, p. 54; La Rocca, *Italy*, p. 28.

[90] Schiaparelli, *Codice*, no. 437, pp. 437–39.

This is exactly the case for a witness who identified himself as a *medicus* in a charter which was produced in or around Asti (South West of Turin in North West Italy) and is still conserved there.[91] It was written in 792, and documented an exchange of land between a priest and a certain Sonderulfus, a royal officer (*gastald*).[92] On line 33 the *medicus* Rotcaus signed as a witness in a cursive minuscule and was therefore literate in a basic way at least, which is notable, as the majority of witnesses in this charter do not sign their own name.[93] Further, apart from the notary who drew up the charter, Rotcaus was the only witness who included his profession. From this it might be concluded that not only was the attribution *medicus* a marker of status but also that it was the key characteristic by which the community identified Rotcaus.

In ninth-century Asti charters the other professions listed include judges, officials, merchants, and an *arsenario*. Rotcaus's status therefore appears to have been closer to that of a profession than a trade.[94] However, given that not all the witnesses of the charter were able to sign their own names, the circles in which Rotcaus was actually moving were less exulted, perhaps neighbours or even former or current patients. Given the absence of any indication of clerical status, it is impossible to be certain where or how Rotcaus was trained — possibly not even in Asti, since no other *medici* are attested in the pre-1000 charters from this city. He was apparently a lay *medicus*, since no clerical status is included, but otherwise we know nothing else about him.

Likewise, it is very difficult to contextualize the *medicu* (*sic*) Radso who participated in a transaction in 821 at a place called Pacilianu in Central Italy, around Siena.[95] He was able to sign his name, as were some but not all of the other witnesses. Unlike Rotcaus, he did also identify himself as a *clericus*. Were *medici* such as Radso or Rotcaus, born, trained, and buried in such places, or were they partly peripatetic? We do not even know if they lived in the places in which they witness charters, or had come there to market or to visit patients. One would presume that the majority of *medici* were based in urban centres,

[91] Archivio Capitolare, pergamene sparse, Liber I anniversariorum (cassetta 1, no. 3), edited in *ChLA*, 27, no. 836, pp. 107–09.

[92] *ChLA*, 27, no. 836, pp. 107–09.

[93] *ChLA*, 27, line 33. The only other witness who signs his own name unaided is Petrus on line 34.

[94] *ChLA 2nd ser.*, 56. See for example Asti, Archivio capitolare, Pergamene dal 775 al 1002, I 4 (Iura Ecclesie mazzo 26, n. 3), dated 814, p. 14 lines 2 and 3, and Perg. I 17 (31 n. 5) p. 52 line 31.

[95] *ChLA 2nd ser.*, 62, no. 5, pp. 30–31.

where there were more potential patients, even if they made house visits to rural patients. We also do not know if their training and status was lower than that of their colleagues in more important cities.

It is certainly likely that there was a link between the status of the city and that of the *medicus*. The ancient town of Verona, now in the province of Veneto, had retained its importance under the successive Ostrogothic, Lombard and Carolingian regimes, with new buildings and palaces.[96] In mid-ninth-century Verona a certain Ragibertus *medicus* was called as a prominent member of the local community to participate in a legal judgement. He was one of the many witnesses present in 854 when, further to a previous judgement, Eufrasia, abbess of St Maria puellarum in Verona, formerly declared her convent to be subject both to the patriarch of Aquileia, whose *missus*, Teudemarius, was also present, and to the Abbot of St Maria in Organo.[97] Of those listed, apart from Ragibertus no professions were given unless the person concerned was either an ecclesiastic or an officer of the Carolingian legal and administrative structure such as a *sculdasius*. Further, it is clear that many present were not listed individually, since the document stated that good men and citizens were also present. To be named in this document, therefore, was an honour, and places Ragibertus among the leading citizens of Verona. Was this by virtue of his profession, however, and/or family connections about which we are ignorant? Unfortunately since this was not a conventional charter, but a record of an event, witnesses did not sign for themselves. It is also notable that Ragibertus was not given a clerical status, but we do not know if this was for the sake of brevity or because he had none.

It would appear that Ragibertus may have had some connection with the monastery of St Maria in Organo since he witnessed another case involving the monastery some eight years after the dispute between the convent and monastery of St Maria. In this instance Abbot Rumaldus of St Maria in Organo declared himself ready to pay the *rogator* of the deceased bishop of Verona, Rimbertus, for property given by Bishop Audo to the monastery for the good of his soul. Rimbertus, however, had refused payment.[98] As before, Ragibertus was described as a *medicus* by the scribe in the body of the charter's text, but simply signed his name in his own hand, with no indication of profession, at the base of the charter with the other witnesses.[99]

[96] F. Bougard, 'Public Power and Authority', in *Italy in the Early Middle Ages, 476–1000*, ed. by C. La Rocca (Oxford, 2002), pp. 34–58 (p. 47).

[97] *ChLA 2nd ser.*, 59, no. 19, pp. 99–101.

[98] *ChLA 2nd ser.*, 59, no. 26, pp. 122–23.

[99] *ChLA 2nd ser.*, 59, no. 26, pp. 122–23.

Another strategically important city in early medieval Northern Italy, lying between Parma and Milan, is Piacenza. In 864, the priest Adremundus, son of a certain Adellardus 'clericus et medico' (*sic*) sold a house with land outside the walls of Piacenza near the gate of San Antonino to Ioannes, *canavarius* (housekeeper/provisions master) of San Antonino.[100] Given its location, Ioannes possibly acquired the house and land either for himself or family members to live in. It is notable in this transaction that Adremundus was the only clerical participant in this charter and also the only one to sign his own name.[101] Again scribal practice is significant here as in this charter virtually all the participants are identified in terms of whose son they are, and it is only through this that we even know of the existence of the cleric and *medicus* Adellardus in Piacenza. Further, as in Gumprandus's 817 Lucca charter discussed below, the term *medico* rather than *medicus* is used, suggesting that, rather than a scribal error, this is a contemporary, proto-Romance term for doctor in ninth-century Italy (and indeed the modern Italian term for doctor is *medico*).

As in the case of Eugenius in sixth-century Ravenna, Adremundus does not appear to have followed in his father's footsteps and become a *medicus* himself. Instead he has pursued a career in the church, becoming a *presbyter*, a higher clerical status than his father. Whether the house Adremundus sold was originally his father's property, we cannot tell, but the fact that Adremundus was both literate and had surplus land and property to sell indicates that his family were, in contemporary local terms at least, reasonably well off. The lay witnesses, however, who were not literate (but may nevertheless have owned land and been influential locally) suggest that Adremundus was probably moving in local small landowner circles rather than anything more exulted, and may indeed have been a local priest, although if he was, no specific church is mentioned.

Nearly forty years later, on 1 August 898, again in Piacenza, a Leoprandus 'presbiter et medicus' played an active role in a court judgement (*placitum*) as he presented, together with his *advocatus*, a charter to the court to prove that he was entitled to the usufruct of his friend the layman Adelprandus's property.[102] The charter at the centre of the controversy, dated 892, was cited in the judgement. In this earlier charter Leoprandus's name was obviously promi-

[100] *ChLA 2nd ser.*, 65, no. 5, p. 28.

[101] *ChLA 2nd ser.*, 65, no. 5, p. 29, line 24. For the other witnesses, see lines 25–28.

[102] Manaresi, *I placiti del 'regnum Italiae'*, p. 398. For the ambiguity of the term *advocati* see J. Brundage, *The Medieval Origins of the Legal Profession: Canonists, Civilians and Courts* (Chicago, 2008).

nent as the recipient of Adelprandus's donation, but he was designated 'diaconus et medicus' rather than 'presbiter et medicus'.[103] Between 892 and 898 Leoprandus had therefore obviously progressed up the ecclesiastical hierarchy to become a priest. This is significant because Leoprandus is also the only *medicus* I have found to date in the surviving pre-1000 Northern Italian charter evidence who was described as a *presbiter*. By 898 was he a priest attached to a specific church who also practiced medicine among his parishioners, or was he a member of the episcopal household? The scribe placed the attribution 'presbiter' before 'medicus' but to privilege ecclesiastical over secular status is to be expected. However, to progress from deacon to priest Leoprandus would have to have been attached to an ecclesiastical institution of some kind. Whether he remained in the church to continue his medical education, or was a *medicus* who *then* entered holy orders, it is impossible to say. Certainly the two professions do not appear to be incompatible in the eyes of the scribe at least, and by extension presumably also the local community. Whatever Leoprandus's precise role in the community, he was obviously wealthy enough to afford to hire a lawyer.

It would certainly be an over generalization, however, to assume that all or even the majority of *medici* in Piacenza (or elsewhere) in the ninth and tenth centuries were in clerical orders. In Caorso, in what is now the province of Piacenza, in 860 an apparently lay doctor, a 'Iohannes medicus' acted as a witness to a small land transaction. Iohannes was the only *medicus* apart from Gaidoald of Pistoia in the evidence surveyed in this chapter who did not sign his own name. Since none of the witnesses signed their own names, however, it is likely that this relates to scribal practice or, most probably, to the circumstances in which the charter was drawn up rather than being a reliable indicator alone of the literacy or otherwise of the witnesses.

Could You Just Sign This for Me John? The 'Medici' of Lucca

Like Verona in the North East, Lucca, in Tuscany, was an important city in Lombard Italy: it was a ducal seat, and therefore an administrative centre.[104] The bishop of Lucca also played a key — and growing — role in Lombard and Carolingian rule.[105] Lucca is also notable in having more attestations of *medici*

[103] Manaresi, *I Placiti*, p. 398.

[104] Stoffella, 'Crisi e trasformazioni'.

[105] Stoffella, 'Crisi e trasformazioni', especially pp. 5 and 22.

than anywhere else in early medieval Italy North of Rome: three in the second half of the eighth century and five more in just the opening four decades of the ninth century.[106] However, Lucca also has one of the largest and best preserved early medieval charter collections, so it is possible that other major centres had a similar number of *medici* active in the same time period. The big advantage of such a well-preserved collection, though, is that allows us, uniquely, as I shall show, to trace one *medicus* called Iohannes in no less than fourteen charters over the space of twenty-four years.

The first evidence we have of *medici* active in the city is Adelpert, who witnessed a donation for the sake of a certain Alateus's soul in 777 to the church of St Michele, which he himself had built.[107] He signed his own name, although the charter now survives only in a copy. Significantly, he is the only witness who identifies himself by his profession, and he would appear to be a lay medicus.

He was obviously not the only *medicus* active in the city during this period, as a Wito 'clericus et medicus' is mentioned in two documents in 788 and 797.[108] In the first, he is mentioned only in passing in relation to the location of various parcels of land being sold, and described simply as a 'clericus'.[109] In the 797 charter it is his son, Autchis who is witnessing a donation to the church of St Salvatore in Lucca: he is described as 'filio Witi clerici medici' to distinguish him from another Autchis in the same charter.[110] What is surprising, however, is that the son does not sign his own name, but merely makes his mark. Being the son of a clerical *medicus* is therefore no guarantee of even basic writing skills in offspring. Neither does Autchis appear to have followed his father into a career in either the Church or medicine. An Autpertus 'clericus et medicus' does himself witness two documents, one in 786 and a second in 811.[111] Both

[106] 777 Adelpert medicus, *ChLA*, 36, no. 1059; 786–811 Autpertus clericus et medicus, *ChLA*, 38, no. 1102 and *ChLA 2nd ser.*, 73, no. 39; 788–97 Wito clericus et medicus, *ChLA*, 40, no. 1162 and *ChLA*, 38, no. 1117; 816–40 Iohannes clericus et medico (*sic*) *ChLA 2nd ser.*, 74, nos 17, 27 and 43 (see p. 146 on discussion whether it is Iohannes' signature where he signs himself without the qualifier medico); *ChLA 2nd ser.*, 75, nos 6, 11, 12, 21, 22, 29, *ChLA 2nd ser.*, 76, nos 3 and 34, *ChLA 2nd ser.*, 77, nos 1, 4 and 34; 824 Gunpertus medicus *ChLA 2nd ser.*, 75, no. 30; 831–43 Bonifridus clericus et medicus *ChLA 2nd ser.*, 76, no. 31; *ChLA 2nd ser.*, 77, no. 49; *ChLA 2nd ser.*, 78, no. 12.

[107] *ChLA*, 36, no. 1059, p. 51 line 14.

[108] *ChLA*, 38, no. 1117 and *ChLA*, 40, no. 1162.

[109] *ChLA*, 38, no. 1117, p. 70, line 6.

[110] *ChlA*, 40, no. 1162, p. 23 line 16.

[111] *ChLA*, 38, no. 1102 and *ChLA 2nd ser.*, 73, no. 39.

charters concern donations. The witnesses of the 786 charter are predominately clerical, and all but two sign their own names.[112] In the second charter, Lucca, Archivio arcivescovile, Diplomatico, no. 390 (++K16), an original written on 15 August 811, the main protagonist is a layman.[113] A certain Odolpertus had built on his land a church dedicated to Jesus Christ and the Virgin Mary and he now wished to endow it with land and houses. Odolpertus and his heirs reserved the right, however, to nominate a priest to serve at the church and to pray for the founder and his family. The charter was witnessed by five men including Autpertus as well as the donor and the notary. Unusually, all involved in this transaction sign their own names, albeit with varying degrees of finesse. The lay donor of this charter, Odolpertus, wrote in a large untidy hand that was either quite unpractised or a bit shaky due to age or infirmity. He is followed by the priest Rachiprandus (*presbyter* of the church concerned, perhaps?), the layman Vuiliprandus, followed by Autpertus, who identified himself as a 'clericus et medicus' and two further laymen, Ilmerandus and Lanfridus. The notary, another Richiprandus, was a sub-deacon.

What do these two charters therefore tell us about the social circles in which Autpertus was moving? Of all the witnesses it was arguably the *medicus* Autpertus who in either charter wrote in the most careful, practiced hand, correctly using ligatures such as 'te', 'ri', and 'et'.[114] Like the other witnesses, he wrote in a pre-carolingian Italian minuscule and therefore appears to have been educated in the region rather than North of the Alps, but, to judge the quality of the script, to a higher standard than some of the other witnesses. Autpertus also identified himself as a 'clericus', a general term that indicates that he was enrolled in the lower orders of the church, in what capacity exactly we do not know. Unlike many charters, there does not appear to be any family relationship in either charter between the donor and witnesses. We have to assume, therefore, that the witnesses, including Autpertus, were, in the case of the 811 charter, either neighbours or friends of Odolpertus. Autpertus may therefore have lived nearby and/or been the local doctor. In the case of the 786 charter since the majority of those involved were clergy, perhaps the link was more ecclesiastically based. In both charters the fact that virtually all protagonists/witnesses could sign their own names indicates that all were of at least middling status. Odolpertus, the donor in the 811 charter, was obviously wealthy enough

[112] *ChLA*, 38, no. 1102, p. 28, lines 33–37.

[113] *ChLA*, 38, no. 1102, and *ChLA 2nd ser.*, 73, no. 39, pp. 130–32.

[114] *ChLA 2nd ser.*, 73, no. 39, p. 130.

to build and endow a church, but the endowment was relatively modest and he could therefore be characterized as comfortably off rather than enormously wealthy. It is in such circles that our *medicus* Autpertus was moving.

The Lucchese cleric and *medicus* Bonifridus may have been moving in slightly more influential circles, possibly connected with the bishop: in 831 he signed what was effectively a rental agreement.[115] In return for presenting the bishopric's representative with a quarter of the harvest (including wine) *per annum*, Bonifridus, for as long as he lived, obtained the usufruct on a house with courtyard, and land and other properties at *Colonna di Buriano*, near what is now the Tuscan coastal town of Castiglione della Pescaia, in the Maremma.[116] He signed the charter in a clear, rounded and confident hand, using abbreviations for 'clericus', 'cartulam', 'subscripsi', and the ligatures 'et' and 'ct'.[117] All the other witnesses were able to sign their own names and included a 'scavinus' (Carolingian legal official) called Donusdei.[118] In 841 he sublet another property and land in Cune which he himself had received from Bishop Berengarius.[119] Business presumably continued to be good as in 843 Bonifridus bought outright, for the sum of a hundred *soldi*, a further house and lands in Vacculi: his retirement plan, perhaps?[120]

Over two decades earlier, but also in Lucca, on the 9 July 817 the priest Gumprandus was, like Odolpertus above, making arrangements for the church he had founded, this time dedicated to the saints Martin and George.[121] Another connection between Odolpertus's and Gumprandus's charters is that both were witnessed by the priest Rachiprandus, who appears to have been a popular witness for Lucchese charters.[122] Otherwise, the witnesses were different, but again were a mixture of laymen and ecclesiastics: Fluripertus, Floripandus, and Daiprandus appear to have been from the laity, and no profession is given, while Gunfridus was a cleric and Periteus the brother of the

[115] Lucca, Archivio arcivescovile, Diplomatico, no. 534 (*E 87), *ChLA 2nd ser.*, 76, no. 31, pp. 114–17.

[116] *ChLA 2nd ser.*, 76, no. 31, p. 115, n. 2.

[117] *ChLA 2nd ser.*, 76, no. 31, p. 117, line 24.

[118] *ChLA 2nd ser.*, 76, no. 31, p. 117, line 31.

[119] *ChLA 2nd ser.*, 77, no. 49 pp. 150–51.

[120] *ChLA 2nd ser.*, 78, no. 12, pp. 41–42.

[121] Lucca, Archivio arcivescovile, Diplomatico no. 428 (+N 26), *ChLA 2nd ser.*, 74, no. 27 pp. 99–101.

[122] *ChLA 2nd ser.*, 73, nos 5, 25 and 35.

donor.[123] Gunfridus and Periteus were descendents of Sundipert, brother of the Lucchese bishop after whom Periteus was named: Stoffella argues that charters are significant in that they show how elites and their families sought to regroup and form new associations in the new, post-Lombard era as part of the Carolingian Empire.[124] Among these a certain Iohannes signed himself as 'clericus et medico' (*sic*). Fluripertus and Periteus did not sign their own names, but otherwise all other witnesses are present and literate. In Iohannes' case, his letters were simply but competently formed.

What is particularly striking, however, is that this *medicus* Iohannes appears to have been something of a 'professional' witness since he appears in up to thirteen other surviving Lucchese charters between 816 and 840, several with connections to the episcopate of Lucca.[125] In two of these, however, Iohannes only signed himself as 'clericus' without the qualifier 'et medico' (*sic*).[126] This is a stark reminder that the number of *medici* or indeed any other profession in our documents is entirely dependant on both scribal customs and also perhaps on how a witness felt like describing themselves on a particular day (or in a particular social context). It is significant however, that the witnesses in the two charters where Iohannes did not identify himself as a *medicus* (listed in italics in the chart) were overwhelmingly lay, whereas in the other charters he was involved in there was a stronger clerical presence in the witness list. This suggests that Iohannes was consciously deploying two versions of occupational identity. The use of the qualifiers 'clericus' and 'clericus et medico' allowed Iohannes to distinguish himself, both practically (in the absence of surnames in this period) but also socially, from the other witnesses. It is also possible that his medical status was relevant in those charters where he signed himself 'clericus et medico' because the witnesses or protagonists included patients or employers of Iohannes.

Certainly there are a cluster of individuals who appeared in more than one charter alongside Iohannes who may have been colleagues or perhaps even friends or patients (see Table 3). The notary Gundelprandus was scribe for two of the charters Iohannes witnesses, and was a witness himself for another in

[123] *ChLA 2nd ser.*, 74, no. 27, p. 102.

[124] Stoffella, 'Crisi e trasformazioni', pp. 28 and 29.

[125] *ChLA 2nd ser.*, 74, no. 17 and probably also no. 43 (see p. 146 on this point); *ChLA 2nd ser.*, 75, nos 6, 11 12, 21, 22, 29; *ChLA 2nd ser.*, 76, nos 3 and 34; *ChLA 2nd ser.*, 77, nos 1, 4 and 34.

[126] *ChLA 2nd ser.*, 74, nos 17 and 43.

Table 3. Iohannes' social circle.

	Iohannes clericus et medicus	Gundel-prandus notarius	Petrus Bishop of Lucca	Anspald clericus	Petrus clericus notarius
April 816 no. 17	Witness				
July 817 no. 27	Witness	Scribe			
Sept 819 no. 43	Witness	Witness			
Sept 821 no. 6	Witness		Leaser	Witness	Scribe
6 Dec 822 no. 11	Witness			Witness	
16 Dec 822 no. 12	Witness		Gives permission for exchange		Witness
Nov 823 no. 21	Witness		Leaser		
Jan 824 no. 22	Witness	Scribe			Witness
April 824 no. 29	Witness		Leaser		Scribe
4 Feb 827 no. 3	Witness		Buyer	Witness	
30 Oct 832 no. 34	Witness				Scribe

Table 4. Status of principal protagonists of charters involving the *medicus* Iohannes.

	Status Seller/donor/leaser	Status Recipient/buyer/leasee
April 816 no. 17	Bishop	Church
July 817 no. 27	Priest	Lay
Sept 819 no. 43	Priest	Lay
Sept 821 no. 6	Bishop	Church
6 Dec 822 no. 11	Priest	Lay
16 Dec 822 no. 12	Bishop	Lay
Nov 823 no. 21	Bishop	Lay
Jan 824 no. 22	Priest	Lay
April 824 no. 29	Bishop	Bishop
4 Feb 827 no. 3	Priest	Church
Oct 832 no. 34	Cleric	Church
8 May 835 no. 1	Cleric	Undefined
9 June 836 no. 4	Deacon	Bishop
28 Jan 839–27 Jan 840 no. 34	Priest	

which Iohannes was involved.[127] This in itself may be coincidence, given that Gundelprandus was a Lucchese notary and Iohannes a fairly regular witness. However, the more marked corollaries are between Iohannes, a cleric and notary called Petrus, and Bishop Petrus of Lucca. The Petrus who identified himself as 'clericus notarius' was scribe for three of the charters Iohannes signed, and also witness for two more alongside the *medicus*.[128] Petrus appears to have been a notary closely associated with the episcopal see of Lucca. All the charters he drew up involved either the Bishop himself, or priests/clergy.[129] He was also the scribe for the *medicus* and *clericus* Bonifridus's charter of 831, discussed above. Further, the majority of charters where Petrus *clericus notarius* acted as a witness involved the bishopric either directly or indirectly as several involve the baptismal church of St Maria di Sesto.[130]

Significantly, of the five charters involving Bishop Petrus of Lucca and Iohannes, at three of these the notary and cleric Petrus was also present, twice as a scribe and once as a witness (see Table 3). An Anspald cleric also appeared in three charters with Iohannes, two of which, written in September 821 and February 827, also involved the two Petrus's.[131] With the exception of Gundelprandus, therefore, all the participants who appear in more than one charter with Iohannes were clergy. Apart from the Bishop, however, Anspald, Iohannes and the other Petrus were all in lower clerical orders. Only Anspald did not combine being a *clericus* with being a *notarius* or *medicus* like Iohannes and Petrus.[132] A bishop would have had several clergy working for him at the

[127] July 817, *ChLA 2nd ser.*, 74, no. 27; January 824, *ChLA 2nd ser.*, 75, no. 22; September 819, *ChLA 2nd ser.*, 74, no. 43 (witness).

[128] September 821, *ChLA 2nd ser.*, 75, no. 6; December 822, *ChLA 2nd ser.*, 75, no. 12 (witness); October 832, *ChLA 2nd ser.*, 76, no. 34; January 824, *ChLA 2nd ser.*, 75, no. 22 (witness); April 824, *ChLA 2nd ser.*, 75, no. 29.

[129] *ChLA 2nd ser.*, no. 49; *ChLA 2nd ser.*, 75, nos 9, 10, 11, 19, 24, 27, 28, 37, 38, 40, 43, 45.

[130] *ChLA 2nd ser.*, 75, nos 5, 12, 16, 22, 31, 46, 47. The priests of Baptismal churches were chosen by the *populus* but were attached to the bishopric and paid tax to the episcopacy. Langeli argues, however, that there was a danger of them slipping into lay control. Perhaps one way to prevent this was have a clerical notary such as Petrus witness charters relating to the church to maintain control? See C. Azarra, 'Ecclesiastical Institutions', in *Italy in the Early Middle Ages, 476–1000*, ed. by C. La Rocca (Oxford, 2002), pp. 85–101 (pp. 92–93).

[131] Sept 821, *ChLA 2nd ser.*, 75, no. 6. Anspald is another serial witness — he also witnesses charter numbers 5, 7, 26, 28 and 39 in the same volume.

[132] An Anspald, cleric and lawyer (*advocatus*) for the bishopric crops up in a charter of 820 at Lucca, but since he does not sign this, we have no way of knowing of this is the same Anspald or not. See *ChLA 2nd ser.*, 74, no. 49, p. 164.

episcopal palace: should we see Iohannes, Anspald, and Petrus as part of this retinue? Certainly some connection between these four men is possible but what that link was exactly is difficult to know for sure: it is even conceivable that they trained together.

If we put aside the witnesses and turn to the status of the main protagonists in the charters Iohannes witnesses, for one half of the transactions, one principal protagonist was lay, the other clerical or a church. The other half of the transactions listed were exclusively ecclesiastic (see Table 4). It might be assumed from this that Iohannes was primarily moving in, and connected with, clerical circles. However, he invariably signed as a witness for the lay leasee or donor. Further, critically, the early medieval charters which have survived have done so largely because the land they relate to came into episcopal or monastic hands at some point in its history. Therefore, although some exclusively early medieval Italian lay charters survive which document land that was only given to the Church at a later stage, the majority involve representatives of churches, bishoprics, or monasteries. In the case of Lucca, the early medieval charters were preserved in the episcopal archives.[133] This may very well explain the frequency with which the Bishops of Lucca appear in the charters Iohannes witnessed.[134]

Was Iohannes perhaps popular as a witness because he had links in both clerical and lay circles, and indeed, epitomizes the 'fuzziness' of boundaries between the two? After all, many families compromised a mixture of lay and clerical, and sometimes monastic members, and as these charters show, transactions were frequent. It could of course be argued that Iohannes was called primarily as a clerical witness: if that is how he saw himself, however, there would have been no need for him to add the qualifier 'medico'. Alternatively, rather than simply being chosen, did he himself also actively seek to witness at least one charter a year in order to cultivate new or existing clients?

If this is the case, was this an unusual strategy or was he a particularly in-demand witness, whether because of his possible episcopal connections or professional standing? It is certainly possible that there was something unusual about Iohannes' witnessing activities, as the two other doctors appearing in early ninth-century Lucchese charters, Autpertus and Gunpertus were attested only once each. In the case of Autpertus, he signed himself, similarly to

[133] Bartoli Langeli, 'Private Charters', p. 206.

[134] Apart from Bishop Petrus, the name of his predecessor Bishop Iocabus appears in the very first charter for which we have Iohannes' signature. See Lucca, April 816, *ChLA 2nd ser.*, 74, no. 17.

Iohannes, as 'clericus et medicus'.[135] This is some five years before Iohannes witnessed his first surviving charter. Interestingly, though, Gunpertus witnessed a charter, like Iohannes, in April 824 in Lucca. Further, like many of the charters Iohannes signs, the charter concerned was a leasehold agreement between the bishopric and one Agimondo.[136] Unlike Iohannes, however, Gunpertus gave no clerical status: he simply signed himself as 'medicus'. Further, his hand is described by the editors of *Chartae Latinae antiquiores* as 'a simple script, uncertainly drawn', whereas Iohannes' was 'sufficiently expert'.[137] Even within the same decade in the same city, therefore, the training, education and social circles in which *medici* were circulating could differ, and there is no straight trajectory from lay to clerical *medici* either.

For example, as the cleric and *medicus* Iohannes' witnessing career was drawing to a close, an apparently lay *medicus*, Auripertus's, begins, again in Lucca: he is involved in five legal transactions between 838 and 849,[138] His signs with a practiced hand, but we can only speculate as to precisely where and how he received his training.[139]

Conclusions: The Origins, Training, and Status of 'Medici' in Early Medieval Northern Italy

The evidence is often frustratingly elusive and fluid due to the divergence of scribal practice which can have such a dramatic impact both on the number of *medici* included and whether an ecclesiastical designation was noted or not. The numbers of cited medical practitioners are also relatively small compared to the thousands of witnesses, donors and recipients recorded in the charter and judgement evidence: I have found nineteen to date in published pre-tenth-century Northern and Central Italian records of legal transactions. This might be seen as supporting Baader's gloomy assumptions about the state of medi-

[135] *ChLA 2nd ser.*, 73, no. 39, p. 131.

[136] *ChLA 2nd ser.*, 75, no. 30, p. 107.

[137] 'Una scrittura semplice a tratta incerta', *ChLA 2nd ser.*, 75, no. 30, p. 106; 'sufficientemente esperta', *ChLA 2nd ser.*, 75, no. 29, p. 104.

[138] 838, *ChLA 2nd ser.*, 75, no. 20; January and April 844, *ChLA 2nd ser.*, 76, nos 19 and 28; 847 and 849, *ChLA 2nd ser.*, 77, nos 25 and 43.

[139] A. Castagnetti discusses Auripertus's career in more detail, including a possible later imperial link — see A. Castagnetti, 'Medici nella Tuscia Longobarda e Carolingia', *Studi Storici Luigi Simeoni*, 62 (2012), 19–32 (pp. 28–31).

cine and healthcare in early medieval Europe.[140] However, as an elite trade one would not expect to find hundreds, and as I have shown above, quite apart from the loss of many charters and judgements, *medici* are likely to have been 'under-reported' in documents where statuses were rarely or irregularly given. Given these important caveats, nineteen is, in early medieval terms, a significant number. Unlike Southern Italy, all the doctors attested in the surviving charters were Christian males.[141]

Perhaps most strikingly, though, nowhere in the charter or other legal evidence for early medieval Northern Italy did the term 'monachus et medicus' ever appear. This supports Zettler's work in the late 1990s.[142] He demonstrates, even for the evidence in what is now Switzerland — on which the argument for the early medieval *Monchsarzt* is often principally based — that those *medici* in monastic *Books of Memory* do not appear in the corresponding lists of monks' professions to a life of chastity, poverty, and obedience. Therefore their designation as monk-doctors is not borne out by the evidence. This is not to say that large monasteries did not have monks who practiced medicine (and yet whom may not have characterized themselves as *medici*). Conversely *medici* could conceivably be attached to, or even living at, their institution, but they might not actually have been fully-professed monks. After all, there is a separate doctor's house towards the edge of the enclosure on the ambitious plan for the famous monastery of St Gallen in present day Switzerland which indicates that the *medicus*, whatever their status, did not necessarily live communally with the other monks, and therefore may have been a *clericus* or *presbyter* rather than a fully fledged monk.[143]

140 Baader, 'Early Medieval Latin Adaptations'.

141 See the appearance of a female lay *medica* called Anna from Balusano in Naples in a charter of 923: *Regesta Neapolitana*, in *Monumenta ad Neapolitani Ducatus Historiam Pertinentia*, ed. by B. Capasso, 2 vols (Napoli, 1881–92), III, doc. 23. The son of the Jewish *medicus* Jude appears in a Salernitan charter of 1004, and Jewish doctors were recorded in Amalfi, and, to the South East, Bari: B. Kreutz, *Before the Normans: Southern Italy in the Ninth and Tenth Centuries* (Philadelphia, 1991), p. 145l, *Codex Cavensis* IV, doc. 567; N. Ferorelli, *Gli Ebrei nell'Italia meridionale dall'eta romana al'secolo XVIII* (Torino, 1915), p. 39; A. Sharf, *The Universe of Shabbetai Donnolo* (Warminster, 1976), all cited in Skinner, *Health and Medicine*, p. 81.

142 A. Zettler, 'Exkurs1: zu den Klosterärzten', in *Das Totengedenken der Abtei: Necrologien und Kommemorierte Personen*, ed. by R. Rappmann (Sigmaringen, 1998), pp. 265–78.

143 P. Jung, 'Das Infirmarium im Bauriss des Klosters von St. Gallen vom Jahre 820', *Gesnerus*, 6.1/2 (1949), 1–8.

Of the nineteen attested *medici* I have found to date in the printed pre-900 AD charter evidence for the Italian peninsula north of Rome, eight were also clergy, although with the exception of Leoprandus at the end of the ninth century, all were in lower clerical orders.[144] Could this be a clue as to where at least some of Northern Italy's early medieval doctors were getting their training? Even if monasteries were not home to numerous monk-doctors, they could still provide, particularly at the larger institutions, high-level education, including medical teaching. Certainly monasteries in all areas of Italy, like their counterparts throughout Europe, were assiduously copying everything from large scale Classical and late antique medical texts to simple herbal recipes scribbled on manuscript flyleaves.[145] The central debate is whether education within monasteries was exclusively for monks, or whether, in certain circumstances, it extended to secular clergy or others not intending to take monastic vows. Hildebrandt, in his 1992 monograph on external schools in Carolingian monasteries, argues that first of all clarity is needed on what an external school was: are we looking at a physical building outside or on the edge of the monastery, or within it but for those without a monastic vocation?[146] Hildebrandt also suggests that oblates, those children dedicated to the monastery, and non-oblates, could have been taught in the same building, but possibly at different times.[147] Therefore the type of student as well as the available buildings, are key to this debate. Much attention has focused on the monastery of St Gallen, since on the famous plan attributed to the monastery, a school with residential accommodation was clearly indicated in the outer ring of monastic buildings. Since oblates and monks had their own accommodation within the monastery, Hildebrandt argues that this was a school for those who were not, nor intending to be, monks.[148] This is despite the early ninth-century directive from the Synod of Aachen that monasteries should not teach external pupils.[149] It could therefore be argued that the call was ignored, but the reputation and status of St Gallen

[144] Isidore of Seville, *The Etymologies of Isidore of Seville*, trans. by S. Barney and others (Cambridge, 2006), VII.12, p. 170.

[145] See chapter 3.

[146] M. M. Hildebrandt, *The External School in Carolingian Society* (Leiden, 1992), pp. 2–3 and 6.

[147] Hildebrandt, *The External School*, pp. 2–3. On child oblates see M. de Jong, *In Samuel's Image: Child Oblation in the Early Medieval West* (Leiden, 1996).

[148] Hildebrandt, *The External School*, pp. 9–10.

[149] Hildebrandt, *The External School*, pp. 8 and 12.

may have meant it was a special case. In the reign of Louis the Pious the focus shifted towards episcopal schools, and one of his son Lothar's tasks in Italy was to develop education in the kingdom.[150]

Perhaps reflecting this general trend in the first half of the ninth century, there is evidence that the teaching of medical knowledge may have taken place outside a monastic context: an 805 Carolingian capitulary at Thoinville orders the teaching of 'physica' at cathedral schools in the Empire.[151] 'Physica' is translated as 'natural philosophy', which could be interpreted as theoretical texts about the workings of the natural world rather than the practice of medicine. However, in a mid-ninth-century letter from Bischop Ermenrich of Passau to abbot Grimald of St Gallen, 'physica' is divided into the study of 'arithmeticam, astronomiam, astrologiam, mechanitiam, medicinam, geometricam, musicam'.[152] We do not know of course exactly what was taught in the section of the curriculum on medicine, or to what extent the capitulary on the teaching of *physica* in cathedral schools was implemented in Northern Italy (or indeed was already underway in this region before 805). We do know that schools for the clergy existed in places such as Verona, Pavia, and Arezzo.[153] At such schools, however, teaching may have been far more modest, aimed at providing clergy only with the necessary knowledge of their faith in order to carry out their duties in churches effectively.[154] If this was the case, however, where were clerics such as Autpertus or Iohannes of Lucca, literate and well-thought-of enough in the city to be called as witnesses on a regular basis, being educated? Further, as discussed above, should we envisage them as attached to the episcopal palace or a specific church, and who were their patients, other clergy and/or the laity?

What arguably lay behind the 817 directive against the education of 'externs', that is laymen and the secular clergy, in monasteries, however, is the liminality of clerics: they were part of the ecclesiastical hierarchy, but not bound to a life of either poverty or chastity, despite the Church's strenuous and ongoing efforts throughout the Middle Ages to enforce the latter.[155] Even outside a monastic

[150] Riche, 'L'école', p. 572, and Hildebrandt, *The External School*, pp. 66–67.

[151] C. Brunner, *Über Medizin und Krankenpflege im Mittelalter in Schweizerischen Landen* (Zürich, 1922), p. 6.

[152] MGH Epistola, 5, p. 541 cited in Brunner, p. 6.

[153] M. Pavan, *La crisi della Scuola del IV secolo d.C* (Bari, 1952), p. 558.

[154] On this point see Riche, 'L'école', p. 572.

[155] Hildebrandt, *The External School*, p. 29. R. Reynolds, *Clerics in the Early Middle Ages: Hierarchy and Image* (Aldershot, 1999), particularly 'Clerics in the Early Middle Ages: Hierarchies and Functions', pp. 1–31.

context, however, there was ongoing concern from Carolingian rulers about educating and above all, controlling, the secular clergy. Part of Carolingian ecclesiastical reforms involved encouraging clergy to live communally if not a parish priest.[156] Communal life for clergy was an ancient idea in Christianity, but was pursued with renewed vigour by the Carolingians.[157] In line with this, several capitularies sought to combat the perceived problem of the wandering cleric, suggesting that many enjoyed more freedom of movement than either monarch or ecclesiastical hierarchy felt was desirable.[158] The chief fear appears to have been the possibility that such 'stray' clerics could spread heresy.[159] There was also concern about who was to pay for the education and support of the clergy: in 826 Pope Eugenius decreed that more clergy should not be ordained than could be supported: did the practice of medicine by some clerics ease this situation?[160]

[156] For example, one topic of an Italian capitulary from *c.* 780–90 AD was on how priests and clergy should live according to the norms of the early Church fathers: 'ut sacerdotes et clericus secundum normam priorum patrum vivant', *Capitularia regum Francorum*, I, no. 89, p. 189, p. 370. This was expanded and made much more specific in the Council of 826, presided over by Pope Eugenius II, in which it is envisaged that clergy would have a single refectory and dormitory: 'ubi clerici consistere debeant. Necessaria etenim res existit, ut iuxta ecclesiam claustra constituantur, in quibus clerici disciplines eclesiasticis vacant; itaque omnibus unum sit refectorium ac dormitorium, seu ceterae officinae ad usus clericorum necessariae.' *Capitularia regum Francorum*, I, no. 180, p. 873. On reform and education in general see: R. McKitterick, *The Frankish Church and the Carolingian Reforms 789–895* (Cambridge, 1977); S. Keefe, *Water and the Word: Baptism and the Education of the Clergy in the Carolingian Empire*, 2 vols (Notre Dame, IN, 2002); J. Bertram, *The Chrodegang Rules: The Rules for the Common Life of the Secular Clergy from the Eighth and Ninth Centuries* (Aldershot, 2005).

[157] M. Claussen, *The Reform of the Frankish Church: Chrodegang of Metz and the 'Regula canonicorum' in the Eighth Century* (Cambridge, 2004), pp. 2 and 12–15. See also Bertram, *The Chrodegang Rules*, pp. 1–2.

[158] 'De clericis: nequaquam de ecclesia ad aliam ecclesiam transmigrentur neque recipiantur sine conscientia episcope et litteras commendatitias de cuius diocesia fuerunt, ne forte discordia exinde veniat in ecclesia.' Frankfurt synod 794, *Capitularia regum Francorum*, I, no. 27, p. 76. See also, in the same volume, no. 35, p. 102 which aims to ensure that: 'clerici de civitate ad civitatem non transmigrentur', and no. 93, p. 196, *Capitulare mantuanum secundum, generale*. '2. ut clerici seu monachi vagantes, siue de ipsa parrochia seu aliunde supervenientes, sine consensus episcope a nemine suscipiantur.'

[159] 'Quidam clericorum vel monachorum peregrinantes per diversas vagando provincias et civitates multiplices spargunt errores et inutiles questiones disseminant decipientes corda simplicium.' *Capitularia regum Francorum*, II, p. 122, ch. 21.

[160] Hildebrandt, *The External School*, p. 63.

Whatever the case, for a cleric who was also a *medicus*, the potential for independent practice was clear, and clerical *medici* should therefore perhaps be seen as doubly liminal, poised between the ecclesiastical and lay world. From the pre-900 charter evidence in Northern and Central Italy, although there appears, in the case of Bonifridus and possibly also Iohannes of Lucca, some connection between these *medici* and the bishopric, it is never made explicit, nor do clerical *medici* appear, in the charter evidence which has survived at least, to be attached to a specific church. Further, as mentioned above, apart from the *presbyter-medicus* Leoprandus in Piacenza in 898, all the other attested clerical *medici* in Central and Northern Italy before this date signed themselves using the general term 'clericus', that is, as mentioned above, someone who was identified, or identified themselves as one of those in the myriad lower orders of the Church (such as *lector* or *cantor*).[161] As such they may have been attached to a bishop's palace or church but also possibly — Carolingian reforms not withstanding — lived not communally but in their own house in the local community or attached to a church. The Lucchese cleric and *medicus* Bonifridus is known to us, as discussed above, not least through a charter of 831 in which he leased land and property from the bishop: was this as a reward for loyal service, a sign of his status in the local community, or in order to provide him with a place to live? Was his further acquisition in 843 of a house and property an investment or alternative/replacement home?

We should surely therefore consider the possibility that clerical *medici* had obtained at least part of their education at a monastic or more probably episcopal school, but then lived in individual houses, whether provided by the bishopric or independently, and tended to the community as a whole, not just to other clerics. At least one attested clerical *medicus*, Adellardus of Piacenza, had a family and presumably also owned property, since a son called Adremundus, a *presbyter*, sold a house in 864. The origins of the clergy practicing medicine as a profession rather than just a Christian duty, about which the 1130 Church Council of Clermont was so concerned, may therefore have had deep roots in early medieval Italy.[162]

[161] Bertram, *The Chrodegang Rules*, pp. 4–5.

[162] Mansi, *Sacrorum conciliorum*, 21:438 'Prava autem consuetude, prout accepimus, et detestabilis inolevit, quoniam monachi et regulares canonici post susceptum habitum et professionem factam, spreta bonorum magistrorum Benedicti et Augustini regula, leges temporales et medicinam gratia lucri temporali addiscunt [...].' translation in D. W. Amundsen, 'Medieval Canon Law on Medical and Surgical Practice by the Clergy', *Bulletin of the History of Medicine*, 52 (1978), 22–44 (p. 28).

The fact remains, though, that over half of attested *medici* in pre-tenth-century Northern and Central Italy were apparently lay. While they may have obtained some education from episcopal or even monastic schools, it is likely that they principally received apprenticeship-style training with established *medici*. This may explain why Gunpertus's script was less assured than his clerical colleagues in Lucca, for example. However, several apparently lay *medici*, from Rotcaus in Asti to Ragibertus in Verona, wrote with confidence. Further, how do we know that clerical *medici* were not receiving a similar training? In this respect, training may have changed less from the Roman period than might be assumed: Riddle points out that the majority of Roman doctors were trained via apprenticeships.[163]

Indeed, the principal change for doctors between the Roman and post-Roman period, I argue, was not so much the method of training as their status in local communities and the way in which they were perceived. As we have seen in chapter four, there was relatively little criticism of doctors in hagiographical literature. Further, the charter evidence discussed in this chapter clearly demonstrates the respect with which they were held in their local communities, although we cannot be sure whether this was due to their medical skills or status as educated men. With the exception of the royal physician Gaidoald, all the *medici* involved in charter transactions in early medieval Northern Italy were definitely able to write, at least to the point of being able to sign their own names. Therefore in early medieval terms they should be counted in the ranks of the educated elite, however they obtained this education. In terms of status, Gaidoald stands at the pinnacle as doctor to Lombard kings, and has the wealth to found and endow, however modestly, ecclesiastical institutions. As for the other *medici*, the fact that they were called as witnesses at all signifies their standing in the local community, but the status of other participants in the charters suggests that in general *medici* moved in modestly well-off circles — which presumably include their paying patients — within their immediate locality rather than on a grander stage. Participating in charters may indeed have been one way for early medieval Northern Italian *medici* to cement their relationship with existing patients or to raise their profile to acquire new clients. Before the age of doctors' notes or certificates proving qualifications or training, doctors were defined and validated by the communities in which they worked.

[163] J. Riddle, 'Theory and Practice in Medieval Medicine', *Viator*, 5 (1974), 157–84 (p. 159).

Conclusion

It is a well-worn truism that everything in life is relative. This is particularly apt for the source material for early medieval Europe — in comparison to our High Medieval or Early Modern colleagues our haul of original charters, letters, manuscripts, or physical artefacts or remains will always be poor. Early medievalists have no choice but to drain every possible drop of significance out of the source material they have, however unpromising it might at first appear! However, when comparing the quantity, quality, and range of sources between regions or kingdoms for the early Middle Ages, it is undeniable that the Italian peninsula has an embarassment of riches. Hundreds of original charters, from the sixth century onwards, is a haul Anglo-Saxonists could only dream about, for example. Similarly, the ability to compare multiple law codes, all, ostensibly at least, in force in one geographical region simultaneously, is a unique resource.

The key question, therefore, is whether the picture of healthcare and medicine in early medieval Italy North of Rome which I have outlined in this book is unique, or follows a pattern that would have been repeated across Western Europe, surviving sources allowing. Certainly one would expect many similarities, given that Western late antique and medieval medicine all followed the same basic ancient precepts and theories, albeit with Old English recipes and traditions thrown in for Anglo-Saxon England.[1] Furthermore, even given the difficulties of travel in the early Middle Ages, men, women, goods, and ideas moved with surprisingly frequency across physical and political boundaries. After 774 AD much of Italy was unified, politically at least, with the Carolingian Empire north of the Alps. Yet, we do not see any marked change in approach with regard to health, illness, or the way doctors were portrayed after this date.

[1] A good overview is A. Meaney, 'The Practice of Medicine in England about the Year 1000', *Social History of Medicine*, 13 (2000), 221–37.

This would suggest that medical traditions and attitudes to health were relatively little affected by a change in political overlords.

Indeed, as I have shown in Chapter one, despite differences in emphasis, lawmakers from all traditions on the peninsula — Roman, Lombard, and Ostrogothic — sought, however ineffectually, to integrate and protect the sick and impaired in society. The backbone of early medieval treatments in Northern Italy, though, as surely was also the case elsewhere throughout Western Europe, were the innumerable medical and herbal recipes copied everywhere from psalter flyleaves to large compendia. What is less clear is to what extent this represents a hidden oral transmission of such recipes, or, in contrast, was a separate learned tradition. Certainly, whatever the comprehensibility and literacy issues, many of the remedies, from Italy to Anglo-Saxon England, could have been made in the more affluent home, albeit by someone with experience who could fill in for themselves any gaps in some of the recipes with regard to quantities, plant identification or techniques.

In contrast, surgery, even by 'experts' was considered with trepidation by most medical writers and probably patients alike. Texts discussing surgery were far less numerous, again a trend reflected more broadly in Europe, learned anatomical texts excepted, and even treatises on bleeding were not perhaps quite as ubiquitous as might be assumed.[2] On the other hand, it is not hard to see why dietitic advice remained enduringly popular both sides of the Alps: it was an non-invasive, cost-effective method of both preventing and treating illness. I therefore analysed archaeological and archeo-botanical data from early medieval Northern Italy in order to provide a context for the dietitic advice and medical recipes. The diet of communities was largely dependent on geographical location and social status rather than dietitic advice, but wealthy individuals and communities (including monasteries) took full advantage of the range of foodstuffs recommended in such texts. The nuns of St Guilia, for example, apparently had access to a similar range of food types as that envisaged by the compilers of the St Gallen monastic plan in what is now Switzerland. Status was arguably the key factor in diet, not geographical location or political affiliation.

For the poor, on the other hand, the precise location of a settlement was vital, and diet could vary from valley to valley, let alone between regions or kingdoms. Basic foodstuffs and accommodation could, however, also be sought at the many *xenodochia* dotted throughout Northern Italy, one of the institu-

[2] On anatomical terminology in early medieval manuscripts, see Glaze, 'The Perforated Wall', pp. 132–43; for a list of pre-twelfth-century medical manuscripts recorded in contemporary library catalogues see Glaze, 'The Perforated Wall', pp. 268–96.

tions I analysed in Part II on people and places of healing. *Xenodochia* were by no means restricted to Italy alone, but were particularly numerous due to the number of pilgrims passing through Northern Italy towards Rome and beyond. The charter and legal evidence suggests, however, that the impact of these hostels was often ineffectual and minimal, and that their revenues were vulnerable to appropriation. They also varied widely in terms of size, degree of organization, and the services they offered: there was a world of difference between a bustling pilgrim-centred hostel in Lucca, for example, and a small rural *xenodochium* converted from a private dwelling. For all the concerns about the physical condition of many *xenodochia* buildings and their often poor or corrupt management, however, *xenodochia* continued to be viewed as an expression of piety and concern for the traveller and needy.

The lay household, in contrast, was a *locus* about which legal, penitential, and other writers felt much more ambivalent. It was where the vast majority of care for the sick took place, and could even contain a household shrine to a particular saint. Simultaneously, however, it was also potentially the location for superstituous and unregulated supernatural and medical practices to aid healing or control fertility. This again would appear to have been a shared European concern. However, although Italy, even today, has an extraordinarily rich hagiographic and architectural religious heritage, many early medieval saints' lives from Northern Italy do not even mention healing. Perhaps ubiquity and familiarity do breed contempt, since the Northern Italian evidence suggests that saints' lives were not usually written to promote healing cults, and that journeys to healing shrines outside the home were a great and unusual event rather than the primary response to illness or impairment. Whether, in this regard, early medieval Italians differed in outlook to their neighbours north of the Alps requires further research.

For those in Northern Italy who could afford it or had an employer prepared to provide it, a doctor (*medicus*) would be called as a first response if home remedies were believed to be indequate or had proved ineffective. This tradition was particularly strong in Italy, perhaps due to its deeply embedded Roman heritage. North of the Alps *medici* can be found in early medieval charter transactions, but much more rarely.[3] In contrast, I have documented

[3] For example, John Contreni found only one mention of a *medicus* in a charter in his study of medicine during the reign of the ninth-century king Charles the Bald, and concluded that educated laymen were the norm. See J. Contreni, 'Masters and Medicine in Northern France during the Reign of Charles the Bald', in *Charles the Bald: Court and Kingdom*, ed. by M. Gibson and J. Nelson (Aldershot, 1990), pp. 267–82.

to date in printed sources alone nineteen *medici* participating in legal transactions between 572 and 900 AD in Northern Italy, of which few have been discussed in any detail previously by historians. Of these, eleven were apparently lay doctors. Thanks to the number of original documents I was also able to demonstrate, principally through examination of original signatures, that all but one were certainly able to write. Some hands were extremely practiced, and although reading and writing were considered separate skills, the majority were likely to have been able to read too.

This therefore provides a whole new context for manuscripts and recipe fragments produced in Northern Italy before 900 AD with which I originally began my research. While the scale and cost of large medical compendiums preclude all but the wealthiest monastic, lay or episcopal owners, this is not necessarily the case for smaller scale manuscripts containing medical material, or where a recipe has been scribbled into the margins of a book.

In early medieval Northern Italian Italy, therefore, it is not the leech, or even the saint, who is king, but the doctor and 'self-help' medical recipes. Potion makers, wisewomen, and local healers are also likely to have been a feature, but evidence is much more scant. I do not believe, however, that we are simply at the mercy of the surviving source material: doctors were prominent in legal transactions throughout early medieval Italy because they were prominent in local society, and many more have become hidden to us if their profession was not recorded by the scribes, or the charters they witnessed no longer survive. In the same way the medical recipes that are still preserved today are only the tip of iceburg, and bear witness to the lively blend of the Classical and the contemporary in early medieval Northern Italy which *do* make it a unique, and uniquely rich, region to study for the history of medicine and healthcare.

Bibliography

Manuscripts and Archival Documents

Barcelona, Biblioteca de la Universidad, 228
Berlin, Deutsche Staatsbibliothek, Hamilton 290
——, Phillipps 1831
Berne, Stadt-und Hochschulbibliothek, Codex A.92 XV
Cesena, Biblioteca Comunale Malatestiana, Codex Sinistro XXI
Città del Vaticano, Biblioteca Apostolica Vaticana, MS Palatini latini 187
——, MS Urbinates latini 293
——, MS Vaticani latini 5751
——, MS Vaticani latini 5763
——, MS Vaticani latini 5951
Darmstadt, Hessiche Landes-u. Hochschulbibliothek, 895
Exeter, Cathedral Library, MS 3519
Firenze, Biblioteca Medicea Laurenziana, Plutei LXXIII codex 1
Halberstadt, Bibliothek des Domgymnasiums, s.n.
Karlsruhe, Badische Landesbibliothek, Cod. Reichenau 120
——, Cod. Reichenau 229
Karlsruhe, Staatsbibliothek, MS Augiensis Pergament 120
——, MS Augiensis Pergament 229
Leiden, Bibliotek der Rijks-Universiteit, Codex Vossiani Latini q. 33
London, British Library, MS Additional 5412
——, MS Harley 5792
Merseburge, Dombibliothek, 103
Milano, Biblioteca Ambrosiana, C105
——, G 108
——, L 28
Modena, Archivio Capitolare, O.I.11

——, O.I.17
München, Bayerische Staatsbibliothek, Codices Latini Monacenses 15028
——, Codices Latini Monacenses 29314
——, Codices Latini Monacenses 3853
Napoli, Biblioteca Nazionale Vittorio Emanuele III, Latin 2
Novara, Biblioteca Capitolare, 18 (LXXI)
Oxford, Bodleian Library, 516 (2570)
Piacenza, Archivio capitolare di S. Antonino, Diplomatico, Atti private, busta 3, n. 370 (formerly C/52)
Paris, Bibliothèque nationale de France, Fonds 2772
——, Fonds 9347
——, Fonds 11219
——, Fonds lat. 1771
——, Fonds nouvelle acquisition latin 281
Sélestat, Bibliothèque municipale, 1 (A)
St Gallen, Stiftsbibliothek, 217
——, 569
——, 751
——, 912
——, 1396
St Petersburg (formerly Leningrad), Saltykov-Scredrin Public Library, MS F.v.I.12
Uppsala, K Universitetsbiblioteket, C. 664 (med. 6)
Vercelli, Biblioteca Capitolare, CXLIII (159)
Verona, Biblioteca Capitolare, LXIII (61)
Wölfenbuttel, Herzog-August Bibliothek, Weissenburg 64

Primary Sources

Acta sanctorum (Brussels, 1643–1940)
Agnellus of Ravenna, *Lectures on Galen's 'De sectis'*, ed. by L. Westerink and others (Buffalo, 1981)
Anthimus, *De observatione ciborum = On the Observance of Foods*, ed. and trans. by M. Grant (Totnes, 1996)
Avitus of Vienne, *Opera*, ed. by R. Peiper, in MGH AA, 6.2 (Berlin, 1883, repr. 1985), pp. 197–294
Benedict of Nursia, *Rule of Benedict*, trans. by C. White (London, 2008)
Caelius Aurelianus, *Akute Krankheiten: Buch I–III; Chronische Krankheiten: Buch IV–V*, ed. by G. Bendz, trans. by I. Pape, 2 vols (Berlin, 1990)
Capitularia regum Francorum, ed. by A. Boretius, MGH Leges sectio, 2, 2 vols (Hannover, 1883); trans. by C. Azzara and P. Moro, eds, *I capitolari italici: storia e diritto della dominazione carolingia in Italia* (Roma, 1998)
Cassiodorus, *Cassiodori Senatoris Variae*, MGH AA, 12, ed. by T. Mommsen, 3 vols (Berlin, 1894; repr. 1981); trans. by S. Barnish, *Cassiodorus: Variae* (Liverpool, 1992)

——, *Variarum Libri XII: De anima*, ed. by A. Fridh (Turnhout, 1973)
Celsus, *De medicina = On Medicine*, trans. by W. G. Spencer, 3 vols (Cambridge, MA, 1935–38)
Chartae Latinae antiquiores, ed. by A. Bruckner and R. Marichal (Olten and Lausanne, 1954–):
Part 25, Italy 6, ed. by A. Bruckner and R. Marichal (1986)
Part 27, Italy 8, ed. by A. Bruckner and R. Marichal (1992)
Part 36, Italy 17, ed. by G. Nicolaj (1990)
Part 38, Italy 19, ed. by M. Palma (1990)
Part 40, Italy 21, ed. by F. Bianchi and M. Palma (1991)
Chartae Latinae Antiquiores, 2nd series, ed. by G. Cavallo and G. Nicolaj (Dietikon-Zurich, 1997–):
Part 54, Italy 26, Ravenna 1, ed. by G. Cavallo and G. Nicolaj (2000)
Part 55, Italy 27, Ravenna 2, ed. by R. Cosma (1999)
Part 56, Italy 28, Piemonte 1, ed. by G. Cavallo and G. Nicolaj (2001)
Part 57, Italy 28, Piemonte 2, ed. by G. Cavallo and G. Nicolaj (2001)
Part 58, Italy 30, Pisa, Volterra, ed. by G. Cavallo and G. Nicolaj (2001)
Part 62, Italy 43, Siena 2, ed. by G. Cavallo and G. Nicolaj (2003)
Part 64, Italy 36, Piacenza 1, ed. by G. Cavallo and G. Nicolaj (2003)
Part 65, Italy 37, Piacenza 2, ed. by C. Mantegna (2004)
Part 67, Italy 39, Piacenza 4, ed. by G. Cavallo and G. Nicolaj (2005)
Part 73, Italy 45, Lucca 2, ed. by G. Cavallo and G. Nicolaj (2003)
Part 74, Italy 46, Lucca 3, ed. by G. Cavallo and G. Nicolaj (2004)
Part 75, Italy 47, Lucca 4, ed. by G. Cavallo and G. Nicolaj (2005)
Part 76, Italy 48, Lucca 5, ed. by G. Cavallo and G. Nicolaj (2007)
Part 77, Italy 49, Lucca 6, ed. by R. Magistrale, C. Gattagrisi and P. Fioretti (2008)
Part 78, Italy 50, Lucca 7, ed. by M. Palma (2009)
Codex Carolinus, in MGH Epistolae, 3, ed. by W. Grundlach (Berlin, 1892; repr. 1994)
Codex Theodosianus, ed. by T. Mommsen and P. Meyer, 3 vols (Berlin, 1905); trans. by C. Pharr, *The Theodosian Code and Novels and the Simondian Constitutions* (Princeton, 1952)
Codice Diplomatico Longobardo, ed. by L. Schiaparelli, 2 vols (Roma, 1929–33)
Codices Latini Antiquiores, ed. by E. A. Lowe (Oxford, 1934–71)
Edictum Theoderici regis, ed. by F. Bluhme, in MGH Leges, 5 (Hannover, 1889; repr. 1987), pp. 145–79
Edictus Rothari, ed. by F. Bluhme, in MGH Leges, 4, ed. by F. Bluhme and A. Boretius (Hannover, 1868; repr. 1984)
Ennodius, *The Life of Saint Epiphanius by Ennodius: A Translation with an Introduction and Commentary*, ed. and trans. by G. M. Cook (Washington, DC, 1942); and ed. and trans. in Italian by M. Cesa, *Ennodio. Vita del beatissimo Epifanio* (Pavia, 1988)
——, *Magni Felicis Ennodi Opera*, MGH AA, 7, ed. by F. Vogel (Berlin, 1885; repr. 1995)
Galen, *Ad glauconem*, ed. by K.-D. Fischer, in *Galenismo e medicina tardoantica: fonti greche, latine e arabe*, ed. by I. Garofolo and A. Roselli (Napoli, 2003), pp. 283–346

——, *Claudii Galeni opera omnia*, ed. by K. G. Kühn, 20 vols (Leipzig, 1821–33; repr. Hildesheim, 1964–65)

——, *Claudii Galeni Pergameni scripta minora*, ed. by G. Helmreich, I. Marquardt, and I. Mueller, 3 vols (Leipzig, 1884–93), III (1893)

——, *Galen: Selected Works*, ed. and trans. by P. Singer (Oxford, 1997)

Gargilii Martialis medicinae, ed. by V. Rose (Leipzig, 1875)

Gregory the Great, *Dialogues*, ed. by A. de Vogüé, 3 vols (Paris, 1978–80); trans. by O. Zimmermann, *The Dialogues of St. Gregory the Great* (New York, 1959)

——, *S. Gregorii Magni Registrum Epistularum*, ed. by D. Norberg (Turnhout, 1982); and previously ed. by P. Ewald and L. Hartmann, *Gregorii I papae Registrum epistolarum*, MGH Epistolae, 1–2 (Berlin, 1887–99)

Gregory of Tours, *Liber in gloria confessorum*, ed. by B. Krusch, in MGH SRM, 1.2 (Hannover, 1885; repr. 1969, 1988), pp. 294–370; trans. by R. Van Dam, *Glory of the Confessors* (Liverpool, 1988)

——, *S. Georgii Florentini Gregorii turonensis episcopi Opera omnia*, in *Patrologiae cursus completus: series latina*, ed. by J.-P. Migne, LXXI (1879)

Halitgar, *De Ordine Peonitentium*, in *Patrologiae cursus completus: series latina*, ed. by J.-P. Migne, CV (1851), cols 649–710

Inscriptiones Christianae Italiae septimo saeculo antiquiores (Bari, 1986–)

Ionae Vitae Sanctorum Columbani, in MGH SRM, 4, ed. by B. Krusch (Hannover, 1905), pp. 1–156

Isidore of Seville, *Etymologiae*, ed. by W. M. Lindsay (Oxford, 1985); trans. by S. Barney and others, *The Etymologies of Isidore of Seville* (Cambridge, 2006); and trans. by P. Throop, *Isidore of Seville's Etymologies* (Charlotte, 2005)

Justinian, *Digest*, ed. by T. Mommsen, in *Corpus Iuris Civilis*, 9th edn, vol. I.2: *Digesta* (Berlin, 1902); trans. by A. Watson, *The Digest of Justinian*, 4 vols (Philadelphia, 1985)

——, *Institutes*, ed. by J. A. C. Thomas, *The Institutes of Justinian, Text, Translation and Commentary* (Oxford, 1975)

Leges Ahistulfi regis, in MGH Leges, 4, ed. by F. Bluhme (Hannover, 1868; repr. 1984); trans. by K. Fischer Drew, *The Lombard Laws* (Philadelphia, 1973)

Leges Alamannorum, in MGH Leges, 3, ed. by J. Merkel (Hannover, 1863; repr. 1993), pp. 1–182; trans. by T. J. Rivers, *Laws of the Alamans and Bavarians* (Philadelphia, 1977)

Leges Liutprandi regis, in MGH Leges, 4, ed. by F. Bluhme (Hannover, 1868; repr. 1984); trans. by K. Fischer Drew, *The Lombard Laws* (Philadelphia, 1973)

Le Liber pontificalis: texte, introduction et commentaire, ed. by L. Duchesne, 2 vols (Paris, 1886–92); trans. by R. Davis, *The Book of Pontiffs (Liber pontificalis): The Ancient Biographies of the First Ninety Roman Bishops to AD 715* (Liverpool, 1989)

Pactus Alamannorum, in MGH Leges, 3, ed. by J. Merkel (Hannover, 1863; repr. 1993)

Paenitentialia minora Franciae et Italiae saeculi VIII–IX, ed. by R. Kottje (Turnhout, 1994)

Passio Apollinaris, in *Sanctuarium sue vitae sanctorum*, ed. by B. Mombritius (Paris, 1910; repr. New York, 1978), I, 116–22

Paul the Deacon, *Historia Langobardorum*, in MGH SRL, ed. by L. Bethmann and G. Waitz (Hannover, 1878); trans. by W. Fouke, *History of the Langobards* (Philadelphia, 1907)

Paulinus, *Vita di S. Ambrogio: introduzione, testo critico e note a cura di Michele Pellegrino*, ed. by M. Pellegrino (Roma, 1961); ed. and trans. by B. Ramsey, *Ambrose* (New York, 1997), pp. 195–218

Quintus Serenus, *Liber medicinalis*, ed. and trans. by R. Pépin (Paris, 1950)

Sacrorum conciliorum nova et amplissima collectio, ed. by J. D. Mansi (Graz, 1961)

Tjäder, J.-O., *Die nichtliterarischen Lateinischen papyri Italiens aus der Zeit 445–700*, 3 vols (Lund, 1954–82)

Venantius Fortunatus, *Vita S. Martini*, Liber IV, ed. by F. Leo, in MGH AA, 4.1 (Berlin, 1881; repr. 1981)

Vita Caesarii episcopi Arelatensis libri duo, in MGH SRM, 3, ed. by B. Krusch (Hannover, 1896; repr. 1995), pp. 433–501; ed. and Italian trans. by E. Bona, *Vita Sancti Caesarii episcopi arelatensis (BHL 1508–1509)* (Amsterdam, 2002)

Secondary Studies

Ageno, F., 'I giorni egiziaci', *Lingua Nostra*, 13.3 (1951), 69–70

Albert, B.-S., *Le Pélerinage à l'époque Carolingianne* (Louvain, 1999)

Amory, P., *People and Identity in Ostrogothic Italy 489–554* (Cambridge, 1997)

Amundsen, D. W., 'Medieval Canon Law on Medical and Surgical Practice by the Clergy', *Bulletin of the History of Medicine*, 52 (1978), 22–44

Arjava, A., *Women and Law in Late Antiquity* (Oxford, 1996)

Arrizabalaga, J., 'Facing the Black Death: Perception and Reactions of University Medical Practitioners', in *Practical Medicine from Salerno to the Black Death*, ed. by L. García-Ballester and others (Cambridge, 1994), pp. 237–88

——, 'Problematizing Retrospective Diagnosis in the History of Disease', *Asclepio*, 54.1 (2002), 51–70

Avesani, R., *La cultura veronese dal secolo IX al secolo XII* (Vicenza, 1976)

Azzara, C., 'Ecclesiastical Institutions', in *Italy in the Early Middle Ages, 476–1000*, ed. by C. La Rocca (Oxford, 2002), pp. 85–101

Baader, G., 'Early Medieval Latin Adaptations of Byzantine Medicine in Western Europe', in *Symposium on Byzantine Medicine*, ed. by J. Scarborough (Washington, DC, 1985), pp. 251–59

Baker, P., 'Roman Medical Instruments: Archaeological Interpretations of their Possible "Non-functional" Uses', *Social History of Medicine*, 17.1 (2004), 3–21

——, 'The Vertebrate Remains from the Longobard and 9th–10thC Occupation of S. Guilia, Brescia', in *S. Giulia di Brescia: gli scavi dal 1980 al 1992, reperti preromani, romani e alto medievali*, ed. by G. P. Brogiolo (Firenze, 1999), pp. 425–49

Balzaretti, R., *The Lands of Saint Ambrose: Monks and Society in Early Medieval Milan* (Turnhout, forthcoming)

Bandera, S., *L'altare d'oro di Sant'Ambrogio* (Milano, 1995)

Bartoli Langeli, A., 'Private Charters', in *Italy in the Early Middle Ages, 476–1000*, ed. by C. La Rocca (Oxford, 2002), pp. 205–19

Bates, D., ed., *Knowledge and the Scholarly Medical Traditions* (Cambridge, 1995)
Beattie, C., A. Maslakovic, and S. Rees Jones, eds, *The Medieval Household in Christian Europe, c. 850–c. 1550: Managing Power, Wealth, and the Body* (Turnhout, 2003)
Beccaria, A., *I codici di medicina del periodo presalernitano* (Roma, 1956)
Bedini, E., and others, 'Paleobiologia del gruppo umano altomedievale della chiesa cimiteriale di Centallo (Cuneo)', in *L'italia centro-settentrionale in eta longobarda: atti del convegno, Ascoli Piceno, 6–7 ottobre 1995*, ed. by L. Paroli (Firenze, 1997), pp. 345–64
Beier, L. M., 'In Sickness and in Health: A Seventeenth-Century Family's Experience', in *Patients and Practitioners: Lay Perceptions of Medicine in Pre-Industrial Society*, ed. by R. Porter (Cambridge, 1985), pp. 101–28
Bertelli, C., ed., *Milano, una capitale da Ambrogio ai Carolingi* (Milano, 1987)
Bertram, J., *The Chrodegang Rules: The Rules for the Common Life of the Secular Clergy from the Eighth and Ninth Centuries* (Aldershot, 2005)
Beumann, H., and W. Schröder, eds, *Die Transalpinen Verbindungen der Bayern, Alemannen und Franken bis zum 10. Jahrhundert* (Sigmaringen, 1987)
Billanovich, G., 'Milano, Nonantola, Brescia', in G. Billanovich and M. Ferrari, 'La trasmissione dei testi nell'Italia nord-occidentale', *La cultura antica nell'occidente latino dal VII all'XI secolo*, Settimane di studio del Centro Italiano di Studi sull'Alto Medioevo, 22 (Spoleto, 1975), pp. 321–52
Bischoff, B., 'Verbreitung der Werke Isidors von Sevilla', in his *Mittelalterliche Studien: Ausgewählte Aufsätze zur Schriftkunde und Literaturgeschichte*, 3 vols (Stuttgart, 1966–81), I (1966), 171–94
——, *Katalog der festländischen Handschriften des neunten Jahrhunderts*, 2 vols (Wiesbaden, 1998–2004)
——, *Latin Palaeography: Antiquity and the Middle Ages*, trans. by D. Ó Cróinín and D. Ganz (Cambridge, 1990)
Blakey, M., T. E. Leslie, and J. Reidy, 'Frequency and Chronological Distribution of Dental Enamel Hypoplasia in Enslaved African Americans: A Test of the Weaning Hypothesis', *American Journal of Physical Anthropology*, 95 (1994), 371–83
Boldsen, J. L., 'Leprosy in the Early Medieval Lauchheim Community', *American Journal of Physical Anthropology*, 135.3 (2008), 301–10
Bonacini, P., 'Giurisdizione pubblica ed amministrazione della giustizia nel territorio piacentino altomedievale', *Civiltà padana: Archeologia e storia del territorio*, 5 (1994), 43–98
Bonfiglioli, B., P. Brasili, and M. G. Belcastro, 'Dento-Alveolar Lesions and Nutritional Habits of a Roman Imperial Age Population (1st–4th C AD): Quadrella (Molise, Italy)', *Homo*, 54.1 (2003), 36–56
Bougard, F., 'Pierre de Niviano, dit le Spolétin, sculdassius, et le gouvernement du comté de Plaisance à l'époque carolingienne', *Journal des savants* (1996), 291–337
——, 'Public Power and Authority', in *Italy in the Early Middle Ages, 476–1000*, ed. by C. La Rocca (Oxford, 2002), pp. 34–58
——, *La justice dans le royaume d'italie: de la fin du VIIIe siècle au début du XIe siècle* (Roma, 1995)

Bowers, B., ed., *The Medieval Hospital and Medical Practice* (Aldershot, 2007)

Boyle, A., and others, *Two Oxfordshire Anglo-Saxon Cemeteries: Berinsfield and Didcot* (Oxford, 1995)

Bremmer, J., and H. Roodenberg, eds, *Gestures in History: A Cultural History of Gestures from Antiquity to the Present* (London, 1991)

Brenk, B., 'Der Kultort, seine Zugänglichkeit und seine Besuche', in *Akten des XII. Internationalen Kongresses für christliche Archäologie, Bonn 22–28 September 1991*, ed. by E. Dassmann and J. Engemann, 2 vols (Münster, 1995), I, 69–122

Brennessel, B., M. Drout, and R. Gravel, 'A Reassessment of the Efficacy of Anglo-Saxon Medicine', *Anglo-Saxon England*, 34 (2005), 183–95

Brickley, M., S. Mays, and R. Ives, 'An Investigation of Skeletal Indicators of Vitamin D Deficiency in Adults: Effective Markers for Interpreting Past Living Conditions and Pollution Levels in 18th and 19th Century Birmingham, England', *American Journal of Physical Anthropology*, 132 (2007), 67–79

——, 'Skeletal Manifestations of Vitamin D Deficiency Osteomalacia in Documented Historical Collections', *International Journal of Osteoarchaeology*, 15 (2005), 389–403

Bridges, P., 'Review of *A Field Guide to Joint Disease in Archaeology*, by J. Rogers and T. Waldron', *American Antiquity*, 61.3 (1996), 630

Brody, S., *The Disease of the Soul: Leprosy in Medieval Literature* (Ithaca, 1974)

Brogiolo, G. P., ed., *S. Giulia di Brescia: gli scavi dal 1980 al 1992, reperti preromani, romani e alto medievali* (Firenze, 1999)

Brogiolo, G. P., and C. Cuni, 'Le sepolture di età longobarda di S. Giulia in Brescia', *Rivista di Studi Liguri*, 54 (1988), 145–58

Brown, P., *Poverty and Leadership in the Later Roman Empire* (London, 2002)

Brown, T. S., 'Byzantine Italy, *c.* 680–*c.* 876', in *The New Cambridge Medieval History*, 7 vols (Cambridge, 1995–2005), II: *c. 700–c. 900*, ed. by R. McKitterick (1995), pp. 320–48

——, 'The Transformation of the Mediterranean 400–900', in *The Oxford Illustrated History of Medieval Europe*, ed. by G. Holmes (Oxford, 1988), pp. 1–62

——, *Gentlemen and Officers: Imperial Administration and Aristocratic Power in Byzantine Italy AD 554–800* (Roma, 1984)

Brown, W., 'When Documents are Destroyed or Lost: Lay People and Archives in the Early Middle Ages', *Early Medieval Europe*, 11.4 (2002), 337–66

Brubaker, L., *Vision and Meaning in Ninth-Century Byzantium: Image as Exegesis in the Homilies of Gregory of Nazianzus of Paris* (Cambridge, 1999)

Brundage, J., *Medieval Canon Law* (London, 1995)

——, *The Medieval Origins of the Legal Profession: Canonists, Civilians and Courts* (Chicago, 2008)

Brunner, C., *Über Medizin und Krankenpflege im Mittelalter in Schweizerischen Landen* (Zürich, 1922)

Büchi, J., *Die Entwicklung der Rezept-und Arzneibuchliteratur*, 3 vols (Zürich, 1982–86)

Bury, M., 'Social Constructionism and the Development of Medical Sociology', *Sociology of Health and Illness*, 8 (1986), 137–69

——, 'Social Constructionism and Medical Sociology: A Rejoinder to Nicolson and McLaughlin', *Sociology of Health and Illness*, 9 (1987), 439–41

Byard, R., and H. Krous, eds, *Sudden Infant Death Syndrome: Problems, Progress, and Possibilities* (London, 2001)

Cabré, M., 'Women or Healers? Household Practices and the Categories of Health Care in Late Medieval Iberia', *Bulletin of the History of Medicine*, 82.1 (2008), 18–51

Cameron, A., *The Mediterranean World in Late Antiquity AD 395–600* (London, 1993)

Cammarosano, P., *Storia dell'Italia medievale: dal VI all'XI secolo* (Roma, 2001)

Canedi, M., *Runica manuscripta: un nuovo alfabeto runico* (Verona, 1983)

Cantino Wataghin, G., E. Destefanis, and S. Uggé, 'Monasteri e territorio: l'Italia settentrionale nell'alto medieovo', in *Sepolture e luoghi di culto in età longobarda: il modello regio: il Congresso Nazionale di Archeologia Medievale*, ed. by G. P. Brogiolo (Firenze, 2000), pp. 311–16

Cantino Wataghin, G., and L. Pani Ermini, *Santuari martiriali e centri di pellegrinaggio in Italia fra Tarda antichita e Alto medioevo, Akten des XII Internationalen Kongresses für christliche Archäologie* (Münster, 1995)

Capasso, B., ed., *Monumenta ad Neapolitani Ducatus Historiam Pertinentia*, 2 vols (Napoli, 1881–92)

Capponi, C., ed., *L'altare d'oro di Sant' Ambrogio* (Milano, 1996)

Carbonelli, G., *Frammento medico del secolo VII: Cod Vat urb lat 293* (Roma, 1921)

Carile, A., ed., *Storia di Ravenna*, 3 vols (Ravenna, 1990–92)

Castagnetti, A., 'Medici nella Tuscia Longobarda e Carolingia', *Studi Storici Luigi Simeoni*, 62 (2012), 19–32

Castiglioni, E., M. Cottini, and M. Rottoli, 'I resti botanici di Santa Guilia a Brescia', in *S. Giulia di Brescia: gli scavi dal 1980 al 1992, reperti preromani, romani e alto medievali*, ed. by G. P. Brogiolo (Firenze, 1999), pp. 401–24

Cattaneo, E., 'La devozione a Sant' Ambrogio', *Archivio ambrosiano*, 27 (1974), 85–110

Cavallo, G., 'La cultura scritta tra antichità tarda e alto medioevo', in *Storia di Ravenna, 2.2 Dall'età bizantina all'età ottoniana: ecclesiologia, cultura e arte*, ed. by A. Carile (Ravenna, 1992), pp. 79–126

——, 'Libri e continuità della cultura antica in età barbarica', in *Magistra barbaritas: I barbari in Italia*, ed. by G. P. Carratelli (Milano, 1984), pp. 603–62

Cavarra, B., 'La cultura medica a Ravenna fra VI e VII secolo', *Medicina nei secoli*, 5.3 (1993), 345–59

Cencetti, G., 'Scriptoria e scrittura nel Monachesimo benedettino', in *Il monachesimo nell'Alto medioevo e la formazione della civiltà occidentale* (Spoleto, 1957), pp. 187–219

Christie, N., *From Constantine to Charlemagne: An Archaeology of Italy AD 300–800* (Aldershot, 2006)

——, *The Lombards: The Ancient Longobards* (Oxford, 1995)

Clark, H. B., and M. Brennan, eds, *Columbanus and Merovingian Monasticism* (Oxford, 1981)

Claussen, M., *The Reform of the Frankish Church: Chrodegang of Metz and the 'Regula canonicorum' in the Eighth Century* (Cambridge, 2004)

Codoñer Merino, C., 'La medicina en algunos manuscritos de Isidoro de Sevilla', in *Isidorus medicus: Isidoro de Sevilla y los textos de medicina*, ed. by A. Ferraces Rodriguez (Coruña, 2005), pp. 65–84

Cohn, S., *The Black Death Transformed: Disease and Culture in Early Renaissance Europe* (London, 2003)

Collins, M., *Medieval Herbals: The Illustrative Traditions* (London, 2000)

Conrad, L., and others, *The Western Medical Tradition 800 BC to AD 1800* (Cambridge, 1995)

Contreni, J., 'Masters and Medicine in Northern France during the Reign of Charles the Bald', in *Charles the Bald: Court and Kingdom*, ed. by M. Gibson and J. Nelson (Aldershot, 1990), pp. 267–82

Cook, H., *The Decline of the Old Medical Regime in Stuart London* (Ithaca, 1986)

Cooper, K., 'Approaching the Holy Household', *Journal of Early Christian Studies*, 15.2 (2007), 131–42

——, *The Fall of the Roman Household: Religion, Gender, and the Household in the Sixth-Century* (Cambridge, 2007)

Cooper, K., and J. Hillner, eds, *Religion, Dynasty and Patronage in Early Christian Rome 300–900* (Cambrige, 2007)

Cosentino, S., 'La figura del medicus in italia tra tardoantico e altomedioevo: Tipologie sociali e forme di rappresentazione', *Medicina nei secoli, arte e scienze*, 9.3 (1997), 361–89

Coturri, E., 'Gli ospedali lucchesi del periodo longobardo', in *Atti del primo Congresso Italiano di storia ospitaliera* (Reggio Emilia, 1957), pp. 148–62

Courcelle, P., *Recherches sur Saint Ambroise: 'Vies' anciennes, culture, iconographie* (Paris, 1973)

Crislip, A., *From Monastery to Hospital: Christian Monasticism and the Transformation of Health Care in Late Antiquity* (Ann Arbor, 2005)

Cruse, A., *Roman Medicine* (Stroud, 2004)

Deichmann, F. W., *Ravenna: Hauptstadt des spätantiken Abendlandes*, 5 vols (Wiesbaden, 1958–89)

Del Panta, L., ed., *La Populazione Italiana dal medioevo a oggi* (Roma, 1996)

Delogu, P., 'Lombard and Carolingian Italy', in *The New Cambridge Medieval History*, 7 vols (Cambridge, 1995–2005), II: *c. 700–c. 900*, ed. by R. McKitterick (1995), pp. 290–319

Demaitre, L., *Leprosy in Pre-modern Medicine: A Malady of the Whole Body* (Baltimore, 2007)

Destefanis, E., *Il monastero di Bobbio in età altomedievale: Ricerche di archeologia altomedievale e medievale* (Firenze, 2002)

Dey, H. W., 'Diaconiae, Xenodochia, Hospitalia and Monasteries: "Social Security" and the Meaning of Monasticism in Early Medieval Rome', *Early Medieval Europe*, 16.4 (2008), 398–422

Drew, K. F., *Law and Society in Early Medieval Europe* (London, 1988)

Dufourcq, A., *Étude sur les Gesta martyrum romains*, 3 vols (Paris, 1900)

Duft, J., *Sankt Otmar: die Quellen zu seinem Leben, lateinisch und deutsch* (Zürich, 1959)

Durliat, J., 'La peste de 6e siècle', in *Hommes et richesses dans l'empire Byzantin*, ed. by C. Abadie-Reynal and others, 2 vols (Paris, 1989–1991), I: *IVe–VIIe siècles* (1989), pp. 107–25

Elsakkers, M., 'Abortion, Poisoning, Magic and Contraception in Eckhardt's *Pactus Legis Salicae*', *Amsterdamer Beiträge zur Älteren Germanistik*, 57 (2003), 233–67

——, 'The Early Medieval Latin and Vernacular Vocabulary of Abortion and Embryology', in *Science Translated: Proceedings of the Leuven Congress 2004*, ed. by M. Goyens, P. De Leuvens, and A. Smet (Turnhout, 2008), pp. 367–403

——, 'Gothic Bible, Vetus Latina and Visigothic Law: Evidence for a Septuagint-based Gothic Version of Exodus', *Sacris Erudiri*, 44 (2005), 37–76

——, 'Inflicting Serious Bodily Harm: The Visigothic Antiquae on Violence and Abortion', *Tijdschrift voor Rechtsgeschiedenis: The Legal History Review*, 71 (2003), 55–63

——, 'Reading Between the Lines: Old Germanic and Early Christian Views on Abortion' (unpublished doctoral thesis, University of Amsterdam, 2010)

Everett, N., 'The Hagiography of Lombard Italy', *Hagiographica*, 7 (2000), 49–126

——, *Literacy in Lombard Italy* (Cambridge, 2003)

Feliu, G., and J. M. Salrach, eds, *Els Pergamins de l'Arxiu Comtal de Barcelona de Ramon Borrell a Ramon Berenguer I* (Barcelona, 1999)

Ferorelli, N., *Gli Ebrei nell'Italia meridionale dall'eta romana al'secolo XVIII* (Torino, 1915)

Ferraces Rodriguez, A., ed., *Isidorus medicus: Isidoro de Sevilla y los textos de medicina* (Coruña, 2005)

Ferrari, M., 'La biblioteca del monastero di S. Ambrogio: episodi per una storia', in *Il Monastero di S. Ambrogio nel Medieovo: convegno di studi nel XII centenario 784–1984* (Milano, 1988), pp. 82–104

——, 'Manoscritti e cultura', in *Milano e i Milanesi prima del mille: X Congresso internazionale di studi sull'alto medioevo* (Spoleto, 1986), pp. 270–73

Fischer, K.-D., 'Ad glauconem', in *Galenismo e medicina tardoantica: fonti greche, latine e arabe*, ed. by I. Garofolo and A. Roselli (Napoli, 2003), pp. 283–346

——, 'Anweisungen zur selbstmedikation von Laien in der Spätantike', *XXX Internationaler Kongress für Geschichte der Medizin* (Düsseldorf, 1988) pp. 867–74

——, 'Der Liber medicinalis des Pseudo-Democritus', in *Tradición e innovación de la medicina latina de la antigüedad y de la Alta Edad Media*, ed. by M. E. Vázquez Buján (Santiago de Compostela, 1994), pp. 45–56

——, 'Der Pseudogalenische Liber tertius', in *Galenismo e medicina tardoantica: fonti greche, latine e arabe*, ed. by I. Garofolo and A. Roselli (Napoli, 2003), pp. 101–32

——, 'Dr Monk's Medical Digest', *The Year 1000: Medical Practice at the End of the First Millennium, Social History of Medicine*, 13.2 (2000), 239–51

——, 'Neues zur Überlieferung der lateinischen "Aphorismen" im Frühmittelalter', *Latomus*, 62.1 (2003), 156–64

——, 'Praenostica — Die Rezeption des Prognostikons im Frühmittelalter', in *La science médicale antique: nouveaux regards*, ed. by V. Boudon-Millot and others (Paris, 1980), pp. 183–220

——, 'Quelques réflexions sur la structure et deux nouveaux témoins de la Physica Plinii' (C- St. Gallen 217 and 751), in *Pline L'ancien: temoin de son temps*, ed. by J. Pigeaud and I. Orozius (Nantes, 1987), pp. 53–65

——, 'Unberücksichtigte Handscriftenfunde zur Überlieferung der Werke des Caelius Aurelianus', in *Le traité des Maladies aiguës et des Maladies chroniques de Caelius Aurelianus: nouvelles approches*, ed. by P. Mudry (Nantes, 1999), pp. 161–70

Fischer, K.-D., and others, eds, *Bibliographie des textes médicaux latins* (Saint-Étienne, 1983)

Fleming, R., 'Bones for Historians: Putting the Body Back into Biography', in *Writing Medieval Biography: Essays in Honour of Frank Barlow*, ed. by D. Bates, J. Crick, and S. Hamilton (Woodbridge, 2006), pp. 29–48

——, *Medicine and the Making of Roman Women: Gender, Nature and Authority from Celsus to Galen* (Oxford, 2000)

Flint, V., 'The Early Medieval Medicus, the Saint — and the Enchanter', *Social History of Medicine*, 2.2 (1989), 127–45

——, *The Rise of Magic in Early Medieval Europe* (Princeton, 1991)

Fornaciari, G., S. Giusiani, and A. Vitiello, 'Paleopatologia del cimitero signorile del castello di monte di croce (1st fase, XI secolo)', *Atti del III Congresso Nazionale di Archeologia Medievale, Salerno* (Salerno, 2003), pp. 716–19

Fouracre, P., and R. A. Gerberding, eds, *Late Merovingian France: History and Hagiography 640–720* (Manchester, 1996)

Frede, M., 'The Method of the So-Called Methodical School of Medicine', in *Science and Speculation: Studies in Hellenistic Theories and Practice*, ed. by J. Barnes and others (Cambridge, 1982), pp. 1–23

French, R., *William Harvey's Natural Philosophy* (Cambridge, 1994)

Garofolo, I., and A. Roselli, eds, *Galenismo e medicina tardoantica: fonti greche, latine e arabe* (Napoli, 2003)

Gasparri, S., 'The Aristocracy', in *Italy in the Early Middle Ages, 476–1000*, ed. by C. La Rocca (Oxford, 2002), pp. 59–84

Gentilcore, D., *Healers and Healing in Early Modern Italy* (Manchester, 1998)

George, J. W., *Venantius Fortunatus: A Latin Poet in Merovingian Gaul* (Oxford, 1992)

Ghiglione, N., 'Il libro nel territorio ambrosiano', in *Milano, una capitale da Ambrogio ai Carolingi*, ed. by C. Bertelli (Milano, 1987), pp. 149–54

Ghignoli, A., 'Su due famosi documenti pisani dell'VIII secolo', *Bulletino dell'Istituto Storico Italiano per il medio evo*, 106.2 (2004), 1–69

Ginatempo, M., 'Corpi e uomini tra scienza e storia: studi di osteo-archeologia umana per l'italia medievale', *Archeologia Medievale*, 15 (1988), 7–64

Giovannini, F., *Natalità, Mortalità e Demografia dell'Italia Medievale sulla Base dei Dati Archeologici* (Oxford, 2001)

Glaze, F. E., 'The Perforated Wall: The Ownership and Circulation of Medical Books in Medieval Europe, *c.* 800–1200' (unpublished doctoral thesis, Duke University, 1999)

Gourevitch, D., 'The Paths of Knowledge: Medicine in the Roman World', in *Western Medical Thought from Antiquity to the Middle Ages*, ed. by M. Grmek (Cambridge, MA, 1998), pp. 125–29

Graesse, J., F. Benedict, and H. Plechl, eds, *Orbis Latinus: Lexikon lateinischer geographischer Namen des Mittelalters und der Neuzeit*, 3 vols (Braunschweig, 1972)

Green, M., 'Bodies, Gender, Health, Disease: Recent Work on Medieval Women's Medicine', *Studies in Medieval and Renaissance History*, 3.2 (2005), 1–46

——, 'Documenting Medieval Women's Medical Practice', in *Practical Medicine from Salerno to the Black Death*, ed. by L. Garcia-Ballester and others (Cambridge, 1994), pp. 322–52

——, 'Flowers, Poisons and Men: Menstruation in Medieval Western Europe', in *Menstruation: A Cultural History*, ed. by A. Shail and G. Howie (Basingstoke, 2005), pp. 51–64

——, 'Women's Medical Practice and Health Care in Medieval Europe', *Signs*, 14.2 (1989), 434–73

——, *Making Women's Medicine Masculine: The Rise of Male Authority in Pre-Modern Gynaecology* (Oxford, 2008)

——, ed., *The Trotula: An English Translation of the Medieval Compendium of Women's Medicine* (Philadelphia, 2002)

Grmek, M., *Diseases in the Ancient Greek World* (Baltimore, 1989)

——, ed., *Western Medical Thought from Antiquity to the Middle Ages* (Cambridge, MA, 1999)

Gröenke, F. D., *Die frühmittelalterlichen lateinischen Monatskalendarien: Text, Übersetzung, Kommentar* (Berlin, 1986)

Guérard, B., *Polyptique de l'abbé Irminon*, 2 vols (Paris, 1844)

Haegar, K., *The Illustrated History of Surgery*, 2nd edn (London, 2000)

Hägele, G., *Das Paenitentiale Vallicellianum, I: Ein oberitalienischer Zweig der frühmittelalterlichen kontinentalen Bussbücher: Überlieferung, Verbreitung und Quellen* (Sigmaringen, 1984)

Hahn, C., 'Narrative on the Golden Altar of Sant'Ambrogio in Milan: Presentation and Reception', *Dumbarton Oaks Papers*, 53 (1999), 167–87

Hamilton, S., *The Practice of Penance, 900–1050* (Woodbridge, 2001)

Härke, H., '"Warrior Graves?" The Background of the Anglo-Saxon Weapon Burial Rite', *Past and Present*, 126.1 (1990), 22–43

Harley, D., 'Rhetoric and the Social Construction of Sickness and Healing', *Social History of Medicine*, 12.3 (1999), 407–35

Harris, W. V., ed., *The Transformations of Urbs Roma in Late Antiquity*, Journal of Roman Archaeology Supplementary Series, 33 (1999)

Hays, J., 'Historians and Epidemics: Simple Questions, Complex Answers', in *Plague and the End of Antiquity: The Pandemic of 541–750*, ed. by L. Little (Cambridge, 2007), pp. 33–58

Helm, J., 'Sickness in Early Christian Healing Narratives — Medical, Religious and Social Aspects', in *From Athens to Jerusalem: Medicine in Hellenized Jewish Lore and in Early Christian Literature*, ed. by S. Kottek and M. Horstmanshoff (Rotterdam, 2000), pp. 241–58

Henderson, J., P. Horden, and A. Pastore, eds, *The Impact of Hospitals, 300–2000* (Oxford, 2007)

Herlihy, D., *Medieval Households* (London, 1985)

Hildebrandt, M. M., *The External School in Carolingian Society* (Leiden, 1992)

Hill, J., and M. Swan, eds, *The Community, the Family, and the Saint: Patterns of Power in Early Medieval Europe* (Turnhout, 1998)

Hillson, S., *Teeth* (Cambridge, 1990)

Hlawitschka, E., *Franken, Alemannen, Bayern und Burgunder in Oberitalien, 774–962* (Freiburg im Breisgau, 1960)

Holder, A., *Die Reichenauer Handscriften*, 3 vols (Leipzig, 1906–18)

Hoover, K. C., and others, 'Exploring the Relationship Between Hypoplasia and Odontometric Asymmetry in Isola Sacra, an Imperial Roman Necropolis', *American Journal of Human Biology*, 17.6 (2005), 752–64

Horden, P., 'The Earliest Hospitals in Byzantium, Western Europe, and Islam', *Journal of Interdisciplinary History*, 35.3 (2005), 361–89

——, 'The Late Antique Origins of the Lunatic Asylum?', in *Transformations of Late Antiquity: Essays for Peter Brown*, ed. by P. Rousseau (Aldershot, 2009), pp. 259–78

——, 'Mediterranean Plague in the Age of Justinian', in *The Cambridge Companion to the Age of Justinian*, ed. by M. Maas (Cambridge, 2005), pp. 134–60

——, 'A Non-Natural Environment: Medicine without Doctors and the Medieval European Hospital', in *The Medieval Hospital and Medical Practice*, ed. by B. Bowers (Aldershot, 2007), pp. 133–45

——, 'Sickness and Healing', in *The Cambridge History of Christianity*, 9 vols (Cambridge, 2005–2009), III: *Early Medieval Christianities, c. 600–c. 1100*, ed. by T. F. X. Noble and J. M. H. Smith (2008), pp. 416–32

——, 'Travel Sickness: Medicine and Mobility in the Mediterranean from Antiquity to the Renaissance', in *Rethinking the Mediterranean*, ed. by W. V. Harris (Oxford, 2005), pp. 179–99

——, 'What's Wrong with Early Medieval Medicine?', *Social History of Medicine*, 24.1 (2011), 5–25

——, *Hospitals and Healing from Antiquity to the Later Middle Ages* (Aldershot, 2008)

Horden, P., and N. Purcell, *The Corrupting Sea: A Study of Mediterranean History* (Oxford, 2000)

Horn, W., and E. Born, *The Plan of St Gall: A Study of the Architecture and Economy of, and Life in a Paradigmatic Carolingian Monastery*, 3 vols (London, 1979)

Humphries, M., *Communities of the Blessed: Social Environment and Religious Change in Northern Italy, AD 200–400* (Oxford, 1999)

Hunter, L., 'Women and Domestic Medicine: Lady Experimenters, 1570–1620', in *Women, Science and Medicine 1500–1700*, ed. by L. Hunter and S. Hutton (Stroud, 1997), pp. 89–107

Ieraci Bio, A. M., 'La cultura medica a Ravenna nel VI secolo', *Atti dell'Accademia Pontaniana*, 43 (1994), 279–308

Il Monastero di S. Ambrogio nel Medieovo: convegno di studi nel XII centenario 784–1984 (Milano, 1988)

Jackson, R., 'A Roman Doctor's House in Rimini', *British Museum Magazine*, 44 (2002), 20–23

——, 'Roman Doctors and their Instruments: Recent Research into Ancient Practice', *Journal of Roman Archaeology*, 3 (1990), 5–27

Jermyn, J., *Alpine Plants of Europe: A Gardener's Guide* (Portland, OR, 2005)

Jolly, K., *Popular Religion in Late Saxon England: Elf Charms in Context* (London, 1996)

Jong, M. de, *In Samuel's Image: Child Oblation in the Early Medieval West* (Leiden, 1996)

Jouanna, J., 'Remarques sur la valeur relative des traductions latines pour l'édition des texts hippocratiques', in *Le Latin Médical: la constitution d'un langage scientifique, réalités et langage de la medicine dans le monde romain*, ed. by G. Sabbah (Saint-Étienne, 1991), pp. 11–26

——, *Hippocrates*, trans. by M. DeBevoise (Baltimore, 1999)

Jung, P., 'Das Infirmarium im Bauriss des Klosters von St. Gallen vom Jahre 820', *Gesnerus*, 6.1/2 (1949), 1–8

Kazhdan, A., 'The Image of the Medical Doctor in Byzantine Literature of the Tenth to Twelfth Centuries', *Dumbarton Oaks Papers*, 38 (1984), 43–51

Keefe, S., *Water and the Word: Baptism and the Education of the Clergy in the Carolingian Empire*, 2 vols (Notre Dame, IN, 2002)

Keiser, R., 'Two Medieval Plague Treatises and their Afterlife in Early Modern England', *Journal of the History of Medicine and Allied Sciences*, 58.3 (2003), 292–324

Kennell, S., *Magnus Felix Ennodius: A Gentleman of the Church* (Ann Arbor, 2000)

Kerff, F., 'Mittelalterliche Quellen und mittelalterliche Wirklichkeit: zu den Konsequenzen einer jüngst erschienenen Edition für unser Bild kirchlicher Reformbemühungen', *Rheinische Vierteljarhsblätter*, 51 (1987), 275–86

Kieckhefer, R., *Magic in the Middle Ages* (Cambridge, 2000)

Köpp, P., *Vademecum eines frühmittelalterlichen Arztes: Die gefaltete lateinische Handschrift medizinischen Inhalts im Codex 217 und in der Fragmentensammlung 1396 der Stiftsbibliothek in St. Gallen* (Aarau, 1980)

Körntgen, L., 'Ein italienisches Bussbuch und seine fränkischen Quellen: das anonyme Paenitentiale der Handschrift Vatikan Archiv. S. Pietro H. 58', in *Aus Archiven und Bibliotheken: Festschrift für Raymund Kottje zum 65. Geburtstag*, ed. by H. Mordek (Frankfurt, 1992), pp. 189–205

Korpela, J., *Das Medizinalpersonal im Antiken Rom: ein sozialgeschichte Untersuchung* (Helsinki, 1987)

Kottje, R., 'Busspraxis und Bussritus', in *Segni e riti nella chiesa altomedievale occidentale*, Settimane di studio del Centro Italiano di Studi sull'Alto Medioevo, 33 (Spoleto, 1987), pp. 369–403

Kottje, R., *Die Bussbücher Halitgars von Cambrai und des Hrabanus Maurus: ihre Überlieferung und ihre Quellen* (Berlin, 1980)

Krautheimer, R., *Corpus Basilicarum Christianarum Romae*, 5 vols (Città del Vaticano, 1937–77)

Kreutz, B., *Before the Normans: Southern Italy in the Ninth and Tenth Centuries* (Philadelphia, 1991)

Kroll, J., and B. Bachrach, 'Sin and the Etiology of Disease in Pre-Crusade Europe', *Journal of the History of Medicine and Allied Sciences*, 41.4 (1986), 395–414

Krützfeld, K., 'Pfeffer als Gewürz und Arzneimittel: Eine Geschichte mit Höhen und Tiefen', *Deutsche Apotheker Zeitung*, 141.51–52 (2001), 42–48
La Rocca, C., ed., *Italy in the Early Middle Ages, 476–1000* (Oxford, 2002)
Lachmund, J., and G. Stollberg, eds, *The Social Construction of Illness: Illness and Medical Knowledge in Past and Present* (Stuttgart, 1992)
Landgraf, E., 'Ein frühmittelalterlicher Botanicus', *Kyklos*, 1 (1928), 114–46
Lanzoni, F., *Le fonti della leggenda di Sant'Apollinare di Ravenna* (Bologna, 1915)
Lawrence, C. H., *Medieval Monasticism: Forms of Religious Life in Western Europe in the Middle Ages* (London, 1984)
Leiber, E., 'Old Testament "Leprosy", Contagion and Sin', in *Contagion: Perspectives from Pre-Modern Soceties*, ed. by L. Conrad and D. Wujastyk (Aldershot, 2000), pp. 99–136
Lewis, C., and C. Short, eds, *A Latin Dictionary* (Oxford, 1969)
Lewis, S., 'Function and Symbolic Form in the Basilica Apostolorum at Milan', *Journal of the Society of Architectural Historians*, 28.2 (1969), 83–98
Leyser, C., '"A Church in the House of the Saints": Property and Power in the Passion of John and Paul', in *Religion, Dynasty and Patronage in Early Christian Rome 300–900*, ed. by K. Cooper and J. Hillner (Cambridge, 2007), pp. 140–62
——, 'Masculinity in Flux: Nocturnal Emission and the Limits of Celibacy in the Early Middle Ages', in *Masculinity in Medieval Europe*, ed. by D. M. Hadley (Harlow, 1999)
——, 'The Temptations of Cult: Roman Martyr Piety in the Age of Gregory the Great', *Early Medieval Europe*, 9.3 (2000), 289–307
Liebescheutz, J., *The Decline and Fall of the Roman City* (Oxford, 2001)
Little, L., 'Life and Afterlife of the First Plague Pandemic', in *Plague and the End of Antiquity: The Pandemic of 541–750*, ed. by L. Little (Cambridge, 2007), pp. 3–32
——, ed., *Plague and the End of Antiquity: The Pandemic of 541–750* (Cambridge, 2007)
Lopez, R., and I. Raymond, *Medieval Trade in the Mediterranean World* (London, 1955)
Loseby, S., 'The Mediterranean Economy', in *The New Cambridge Medieval History*, 7 vols (Cambridge, 1995–2005), I: *c. 500–c. 700*, ed. by P. Fouracre (2005), pp. 605–38
Lucchesi, G., *Note agiografiche sui primi vescovi di Ravenna* (Faenza, 1941)
Maas, M., ed., *The Cambridge Companion to the Age of Justinian* (Cambridge, 2005)
Mackie, G., *Early Christian Chapels in the West: Decoration, Function and Patronage* (Toronto, 2003)
MacKinney, L., *Early Medieval Medicine: With Special Reference to France and Chartres* (Baltimore, 1937)
Maguire, H., 'Magic and Money in the Early Middle Ages', *Speculum*, 74.4 (1997), 1037–54
Malcolm, S., *The Encyclopaedia of Herbs and Herbalism* (London, 1979)
Mallegni, F., and others, 'Su alcuni gruppi umani del territorio piemontese dal IV al XVIII secolo: aspetti di paleobiologia', in *Archeologia in Piemonte*, ed. by M. V. Gambari, L. Mercando, and E. Micheletto (Torino, 1998), III: *Medioevo*, ed. by L. Mercando and E. Micheletto, pp. 233–61
Manaresi, C., *I placiti del 'regnum Italiae'* (Roma, 1955)
Manzi, G., and others, 'Discontinuity of Life Conditions at the Transition from the Roman Imperial Age to the Early Middle Ages: Example from Central Italy Evaluated by

Pathological Dento-Alveolar Lesions', *American Journal of Human Biology*, 11 (1999), 327–41

Mays, S. A., 'A Possible Case of Surgical Treatment of Cranial Blunt Force Injury from Medieval England', *International Journal of Osteoarchaeology*, 16 (2006), 95–103

Mazzini, I., 'I caratteri comuni a tutto: Ippocrate latino tardo-antico e conseguenti considerazioni su alcuni emendamenti al texto', in *I Testi di medicina latini antichi: problemi filologici e storici*, ed. by I. Mazzini and F. Fusco (Roma, 1985), pp. 65–74

Mazzini, I., and N. Palmieri, 'L'école médicale de Ravenne: Programmes et méthodes d'enseignement, langue, hommes', in *Les écoles médicales à Rome*, ed. by P. Mudry and H. Pigeaud (Geneva, 1991), pp. 285–310

McCormick, M., 'Rats, Communications, and Plague: Toward an Ecological History', *Journal of Interdisciplinary History*, 34.1 (2003), 1–25

——, 'Towards a Molecular History of the Justinianic Pandemic', in *Plague and the End of Antiquity: The Pandemic of 541–750*, ed. by L. Little (Cambridge, 2007), pp. 290–312

——, *Origins of the European Economy: Communications and Commerce AD 300–900* (Cambridge, 2002)

McKenna, J. J., and S. Mosko, 'Mother-Infant Cosleeping: Toward a New Scientific Beginning', in *Sudden Infant Death Syndrome: Problems, Progress, and Possibilities*, ed. by R. Byard and H. Krous (London, 2001), pp. 258–74

McKitterick, R., 'Paul the Deacon and the Franks', *Early Medieval Europe*, 8.3 (1999), 319–39

——, *The Carolingians and the Written Word* (Cambridge, 1989)

——, *The Frankish Church and the Carolingian Reforms 789–895* (Cambridge, 1977)

——, *The Frankish Kingdoms under the Carolingians 751–987* (London, 1983)

——, ed., *c. 700–c. 900*, in *The New Cambridge Medieval History*, 7 vols (Cambridge, 1995–2005), II (1995)

McLynn, N., *Ambrose of Milan: Church and Court in a Christian Capital* (Berkeley, 1994)

McNeill, J. T., and H. M. Gamer, eds, *Medieval Handbooks of Penance: A Translation of the Principal Libri Poenitentiales and Selections from Related Documents* (New York, 1938)

McVicar, J., *Jekka's Complete Herb Book* (London, 1994)

Meaney, A., 'The Practice of Medicine in England about the Year 1000', *Social History of Medicine*, 13 (2000), 221–37

——, 'Women, Witchcraft and Magic in Anglo-Saxon England', in *Superstition and Popular Medicine in Anglo-Saxon England*, ed. by D. Scragg (Manchester, 1989) pp. 9–40

Meens, R., 'Children and Confession', in *The Church and Childhood*, ed. by D. Wood (Oxford, 1994), pp. 53–65

——, 'The Frequency and Nature of Early Medieval Penance', in *Handling Sin: Confession in the Middle Ages*, ed. by P. Biller and A. J. Minnis (York, 1998), pp. 35–61

——, 'Penitentials and the Practice of Penance in the Tenth and Eleventh Centuries', *Early Medieval Europe*, 14.1 (2006), 7–21

Mendelson, S., and P. Crawford, *Women in Early Modern England 1550–1720* (Oxford, 1998)

Metzler, I., *Disability in Medieval Europe: Thinking about Physical Impairment during the High Middle Ages, c. 1100–1400* (London, 2006)

Milano capitale dell'impero romano 286–402 D.C. (Milano, 1990)

Mirabella Roberti, M., 'Sepolture privilegiate nelle chiese paleocristiane di Milano', in *L'inhumation privilégiée du IVe au VIIIe siècle en Occident*, ed. by Y. Duval and J.-C. Picard (Paris, 1986), pp. 157–61

Mitchell, J., 'Keeping the Demons out of the House: The Archaeology of Apotropaic Strategy and Practice in Late Antique Butrint and Antigoneia', in *Objects in Context, Objects in Use: Material Spatiality in Late Antiquity*, ed. by L. Lavan, E. Swift, and T. Putzeys (Leiden, 2007), pp. 273–310

Monot, M., and others, 'On the Origin of Leprosy', *Science*, 308.5724 (2005), 1040–42

Moorhead, J., *Theoderic in Italy* (Oxford, 1992)

Morelli, M., and M. Palma, 'Indagine su alcuni aspetti materiali della produzione libraria a Nonantola nel secolo IX', *Scrittura e civilta*, 6 (1982), 23–98

Müller, I., *Humoralmedizin: physiologische, pathologische und therapeutische Grundlagen der galenistischen Heilkunst* (Heidelberg, 1993)

Natale, A., *Il museo diplomatico dell'Archivio di Stato di Milano* (Milano, 1971)

Nicolson, N., and C. McLaughlin, 'Social Constructionism and Medical Sociology: A Reply to M. R. Bury', *Sociology of Health and Illness*, 9 (1987), 107–26

Niederhellmann, A., *Arzt und Heilkunde in den frühmittelalterlichen Leges: Eine wort- und sachekundliche Untersuchung* (Berlin, 1983)

Niermeyer, J., *Mediae latinitatis lexicon minus* (Leiden, 1976)

Nutton, V., 'Archiatri and the Medical Profession in Antiquity', *Papers of the British School at Rome*, 45 (1977), 191–226; repr. in V. Nutton, *From Democedes to Harvey: Studies in the Social History of Medicine* (London, 1988)

——, 'From Galen to Alexander, Aspects of Medicine and Medical Practice in Late Antiquity', in *Symposium on Byzantine Medicine*, ed. by J. Scarborough (Washington, DC, 1985), 1–14

——, 'The Medical Profession in the Roman Empire from Augustus to Justinian' (unpublished doctoral thesis, University of Cambridge, 1970)

——, 'Medicine in Late Antiquity and the Early Middle Ages', in *The Western Medical Tradition 800 BC to AD 1800*, ed. by L. Conrad and others (Cambridge, 1995), pp. 71–88

——, 'Medicine in the Greek World, 800 BC to 50 BC', in *The Western Medical Tradition 800 BC to AD 1800*, ed. by L. Conrad and others (Cambridge, 1995), pp. 11–38

——, 'Roman Medicine 250 BC to AD 200', *The Western Medical Tradition 800 BC to AD 1800*, ed. by L. Conrad and others (Cambridge, 1995), pp. 39–70

——, 'The Seeds of Disease: An Explanation of Contagion and Infection from the Greeks to the Renaissance', *Medical History*, 27.1 (1983), 1–34

——, *Ancient Medicine* (London, 2004)

——, ed., *Pestilential Complexities: Understanding Medieval Plague, Medical History*, Supplement, 27 (London, 2008), pp. 1–16

Oliver, L., *The Body Legal in Barbarian Law* (Toronto, 2011)

Olsan, L. T., 'Charms and Prayers in Medieval Medical Theory and Practice', *Social History of Medicine*, 16.3 (2003), 343–66

Ortalli, J., 'Rimini: la Domus 'del chirurgo', in *Aemilia: La cultura romana in Emilia Romagna dal III secolo a.C. all'eta costantiniana*, ed. by M. Marini Calvani, R. Curina, and E. Leppolis (Bologna, 2000), pp. 512–26

Palmieri, N., 'Nouvelles remarques sur les commentaires à Galien de l'école médicale de Ravenne', in *Docente Natura: Mélanges de médicine ancienne et médiévale offerts à Guy Sabbah*, ed. by N. Palmieri and A. Debru (Saint-Étienne, 2001), pp. 209–46

——, 'Un antico commento a Galeno della scuola medica di Ravenna', *Physis*, 23.2 (1981), 196–295

Palmieri, N., and A. Debru, eds, *Docente Natura: Mélanges de médicine ancienne et médiévale offerts á Guy Sabbah* (Saint-Étienne, 2001)

Paredi, A., 'Paulinus of Milan', *Sacris Erudiri*, 14 (1963), 206–30

——, *Vita e meriti di S. Ambrogio: testo inedito del secolo nono illustrato con le miniature del salterio di Arnolfo* (Milano, 1964)

Patini, F., 'I luoghi di sepoltura dei vescovi Ravennati nel "Liber pontificalis" di Andrea Agnello', *Felix Ravenna*, 98 (1968), 6–12

Pavan, M., *La crisi della Scuola del IV secolo d.C* (Bari, 1952)

Payer, P., *Sex and the Penitentials: The Development of a Sexual Code 500–1150* (Toronto, 1984)

Pellegrino, M., *Paolino di Milano: introduzione, testo critico e note a cura di Michele Pellegrino* (Roma, 1961)

Pelling, M., *Medical Conflicts in Early Modern London: Patronage, Physicians, and Irregular Practitioners 1550–1640* (Oxford, 2003)

Peterson, D. W., 'Galen's Therapeutics to Glaucon and Its Early Commentaries' (unpublished doctoral thesis, John Hopkins University, 1974)

Petrucci, A., 'Book, Handwriting and School', in A. Petrucci, *Writers and Readers in Medieval Italy: Studies in the History of Written Culture*, ed. and trans. by C. Radding (London, 1995), pp. 59–76 (originally published as 'Libro, scrittura e scuola', in *La scuola nell'occidente latino dell alto medioevo* (Spoleto, 1972), pp. 313–38

——, *Medioevo da leggere: guida allo studio delle testimonianze scritte del medioevo italiano* (Torino, 1992)

Petrucci, A., *Writers and Readers in Medieval Italy: Studies in the History of Written Culture*, ed. and trans. by C. Radding (London, 1995)

Petrucci, A., and Romeo, C., *'Scriptores in urbibus': Alfabetismo e cultura scritta nell'Italia altomedievale* (Bologna, 1992)

Peyer, P., ed., *Gastfreundschaft, Taverne und Gasthaus im Mittelalter* (München, 1983)

Picard, J.-C., *Le Souvenir des évêques: sépultures, listes épiscopales et culte des évêques en Italie du Nord des origins au Xe siècle* (Roma, 1988)

Piccinini, L., 'Rune anglosassoni in un codice latino (Archivio Capitolare di Modena, O.I.11)', *Romanobarbarica*, 12 (1992–93), 173–88

Pierce, R. (later McKitterick, R.), 'The "Frankish" Penitentials', in *The Materials, Sources and Methods of Ecclesiastical History: Papers Read at the Twelfth Summer Meeting and the Thirteenth Winter Meeting of the Ecclesiastical History Society*, ed. by D. Baker (Oxford, 1975), pp. 31–39

Pilsworth, C., 'Beyond the Medical Text: Health and Illness in Early Medieval Italian Sources', *Social History of Medicine*, 24.1 (2011), 26–40

——, 'Could You Just Sign This for Me John? Doctors, Charters and Occupational Identity in Early Medieval Northern and Central Italy', *Early Medieval Europe*, 17.4 (2009), 363–88

——, 'Medicine and Hagiography in Italy *c.* 800–1000', *Social History of Medicine*, 13.2 (2000), 253–64

——, 'Representations of Sanctity in Milan and Ravenna, *c.* 400–*c.* 900 AD' (unpublished doctoral thesis, University of Cambridge, 1999)

——, 'Sanctity, Crime and Punishment in the *Vita Walfredi*', *Hagiographica*, 7 (2000), 181–99

Pizarro, J., *Writing Ravenna: The Liber Pontificalis of Andreas Agnellus* (Ann Arbor, 1995)

Pohl-Resl, B., 'Legal Practice and Ethnic Identity in Lombard Italy', in *Strategies of Distinction: The Construction of Ethnic Communities, 300–800*, ed. by W. Pohl and H. Reimitz (Leiden, 1998), pp. 205–19

Pohl, W., 'Invasions and Ethnic Identity', in *Italy in the Early Middle Ages, 476–1000*, ed. by C. La Rocca (Oxford, 2002), pp. 11–33

——, *Le origini etniche dell'Europa* (Roma, 2000)

Pohl, W., and H. Reimitz, eds, *Strategies of Distinction: The Construction of Ethnic Communities, 300–800* (Leiden, 1998)

Prowse, T., and others, 'Isotopic Evidence for Age Related Variation in Diet from Isola Sacra, Italy', *American Journal of Physical Anthropology*, 128 (2005), 2–13

Randsborg, K., *The First Millennium AD in Europe and the Mediterranean: An Archaeological Essay* (Cambridge, 1991)

Rauty, N., *Storia di Pistoia*, I: *Dall'alto medioevo all'età precomunale 406–1105* (Firenze, 1988)

Rawcliffe, C., *Leprosy in Medieval England* (Woodbridge, 2006)

Reggiori, F., 'La lettera di Sant'Ambrogio', in *Antichi tessuti della Biblioteca Ambrosiana*, ed. by A. Capitani d'Arzago (Milano, 1941), pp. 107–16

——, *La basilica di Sant'Ambrogio* (Milano, 1966)

Reynolds, R., *Clerics in the Early Middle Ages: Hierarchy and Image* (Aldershot, 1999)

Riberi, A. M., *S. Dalmazzo di Pedona e la sua abazia (Borgo San Dalmazzo) con documenti inediti* (Torino, 1929)

Richards, A., 'Biological Adaptation to Malaria: Ancient DNA Survey of a Fifth-Century Italian Infant Cemetery' (unpublished master's thesis, University of Manchester Institute of Science and Technology, 1999)

Richards, P., *The Medieval Leper and his Northern Heirs* (Woodbridge, 1977)

Riché, P., *Daily Life in the World of Charlemagne*, trans. by J. A. McNamara (Philadelphia, 1978)

Riddle, J. M., *Contraception and Abortion from the Ancient World to the Renaissance* (Cambridge, MA, 1992)

——, *Eve's Herbs: A History of Contraception and Abortion in the West* (Cambridge, MA, 1997)

——, 'Gargilius Martialis as a Medical Writer', *Journal of the History of Medicine and Allied Sciences*, 39.4 (1984), 408–29

——, 'Pseudo-Dioscorides' *Ex herbis femininis* and Early Medieval Medical Botany', *Journal of the History of Biology*, 14 (1981), 43–81

——, 'Theory and Practice in Medieval Medicine', *Viator*, 5 (1974), 157–84

Roberts, C., and M. Cox, *Health and Disease in Britain* (Stroud, 2003)

Rogers, J., I. Watt, and P. Dieppe, 'Arthritis in Saxon and Mediaeval Skeletons', *British Medical Journal*, 283.6307 (1981), 1668–70

Romanucci-Ross, L., and others, eds, *The Anthropology of Medicine: From Culture to Method* (South Hadley, MA, 1983)

Rouche, M., 'Europe Accumulates its First Gains: Sixth to Ninth Centuries', in *The Cambridge Illustrated History of the Middle Ages*, 3 vols (Cambridge, 1986–97), I: *350–950*, ed. by R. Fossier, trans. by J. Sondheimer (Cambridge, 1989), pp. 474–529

Ruas, M.-P., 'Aspects of Early Medieval Farming from Sites in Mediterranean France', *Vegetation History and Archaeobotany*, 14.4 (2005), 400–15

Ruggini, L., 'Sulla fortuna della Vita Ambrosii', *Athenaeum*, n.s., 41 (1963), 98–110

Russo, G., 'Leggi longobarde nel codice O.I.2 della Biblioteca Capitolare di Modena', in *Longobardi e Lombardia: Aspetti di civilità Longobarda, Atti del 6 congresso internazionale di studi sull'alto medioevo* (Spoleto, 1980), pp. 607–21

Sabbah, G., and P. Mudry, eds, *La Médecine de Celse: aspects historiques, scientifiques et littéraires* (Saint-Étienne, 1994)

Sallares, R., 'Ecology, Evolution and Epidemiology of Plague', in *Plague and the End of Antiquity: The Pandemic of 541–750*, ed. by L. Little (Cambridge, 2007), pp. 231–89

——, *Malaria and Rome: A History of Malaria in Ancient Italy* (Oxford, 2002)

Sannazaro, M., 'Attestazioni di militari e militaria a milano', in *Miles Romanus: dal Po al Danubio nel tardoantico: atti del convegno internazionale, Pordenone-Concordia Sagittaria*, ed. by M. Buora (Pordenone, 2002), pp. 65–80

——, 'Chiese e comunita cristiane rurali nelle fonti epigrafiche dell'italia settentrionale', in *Chiese e insediamenti nelle campagne tra V e VI secolo*, ed. by G. P. Brogiolo (Mantova, 2003), pp. 39–55

Savio, F., 'Due lettere falsamente attribuite a Sant' Ambrogio', *Nuovo Bulletino di Archeologia Cristiana*, 3 (1897), 153–77

——, *Gli antichi vescovi d'Italia dalle orgini al 1300 descritti per regioni. La Lombardia. I. Milano* (Firenze, 1913)

Scalon, C., ed., *Libri e documenti d'Italia: dai Longobardi alla rinascita delle città* (Udine, 1996)

Scarborough, J., ed., *Symposium on Byzantine Medicine* (Washington, DC, 1985)

Scheidel, W., 'Germs for Rome', in *Rome the Cosmopolis*, ed. by C. Edwards and G. Woolf (Cambridge, 2003), pp. 158–76

Schönfeld, W., 'Die Xenodochien in Italien und Frankreich im frühen Mittelalter', *Zeitschrift der Savigny-Stiftung für Rechtsgeschichte, Kanonische Abteilung*, 12 (1922), 1–54

Schott, C., *Lex Alamannorum: Das Gesetz der Alemannen*, 2 vols (Augsburg, 1993)
Schülke, A., 'On Christianization and Grave-Finds', *European Journal of Archaeology*, 2.1 (1999), 77–106
——, *Geschichte des mittelalterlichen Handels und Verkehrs zwischen Westdeutschland und Italien mit ausschluss von Venedig*, 2 vols (Leipzig, 1900)
Sessa, K., 'Domestic Conversions: Households and Bishops in the Late Antique "Papal Legends"', in *The Community, the Family, and the Saint: Patterns of Power in Early Medieval Europe*, ed. by J. Hill and M. Swan (Turnhout, 1998), pp. 79–114
Sharf, A., *The Universe of Shabbetai Donnolo* (Warminster, 1976)
Shrewsbury, J., *A History of Bubonic Plague in the British Isles* (Cambridge, 1971)
Sigerist, H. E., *Studien und Texte zur frühmittelalterlichen Rezeptliteratur* (Leipzig, 1923)
Simonini, R., *'Apulei Liber', Medicinae Varia in codice dell'VIII secolo conservato nell'archivio capitolare della metropolitana di Modena* (Modena, 1929)
——, 'Formulario in "Medicinae Varia" codice Mss. dell'VIII secolo conservato nella Metropolitana di Modena', *Atti e Memorie dell'Accademia di Storia dell'Arte Sanitaria*, 39.6 (1940)
——, *La chiesa Ravennate: splendore e tramonto di una metropole* (Faenza, 1964)
Singer, C., 'The Herbal in Antiquity and its Transmission to Later Ages', *Journal of Hellenic Studies*, 47 (1927), 1–52
Siraisi, N., *Medieval and Early Renaissance Medicine: An Introduction to Knowledge and Practice* (Chicago, 1990)
Skinner, P., 'A Cure for a Sinner: Sickness and Healthcare in Medieval Southern Italy', in *The Community, the Family, and the Saint: Patterns of Power in Early Medieval Europe*, ed. by J. Hill and M. Swan (Turnhout, 1998), pp. 297–307
——, *Health and Medicine in Early Medieval Southern Italy* (Leiden, 1996)
——, *Women in Medieval Italian Society, 500–1200* (Harlow, 2001)
Slack, P., *The Impact of Plague in Tudor and Stuart England* (London, 1985)
Smith, L. W., 'Reassessing the Role of the Family: Women's Medical Care in Eighteenth-Century England', *Social History of Medicine*, 16.3 (2003), 327–42
Soren, D., and N. Soren, *A Roman Villa and a Late Roman Infant Cemetery: Excavation at Poggio Gramignano, Lugnano in Teverina* (Roma, 1999)
Souter, A., *A Glossary of Later Latin to 600 AD* (Oxford, 1949)
Squatriti, P., *Water and Society in Early Medieval Italy, AD 400–1000* (Cambridge, 1998)
Stathakopoulos, D., *Famine and Pestilence in the Late Roman and Early Byzantine Empire* (Aldershot, 2002)
Stiker, H.-J., *A History of Disability* (Ann Arbor, 2000)
Stoclet, A., 'Consilia humana, ops divina, superstitio: Seeking Succor and Solace in Times of Plague, with Particular Reference to Gaul in the Early Middle Ages', in *Plague and the End of Antiquity: The Pandemic of 541–750*, ed. by L. Little (Cambridge, 2007), pp. 135–49
Stoffella, M., 'Crisi e trasformazioni delle élites nella Toscana nord-occidentale nel secolo VIII: esempi a confronto', *Reti Medievali*, 8 (2007); available online <http://www.retimedievali.it> [accessed 10 November 2013]

Stornajolo, C., *Codices Urbinates Latini* (Roma, 1942)
Supino Martini, P., 'Alfabetismo e sottoscrizione testimoniali al documento privato nell'Italia centrale (sec. VIII)', in *Escribir y leer en Occidente*, ed. by A. Petrucci and F. M. Gimeno Blay (Valencia, 1995), pp. 47–61
Szabo, T., 'Xenodochia, Hospitäler und Herbergen — kirchliche und kommerzielle Gastung im mittelalterlichen Italien (7. bis 14. Jahrhundert)', in *Gastfreundschaft, Taverne und Gasthaus im Mittelalter*, ed. by P. Peyer (München, 1983), pp. 61–92
Tapper, R., 'The *materia medica* of Gargilius Martialis' (unpublished doctoral thesis, University of Wisconsin, Wyoming, 1980)
Théodoridès, J., *Histoire de la rage: cave canem* (Paris, 1986)
Tomea, P., 'Ambrogio e i suoi fratelli: Note di agiografia milanese altomedievale', *Filologia Mediolatina*, 5 (1998), 149–232
Totelin, L., 'Old Recipes, New Practice? The Latin Adaptations of the Hippocratic Gynaecological Treatises', *Social History of Medicine*, 24.1 (2011), 74–91
Twigg, G., *The Black Death: A Biological Reappraisal* (London, 1984)
Tyers, T. L., 'Manuscript 3519 Revisited in the Cathedral Library, Exeter: An Analysis of a Medieval Medical Compendium' (unpublished master's thesis, University of Nottingham, 2006)
Udina Martorell, F., ed., *El Archivo Condal de Barcelona en los Siglos IX–X, studio critico de sus fondos* (Barcelona, 1951)
Van Arsdall, A., 'Challenging the "Eye of Newt" Image of Medieval Medicine', in *The Medieval Hospital and Medical Practice*, ed. by B. Bowers (Aldershot, 2007), pp. 195–205
Van Dam, R., *Leadership and Community in Late Antique Gaul* (London, 1985)
——, *Saints and their Miracles in Late Antique Gaul* (Princeton, 1993)
Vázquez Buján, M. E., 'Los Aforismos Hipocráticos', *D'Histoire des Textes*, 23 (1993), 73–94
——, 'Problemas generales de las antiuguas traducciones médicas latinas', *Studi Medievali*, 3rd ser., 25 (1984), 641–80
Voigts, L., 'Anglo-Saxon Plant Remedies and the Anglo-Saxons', *Isis*, 70 (1979), 250–68
Wallis, F., 'The Experience of the Book: Manuscripts, Texts and the Role of Epistemology in Early Medieval Medicine', in *Knowledge and the Scholarly Medical Traditions*, ed. by D. Bates (Cambridge, 1995), pp. 101–26
Ward, B., *Miracles and the Medieval Mind: Theory, Record and Event 1000–1215* (London, 1982)
Watermann, R., *Medizinisches und Hygienisches aus Germania inferior* (Neuss, 1974)
Wear, A., 'Galen in the Renaissance', in *Galen: Problems and Prospects*, ed. by V. Nutton (London, 1981), pp. 229–62
Weißer, C., *Studien zum mittelalterlichen Krankheitslunar* (Pattensen, 1982)
Weston, L. M. C., 'Women's Medicine, Women's Magic: The Old English Metrical Childbirth Charms', *Modern Philology*, 92.3 (1995), 279–93
Wickham, C., 'Rural Society and Economy', in *Italy in the Early Middle Ages, 476–1000*, ed. by C. La Rocca (Oxford, 2002), pp. 118–43
——, *Land and Power: Studies in Italian and European Social History 400–1200* (London, 1994)

Wiechmann, I., and G. Grupe, 'Detection of Yersinia pestis DNA in Two Early Medieval Skeletal Finds From Aschheim (Upper Bavaria, 6th Century AD)', *American Journal of Physical Anthropology*, 126 (2005), 48–55

Will, E., *Saint Apollinare de Ravenna* (Paris, 1936)

Winslow, E. A., *The Cost of Sickness and the Price of Health* (Geneva, 1951)

Wood, D., ed., *The Church and Childhood* (Oxford, 1994)

Wood, I., *The Merovingian Kingdoms, 450–751* (London, 1994)

——, *The Missionary Life: Saints and the Evangelisation of Europe 400–1050* (Harlow, 2001)

Zanetti, U., 'Les Passions des Ss. Nazaire, Gervais, Protais et Celse', *Analecta Bollandiana*, 97 (1979), 69–88

Zattoni, G., 'La data della Passio S. Apollinaris di Ravenna', *Atti delle R. Accademia delle scienze di Torino*, 32 (1904), 364–78 (repr. in G. Zattoni, *Scritti storici e ravennati* (Ravenna, 1975), pp. 115–28)

Zettler, A., 'Exkurs1: zu den Klosterärzten', in *Das Totengedenken der Abtei: Necrologien und Kommemorierte Personen*, ed. by R. Rappmann (Sigmaringen, 1998), pp. 265–78

Index

Page numbers in *italics* refer to figures and tables.

Studies in the Early Middle Ages

All volumes in this series are evaluated by an Editorial Board, strictly on academic grounds, based on reports prepared by referees who have been commissioned by virtue of their specialism in the appropriate field. The Board ensures that the screening is done independently and without conflicts of interest. The definitive texts supplied by authors are also subject to review by the Board before being approved for publication. Further, the volumes are copyedited to conform to the publisher's stylebook and to the best international academic standards in the field.

Titles in Series

Cultures in Contact: Scandinavian Settlement in England in the Ninth and Tenth Centuries, ed. by Dawn M. Hadley and Julian D. Richards (2000)

On Barbarian Identity: Critical Approaches to Ethnicity in the Early Middle Ages, ed. by Andrew Gillett (2002)

Matthew Townend, *Language and History in Viking Age England: Linguistic Relations between Speakers of Old Norse and Old English* (2002)

Contact, Continuity, and Collapse: The Norse Colonization of the North Atlantic, ed. by James H. Barrett (2003)

Court Culture in the Early Middle Ages: The Proceedings of the First Alcuin Conference, ed. by Catherine Cubitt (2003)

Political Assemblies in the Earlier Middle Ages, ed. by P. S. Barnwell and Marco Mostert (2003)

Wulfstan, Archbishop of York: The Proceedings of the Second Alcuin Conference, ed. by Matthew Townend (2004)

Borders, Barriers, and Ethnogenesis: Frontiers in Late Antiquity and the Middle Ages, ed. by Florin Curta (2006)

John D. Niles, *Old English Enigmatic Poems and the Play of the Texts* (2006)

Teaching and Learning in Northern Europe, 1000–1200, ed. by Sally N. Vaughn and Jay Rubenstein (2006)

Narrative and History in the Early Medieval West, ed. by Elizabeth M. Tyler and Ross Balzaretti (2006)

People and Space in the Middle Ages, 300–1300, ed. by Wendy Davies, Guy Halsall, and Andrew Reynolds (2006)

John D. Niles, *Old English Heroic Poems and the Social Life of Texts* (2007)

The Crisis of the Oikoumene*: The Three Chapters and the Failed Quest for Unity in the Sixth- Century Mediterranean*, ed. by Celia Chazelle and Catherine Cubitt (2007)

Text, Image, Interpretation: Studies in Anglo-Saxon Literature and its Insular Context in Honour of Eamonn O Carragain, ed. by Alastair Minnis and Jane Roberts (2007)

The Old English Homily: Precedent, Practice, and Appropriation, ed. by Aaron J. Kleist (2007)

James T. Palmer, *Anglo-Saxons in a Frankish World, 690–900* (2009)

Challenging the Boundaries of Medieval History: The Legacy of Timothy Reuter, ed. by Patricia Skinner (2009)

Peter Verbist, *Duelling with the Past: Medieval Authors and the Problem of the Christian Era, c. 990–1135* (2010)

Reading the Anglo-Saxon Chronicle: Language, Literature, History, ed. by Alice Jorgensen (2010)

England and the Continent in the Tenth Century: Studies in Honour of Wilhelm Levison (1876–1947), ed. by David Rollason, Conrad Leyser, and Hannah Williams (2010)

Early Medieval Northumbria: Kingdoms and Communities, AD 450–1100, ed. by David Petts and Sam Turner (2011)

Conceptualizing Multilingualism in Medieval England, c. 800–c. 1250, ed. by Elizabeth M. Tyler (2011)

Neglected Barbarians, ed. by Florin Curta (2011)

The Genesis of Books: Studies in the Scribal Culture of Medieval England in Honour of A. N. Doane, ed. by Matthew T. Hussey and John D. Niles (2012)

Giselle de Nie, *Poetics of Wonder: Testimonies of the New Christian Miracles in the Late Antique Latin World* (2012)

Lilla Kopár, *Gods and Settlers: The Iconography of Norse Mythology in Anglo-Scandinavian Sculpture* (2012)

R. W. Burgess and Michael Kulikowski, *Mosaics of Time: The Latin Chronicle Traditions from the First Century BC to the Sixth Century AD, vol. I: A Historical Introduction to the Chronicle Genre from its Origins to the High Middle Ages* (2013)

Sacred Sites and Holy Places: Exploring the Sacralization of Landscape through Space and Time, ed. by Sæbjørg Walaker Nordeide and Stefan Brink (2013)

Christine Maddern, *Raising the Dead: Early Medieval Name Stones in Northumbria* (2013)

Landscapes of Defence in Early Medieval Europe, ed. by John Baker, Stuart Brookes, and Andrew Reynolds (2013)

Sara M. Pons-Sanz, *The Lexical Effects of Anglo-Scandinavian Linguistic Contact on Old English* (2013)

Society and Culture in Medieval Rouen, 911–1300, ed. by Leonie V. Hicks and Elma Brenner (2013)

Shane McLeod, *The Beginning of Scandinavian Settlement in England: The Viking 'Great Army' and Early Settlers, c. 865–900* (2014)

Luigi Andrea Berto, *In Search of the First Venetians: Prosopography of Early Medieval Venice* (2014)